THE MENTAL HEALTH AND SUBSTANCE USE WORKFORCE FOR OLDER ADULTS

IN WHOSE HANDS?

Committee on the Mental Health Workforce
for Geriatric Populations

Board on Health Care Services

Jill Eden, Katie Maslow, Mai Le, and Dan Blazer, *Editors*

INSTITUTE OF MEDICINE
OF THE NATIONAL ACADEMIES

THE NATIONAL ACADEMIES PRESS
Washington, D.C.
www.nap.edu

THE NATIONAL ACADEMIES PRESS 500 Fifth Street, NW Washington, DC 20001

NOTICE: The project that is the subject of this report was approved by the Governing Board of the National Research Council, whose members are drawn from the councils of the National Academy of Sciences, the National Academy of Engineering, and the Institute of Medicine. The members of the committee responsible for the report were chosen for their special competences and with regard for appropriate balance.

This study was supported by Contract No. HHSP23320042509XI between the National Academy of Sciences and the Department of Health and Human Services. Any opinions, findings, conclusions, or recommendations expressed in this publication are those of the authors and do not necessarily reflect the views of the organizations or agencies that provided support for the project.

International Standard Book Number-13: 978-0-309-25665-0
International Standard Book Number-10: 0-309-25665-8

Additional copies of this report are available for sale from the National Academies Press, 500 Fifth Street, NW, Keck 360, Washington, DC 20001; (800) 624-6242 or (202) 334-3313; http://www.nap.edu/.

For more information about the Institute of Medicine, visit the IOM home page at: **www.iom.edu.**

Printed in the United States of America

The serpent has been a symbol of long life, healing, and knowledge among almost all cultures and religions since the beginning of recorded history. The serpent adopted as a logotype by the Institute of Medicine is a relief carving from ancient Greece, now held by the Staatliche Museen in Berlin.

Suggested citation: IOM (Institute of Medicine). 2012. *The mental health and substance use workforce for older adults: In whose hands?* Washington, DC: The National Academies Press.

"Knowing is not enough; we must apply.
Willing is not enough; we must do."
—Goethe

INSTITUTE OF MEDICINE
OF THE NATIONAL ACADEMIES

Advising the Nation. Improving Health.

THE NATIONAL ACADEMIES

Advisers to the Nation on Science, Engineering, and Medicine

The **National Academy of Sciences** is a private, nonprofit, self-perpetuating society of distinguished scholars engaged in scientific and engineering research, dedicated to the furtherance of science and technology and to their use for the general welfare. Upon the authority of the charter granted to it by the Congress in 1863, the Academy has a mandate that requires it to advise the federal government on scientific and technical matters. Dr. Ralph J. Cicerone is president of the National Academy of Sciences.

The **National Academy of Engineering** was established in 1964, under the charter of the National Academy of Sciences, as a parallel organization of outstanding engineers. It is autonomous in its administration and in the selection of its members, sharing with the National Academy of Sciences the responsibility for advising the federal government. The National Academy of Engineering also sponsors engineering programs aimed at meeting national needs, encourages education and research, and recognizes the superior achievements of engineers. Dr. Charles M. Vest is president of the National Academy of Engineering.

The **Institute of Medicine** was established in 1970 by the National Academy of Sciences to secure the services of eminent members of appropriate professions in the examination of policy matters pertaining to the health of the public. The Institute acts under the responsibility given to the National Academy of Sciences by its congressional charter to be an adviser to the federal government and, upon its own initiative, to identify issues of medical care, research, and education. Dr. Harvey V. Fineberg is president of the Institute of Medicine.

The **National Research Council** was organized by the National Academy of Sciences in 1916 to associate the broad community of science and technology with the Academy's purposes of furthering knowledge and advising the federal government. Functioning in accordance with general policies determined by the Academy, the Council has become the principal operating agency of both the National Academy of Sciences and the National Academy of Engineering in providing services to the government, the public, and the scientific and engineering communities. The Council is administered jointly by both Academies and the Institute of Medicine. Dr. Ralph J. Cicerone and Dr. Charles M. Vest are chair and vice chair, respectively, of the National Research Council.

www.national-academies.org

COMMITTEE ON THE MENTAL HEALTH WORKFORCE FOR GERIATRIC POPULATIONS

DAN G. BLAZER (*Chair*), J.P. Gibbons Professor of Psychiatry and Behavioral Sciences, Vice Chair for Education and Academic Affairs, Duke University Medical Center, Durham, NC

MARGARITA ALEGRÍA, Director, Center for Multicultural Mental Health Research, Cambridge Health Alliance and Harvard Medical School, Somerville, MA

MARÍA P. ARANDA, Associate Professor; Chair, Older Adult Subconcentration, School of Social Work, University of Southern California, Los Angeles

STEPHEN BARTELS, Director, Dartmouth Centers for Health and Aging, Lebanon, NH

CHRISTINE E. BISHOP, Atran Professor of Labor Economics, Heller School for Social Policy and Management, Brandeis University, Waltham, MA

FREDERIC C. BLOW, Professor and Director, Mental Health Services Outcomes & Translation Section, Department of Psychiatry, University of Michigan; Director, National Serious Mental Illness Treatment Resource Center, Department of Veterans Affairs, Ann Arbor

KATHLEEN C. BUCKWALTER, Professor Emerita, University of Iowa College of Nursing; Codirector, National Health Law and Policy Resource Center, University of Iowa College of Law, Iowa City

CHRISTOPHER M. CALLAHAN, Professor, School of Medicine, Indiana University, Scientist, Regenstrief Institute, Inc., Indianapolis

ANNI CHUNG, President and Chief Executive Officer, Self-Help for the Elderly, San Francisco, CA

GARY L. GOTTLIEB, President and Chief Executive Officer, Partners HealthCare System, Inc., Boston, MA

MICHAEL A. HOGE, Professor of Psychiatry (in Psychology), Yale University School of Medicine, New Haven, CT

OCTAVIO N. MARTINEZ, Executive Director and Clinical Professor, Hogg Foundation for Mental Health, The University of Texas at Austin

WILLARD MAYS, Mental Health and Aging Consultant, Indianapolis, IN, and Past Chair, National Coalition on Mental Health and Aging

PETER V. RABINS, Richman Family Professor, Department of Psychiatry and Behavioral Sciences, Johns Hopkins School of Medicine, Baltimore, MD

MARK SNOWDEN, Associate Professor, Department of Psychiatry and Behavioral Sciences, School of Medicine, University of Washington, Seattle

ROBYN STONE, Senior Vice President of Research, LeadingAge, Washington, DC

Study Staff

JILL EDEN, Study Director
MAI LE, Research Assistant
KATIE MASLOW, Scholar-in-Residence
MATT ALDAG, Mirzayan Fellow (September–December 2011)
AMY ASHEROFF, Senior Program Assistant (through August 2011)
JILLIAN LAFFREY, Board Assistant (from August 2011)
ROGER HERDMAN, Director, Board on Health Care Services

Reviewers

This report has been reviewed in draft form by individuals chosen for their diverse perspectives and technical expertise, in accordance with procedures approved by the National Research Council's Report Review Committee. The purpose of this independent review is to provide candid and critical comments that will assist the institution in making its published report as sound as possible and to ensure that the report meets institutional standards for objectivity, evidence, and responsiveness to the study charge. The review comments and draft manuscript remain confidential to protect the integrity of the deliberative process. We wish to thank the following individuals for their review of this report:

HENRY ACOSTA, Executive Director, National Resource Center for Hispanic Mental Health; Chair, Alliance for Latino Behavioral Health Workforce Development

BARBARA BOWERS, Helen Denne Schulte Professor, Institute on Aging; Associate Dean for Research and Charlotte Jane and Ralph A. Rodefer Chair, School of Nursing, University of Wisconsin–Madison

LOIS K. EVANS, van Ameringen Professor in Nursing Excellence, University of Pennsylvania School of Nursing

MARGARET GATZ, Professor of Psychology, Department of Psychology, University of Southern California

ROBYN L. GOLDEN, Director of Health and Aging, Rush University Medical Center

C. SETH LANDEFELD, Professor of Medicine, Chief, Division of Geriatrics, Director, UCSF-Mt. Zion Center on Aging; Associate Chair for Strategic Planning and Implementation, Department of Medicine

EDWARD O'NEIL, Director and Professor, Center for the Health Professions, University of California, San Francisco

DAVID W. OSLIN, VA Associate Chief of Staff for Behavioral Health Director, VISN 4 MIRECC; Associate Professor, Perelman School of Medicine, University of Pennsylvania

CHARLES F. REYNOLDS, UPMC Endowed Professor in Geriatric Psychiatry; Director, Advanced Center for Interventions and Services Research for Late-Life Depression Prevention; Director, John A. Hartford Center for Excellence in Geriatric Psychiatry, University of Pittsburgh, Western Psychiatric Institute and Clinic (WPIC)

WILLIAM A. VEGA, Provost Professor; Director, Edward R. Roybal Institute on Aging, School of Social Work, University of Southern California

TERI FOX WETLE, Associate Dean of Medicine for Public Health and Public Policy; Professor of Medical Science, Department of Public Health, Brown University Medical School

NANCY L. WILSON, Assistant Professor, Department of Medicine, Section of Geriatrics; Assistant Director, Huffington Center on Aging; Assistant Professor, Center for Medical Ethics and Health Policy, Baylor College of Medicine

Although the reviewers listed above have provided many constructive comments and suggestions, they were not asked to endorse the conclusions or recommendations, nor did they see the final draft of the report before its release. The review of this report was overseen by **Mary E. Tinetti** of the Yale University School of Medicine and **Nancy E. Adler** of the University of California, San Francisco. Appointed by the National Research Council and the Institute of Medicine, they were responsible for making certain that an independent examination of this report was carried out in accordance with institutional procedures and that all review comments were carefully considered. Responsibility for the final content of this report rests entirely with the authoring committee and the institution.

Preface

The burden of mental illness and substance use disorders in older adults in the United States borders on a crisis. Yet, this crisis is largely hidden from the public and many of those who develop policy and programs to care for older people. In contrast, concerns about the physical health care needs of the growing number of older Americans abound, even in the face of exploding Medicare costs and the federal budget deficit. Concerns about how to meet these needs led Congress to commission a report from the Institute of Medicine (IOM) on the physical health care needs of this population and the geriatric health care workforce required to meet them, resulting in the 2008 IOM report *Retooling for an Aging America: Building the Health Care Workforce*.

Following the release of the 2008 report, Congress wisely recognized the largely hidden crisis of mental health and substance use disorders in older adults and commissioned the IOM to convene a committee to study and report on the workforce needed to care for these older Americans. I was privileged to chair the committee that developed this report. The IOM assembled an outstanding committee with broad-ranging expertise, demographic and disciplinary diversity, total dedication to the project, and willingness to work hard to gather the relevant evidence, draft the report, and formulate recommendations. Our committee was supported by an exceptional team from the IOM, including Roger Herdman, Jill Eden (our guiding force as study director), Katie Maslow, Mai Le, Jillian Laffrey, Matt Aldag, and Amy Asheroff.

The task of caring for vulnerable older adults with mental health and substance use conditions is complex, and different disciplines hold divergent views about the best approaches to accomplish the task. Yet, our committee recognized from the outset that we must learn from each other and the consumers, mental health and substance use service providers, and government and private program administrators who shared their perspectives and experience with us, and work as a team to develop recommendations that cut across disciplines and other barriers to enhance the geriatric mental health and substance use workforce.

Overarching themes run through our report and recommendations. First, the public health impact of mental illness and substance use in older adults is significant, but responsibilities for programs and policies to develop and support the workforce that is needed to relieve this burden are not effectively distributed across federal government agencies. The federal government can gain efficiencies and effectiveness by clear assignment and coordination of responsibilities for geriatric mental health and substance use workforce development across agencies. Second, available data about the service needs of these older adults are not adequate to guide future workforce development. More comprehensive and timely data are needed for this purpose. Third, many opportunities that exist in current federal programs have not been fully leveraged for the development and support of the geriatric mental health and substance use workforce. The necessary resources to ensure a viable workforce may be derived in large part from these programs. Fourth, training in essential competencies for the care of older adults with mental illness and substance use disorders must be provided across the workforce if it is to meet the challenges it faces and will face in the future. Finally, new models of care must be put into place. Some of these models have been developed and demonstrated to be effective, and some remain to be developed.

It is with pleasure that we present this report.

Dan G. Blazer, *Chair*
Committee on the Mental Health
Workforce for Geriatric Populations

Acknowledgments

The committee and staff are indebted to a number of individuals and organizations for their contributions to this report. The following individuals provided testimony to the committee:

Moe Armstrong, Founder, Vet to Vet
Carol Colleran, Retired Director of Public Policy and National Affairs, Hanley Center—Addiction Counselor
Mary Ellen Copeland, Wellness Recovery Action Planning (WRAP)
Tim Engelhardt, Director, Demonstration Program, Centers for Medicare & Medicaid Services (CMS) Federal Coordinated Health Care Office (Duals Office)
Stephen Ferrante, Director, Aging Academy, Florida Atlantic University—Screening, Brief Intervention, and Referral to Treatment (SBIRT) Model for Older Adults with Substance Use Problems
Robyn Golden, Director of Older Adult Programs, Rush University Medical Center
Enid Hunkeler, Senior Scientist and Codirector, Inter-Divisional Depression Initiative, Kaiser Permanente Northern California Division of Research
Julie Jensen, Program Manager, Older Adult Services, HEROS Program, Good Samaritan Behavioral Health, Puyallup, WA—Gatekeeper Model

Kathy Kuhn, Director of Workforce Development, Institute for Geriatric Social Work, Boston University—Social Workers, Case Managers, and Outreach Workers
Harold Pincus, Codirector, Irving Institute of Clinical and Translational Research and Professor, Department of Psychiatry, Columbia University
Patrick J. Raue, Associate Professor of Psychology in Psychiatry, Weill Cornell Medical College—Home Care Nurses
Marian Scheinholtz, Public Health Advisor, Community Support Programs Branch, Substance Abuse and Mental Health Services Administration (SAMHSA)
Michael Schoenbaum, Senior Advisor for Mental Health Services, Epidemiology, and Economics, Office of the Director, National Institute of Mental Health (NIMH)—Providing Depression Care in a Primary Care Setting—IMPACT
Bernadette Seifert, Coordinator of Older Adult Services, National Alliance on Mental Illness, New Hampshire
Dan Timmel, Medicaid Long-Term Care Policy Analyst, CMS Disabled and Elderly Health Programs Group
Jurgen Unutzer, Professor, University of Washington Department of Psychiatry

We also extend special thanks to the following individuals who were essential sources of information, generously giving their time and knowledge to further the committee's efforts.

Scott Barstow, American Counseling Association
Carlos Blanco, Columbia University College of Physicians and Surgeons
Kipling M. Bohnert, Department of Veterans Affairs
Alice Bonner, CMS
Elizabeth Bragg, American Geriatrics Society
Shubing Cai, Brown University
David Chambers, NIMH
Robin E. Clark, University of Massachusetts Medical School
Teresa A. Coughlin, Urban Institute Health Policy Center
Nicholas Croce, Jr., American Psychiatric Nurses Association
Paola Daly, American Academy of Physician Assistants
Chris deVries, American Association for Geriatric Psychiatry
Deborah DiGilio, American Psychological Association
Meredith Eisenhart, Council on Social Work Education
Jovier Evans, NIMH

James Finley, American Mental Health Counselors Association
Beth Han, Center for Behavioral Health Statistics and Quality, SAMHSA
Rodney Harrell, AARP
Seiji Hayashi, Bureau of Primary Health Care
Jennifer Hohman, American Academy of Physician Assistants
Bob Hornyak, Administration on Aging
Gail Hunt, National Alliance for Caregiving
Jill Kagan, ARCH National Respite Network and Resource Center
William Lang, American Academy of Colleges of Pharmacy
Katharine Levit, Thomson Reuters
Lydia W. Li, University of Michigan School of Social Work
Cherry Lowman, National Institute on Alcohol Abuse and Alcoholism
Linda Lysoby, National Commission for Health Education Credentialing
Tami Mark, Thomson Reuters
Kristi Martinsen, Office of Rural Health Policy
Paul Moore, Health Resources and Services Administration (HRSA)
Vincent Mor, Brown University
Tom Morris, Office of Rural Health Policy
Mariquita G. Mullan, HRSA
Charlotte Mullican, Agency for Healthcare Research and Quality (AHRQ)
Tim Nanof, American Occupational Therapy Association
George Neiderhe, NIMH
Toru Okura, Bajikoen Clinic, Tokyo, Japan
Eunice Park-Lee, National Center for Health Statistics, Centers for Disease Control and Prevention
Alex Ross, HRSA
M. Katherine Shear, Columbia University School of Social Work
Susie Sherman, American Geriatrics Society
Shannon Skowronski, Administration on Aging
Jennifer Solomon, Center for Substance Abuse Prevention, SAMHSA
Anita Soni, AHRQ
Rebecco Spitzgo, National Health Service Corps
Melinda Anne Stanley, Baylor College of Medicine
Leonila Vega, Direct Care Alliance
Gil Weidenfeld, Annapolis, MD
Joan Weiss, Bureau of Health Professions, HRSA
Tracy Whitaker, National Association of Social Workers
Nancy L. Wilson, Baylor College of Medicine
Li-Tzy Wu, Duke University Medical Center

Funding for this study was provided by the Office of the Assistant Secretary for Planning and Evaluation (ASPE). The committee appreciates the opportunity and support extended by ASPE for the development of this report.

Finally, many within the Institute of Medicine were helpful to the study staff. We would like to thank Clyde Behney, Laura Harbold DeStefano, William McLeod, Abbey Meltzer, Vilija Teel, Lauren Tobias, and Sarah Ziegenhorn.

Contents

APPENDIXES

Boxes, Figures, and Tables

Summary

Boxes

Chapter 1

Boxes

Figure

Tables

Chapter 2

Boxes

Tables

Chapter 3

Boxes

Figures

Tables

Chapter 4

Boxes

Tables

Chapter 5

Boxes

Summary[1]

The aging of America has and will continue to have profound consequences for the nation's economy and society for years to come. The U.S. Census Bureau projects that the number of adults age 65 and older will increase from 40.3 million to 72.1 million between 2010 and 2030. Service providers, health care researchers, workforce experts, demographers, and others have long warned policy makers that with the aging of the baby boomer population, the nation faces a "silver tsunami" with the potential to overwhelm the nation's health care system. Similar calls have been made to address the nation's inadequate training and shortages of personnel for mental health and substance use (MH/SU) care. A health care workforce that is not prepared to address either MH/SU problems or the special needs of an aging population is a compelling public health burden.

In 2008, the Institute of Medicine (IOM) issued a report, *Retooling for an Aging America: Building the Health Care Workforce*, which highlighted the urgency of expanding and strengthening the geriatric health care workforce to meet the demands of our rapidly aging and changing population. The following year, Congress mandated that the IOM undertake a complementary study focusing on the geriatric MH/SU workforce needs of the nation. Thus, the IOM entered into a contract with the Office of the Assistant Secretary for Planning and Evaluation in the U.S. Department of Health and Human Services (HHS). The IOM Committee on the Mental

[1]This summary does not include references. Citations for the findings presented in the Summary appear in subsequent chapters.

Health Workforce for Geriatric Populations was appointed in early 2011 to carry out the charge. The 16-member committee included experts in geriatric psychiatry, substance use, social work, psychology, nursing, direct care, epidemiology, workforce development, labor economics, long-term care, health care delivery and financing, and health care disparities.

The committee's core charge was to assess the MH/SU needs of adults age 65 and older and to recommend how the nation should prepare the MH/SU workforce to meet these needs (Box S-1). The committee focused on the full spectrum of workers who are engaged in the detection, diagnosis, treatment, care, and management of MH/SU conditions in older adults—ranging from personnel who may have minimal education to specialty professionals with the most advanced psychiatric and neurological training. This includes

- MH/SU specialists such as general psychiatrists, psychologists, social workers, psychiatric nurses, and substance use counselors who may provide services to patients of any age;
- primary care providers, such as general internists, family medicine practitioners, advanced practice registered nurses, and physician assistants who may provide services to patients of any age (but may have daily contact with older adults who have MH/SU conditions);
- primary care providers with specialized training in the care of older adults, such as geriatricians and geriatric nurses;
- MH/SU providers with specialized training in the care of older adults, such as geriatric psychiatrists, gerontological nurses, geropsychologists, and gerontological social workers;
- direct care workers (DCWs) who, with minimal training, are employed to provide supportive services either in facilities or in the home;
- peer support providers who, with special training, teach peers the skills and behaviors to self-manage their mental illness; and
- informal caregivers such as family members, friends, and volunteer community members with the potential to identify and support older adults who may need MH/SU services.

The committee limited its scope in accordance with the sponsor's suggestions. The study's target population was older adults who have a prevalent MH/SU condition for which there were sufficient data for study (including the behavioral and psychiatric symptoms of dementia). The principal diagnoses of Alzheimer's disease and other dementias, intellectual disability, and autism spectrum disorder were excluded. Also out of scope were the effectiveness of individual therapeutic interventions,

BOX S-1
Charge to the IOM Committee on the Mental Health Workforce for Geriatric Populations

At the request of the U.S. Department of Health and Human Services' Office of the Assistant Secretary for Planning and Evaluation, the Institute of Medicine (IOM) will convene an ad hoc committee to determine the mental and behavioral health care needs of the target population—the population of Americans who are age 65 years and older—and then make policy and research recommendations for meeting those needs through a competent and well-trained mental health workforce, especially in light of the projected doubling of the aged population by 2030.

The committee will

- Provide a systematic and trend analysis of the current and projected mental and behavioral health care needs of the target population.
- Within the target population, consider the special needs of growing ethnic populations, of veterans with posttraumatic stress disorder, and of persons with chronic disease.
- Weigh the impact of improved diagnostic techniques, of addressing mental health issues as part of effective chronic disease management, and of the implementation of the federal mental health parity law on meeting the mental health needs of the target population.

When making recommendations, the committee will consider forces that shape the health care workforce, such as education, training, modes of practice, and the financing of public and private programs.

tobacco use (as a substance use condition), and workforce issues related to caregivers' needs.

A VULNERABLE AND UNDERSERVED POPULATION

Current and Future Prevalence of MH/SU Conditions Among Older Adults

MH/SU conditions in older people are associated with a wide range of negative effects, including emotional distress, functional disability, reduced physical health, increased mortality, suicide, high rates of hospitalization and nursing home placement, and high costs. The committee identified 27 MH/SU conditions that can have substantial negative effects on a person's emotional well-being, functional and self-care abilities, and quality of life (Box S-2). Although available data do not support definitive prevalence estimates, the committee concluded that at least 5.6 million to 8 million older adults have one or more of these conditions—about 14 to 20 percent of the overall elderly population. Depressive disorders and dementia-related behavioral and psychiatric symptoms are the most prevalent. Serious mental illness—including schizophrenia and bipolar disorder—is less common, but has significant implications for the workforce and care delivery.

Many older adults who have MH/SU conditions also have acute and chronic physical health conditions, and some have cognitive and functional impairments. The interaction of physical health conditions, cognitive and functional impairments, and MH/SU conditions is a defining feature of the geriatric mental health and substance use fields and has critical implications for the workforce. The interaction of these conditions also results in difficult caregiving situations for families, physicians, and other health care professionals, and residential care and home- and community-based service providers. For example:

- Age-related changes in the metabolism of alcohol and drugs, including prescription drugs, can cause or exacerbate alcohol and drug use conditions and increase an older person's risk of dangerous overdoses, even for people who have used alcohol and drugs at the same dose and frequency for many years without serious negative effects.
- Loss and grief are common in old age. The death of a spouse, partner, close relative, or friend can trigger or exacerbate depression and lead to severe, debilitating symptoms. Providers may find it difficult to distinguish major depression and grief when a patient is in the midst of a significant loss.
- Medications to treat common acute and chronic physical health conditions in older people can cause and exacerbate MH/SU conditions and, conversely, medications to treat MH/SU conditions can cause or worsen their physical health conditions.
- Cognitive and functional impairments can complicate the detection and diagnosis of MH/SU conditions. Cognitive impairment can also reduce an older person's ability to comply with treatment recommendations, including medications prescribed for the person's MH/SU and physical health conditions.

BOX S-2
Geriatric Mental Health and Substance Use Conditions Addressed in This Report

DSM-IV-TR Mental Disorders
- Adjustment disorder
- Anxiety disorders (including posttraumatic stress disorder)
- Bipolar disorder
- Depressive disorders
- Personality disorders
- Schizophrenia
- Substance-related disorders (including alcohol dependence and abuse, drug dependence and abuse)

Other Conditions
- Anxiety symptoms
- At-risk drinking or drug use
- Behavioral and psychiatric symptoms of dementia
- Complicated grief
- Fear of falling
- Hoarding
- Minor depression (depressive symptoms)
- Severe domestic squalor
- Severe self-neglect
- Suicidal ideation, plans, or attempts

NOTE: DSM-IV-TR mental disorders are defined by explicit criteria in the *Diagnostic and Statistical Manual of Mental Disorders*, Fourth Edition-Text Revision.

These unique characteristics of geriatric MH/SU create important requirements for workforce competencies, including the ability to detect possible MH/SU conditions in older people with coexisting physical health conditions and cognitive and functional impairments; ability to diagnose the conditions or knowledge about how to refer the person for a diagnostic evaluation; and ability to adapt treatments and ongoing management to accommodate the coexisting conditions.

Several demographic trends—growing population diversity, change in the makeup of the older population and characteristics of the baby boomer cohort—are likely to affect the prevalence of MH/SU conditions and the need for services in the coming decades. The U.S. Census Bureau projects that, from 2010 to 2030, the proportion of whites in the older population will decrease from about 80 to about 71 percent, reflecting sizable increases in the black and Hispanic/Latino older population. During the same period, the black older adult population is expected to increase by about 115 percent, and the Hispanic/Latino older adult population by more than 200 percent. By 2030, blacks will constitute about 10 percent of the older population, and Hispanic/Latinos about 12 percent.

Although there are only limited prevalence data for subgroups of older adults with MH/SU conditions, some analyses suggest important differences among racial and ethnic groups. The proportions of different age cohorts within the 65-and-older age group are also changing and are likely to have implications for the types of MH/SU services that are needed. For example, as the group ages 75-84 grows, dementia and associated psychiatric symptoms will become more prevalent.

As the baby boomers age, the rates of use of illicit drugs appear likely to increase. One recent report by the Substance Abuse and Mental Health Services Administration (SAMHSA), for example, found that illicit drug use nearly doubled among people ages 50-59 between 2002 and 2007, increasing from 5.1 percent in 2002 to 9.4 percent in 2007. This included an increase in marijuana use from 3.1 to 5.7 percent and nonmedical use of prescription drugs from 2.2 to 4 percent.

Adverse drug reactions may also be on the rise. According to SAMHSA, 61 percent of the 1.1 million emergency department visits for adverse drug reactions involved a person age 65 or older in 2008, and nearly a fourth of these emergency visits involved central nervous system drugs, including narcotic and nonnarcotic pain relievers.

Use of MH/SU Services

Older adults have been less likely to use MH/SU services compared with younger people with similar conditions. Older adults have also been less likely to use services provided in specialty settings, such as psychiatric hospitals, mental health clinics, and substance use treatment centers, and more likely to use MH/SU services provided in general medical care, residential care, and community-based service settings. In comparison with the current generation of older people, the baby boom generation has had higher average rates of mental health service use throughout their lives, and it is possible they will continue this pattern of service use as they grow older.

THE GERIATRIC MH/SU WORKFORCE: TOO FEW AND NOT PREPARED

Questions about the relationship between the demand for services and the supply emerge naturally in any discussion of workforce issues. It might seem straightforward to translate data on illness prevalence into estimates of service need and then, in turn, to estimates of required workforce supply. However, such efforts have always been fraught with methodological challenges and serious questions about the validity of the estimates that have been generated.

Data on the geriatric MH/SU workforce are even more elusive because the majority of workers who provide services to the geriatric population do not have recognized credentials in this specialty, and are thus more difficult to count, track, and analyze. Nevertheless, the committee finds that the sheer number of providers entering, working in, and remaining in the fields of primary care, geriatrics, mental health, substance use, and geriatric MH/SU is disconcertingly small.

Geriatric MH/SU specialists are an essential part of the interdisciplinary team because they are the most experienced and best equipped to consult and provide care for serious mental illnesses. With shifting models of care and the changing roles of different professions, it is not possible to estimate with great precision how many geriatric MH/SU specialists will be necessary to serve the geriatric population. However, the rate of specialized providers entering the workforce is dwarfed by the pace at which the population is growing. For example, the number of available fellowships in geriatric psychiatry has remained relatively stagnant since the 1990s, while the number of geriatric psychiatry fellows filling available slots decreased by half. This decline, juxtaposed with the predicted doubling of the geriatric population in the next 20 years, will make it increasingly difficult to rely solely on highly trained specialists to meet the MH/SU needs of older adults.

Training

General providers at all levels should be aware of the signs and symptoms of MH/SU conditions, and be able to respond appropriately within their level of training and scope of practice. However, few professions have mandated curricular standards related to MH/SU in geriatric patients. Where there is curriculum, it is unclear how and to what extent the concepts are applied in the classroom or in practical training. The prevalence of co-occurring conditions in the elderly and the shift toward collaborative models of care make interprofessional training essential to overall training in geriatric MH/SU care. The increasing racial, ethnic, and linguistic diversity of the geriatric population also makes cultural competence imperative. To what extent these aspects of care are being integrated into training and education is also unclear.

Barriers to Growing the Workforce

The barriers to growing and strengthening the geriatric MH/SU workforce are fundamental and entrenched in the systems and programs of numerous public and private entities—including multiple HHS and other federal agencies, professional organizations, medical and professional training institutions, credentialing and accreditation organizations, licensing bodies, service systems, payers, and research institutions (Box S-3). Recent efforts to augment training show that even when provided opportunities to specialize in geriatric MH/SU, students often do not choose to pursue it. This underscores the importance of simultaneously providing more training opportunities, guidance, mentorship, positive experiences, and financial incentives. Building up one of these

BOX S-3
Key Barriers and Issues Related to and Strengthening the Geriatric MH/SU Workforce

Defining the Geriatric MH/SU Workforce

- The geriatric MH/SU workforce is made up of many types of providers. Workforce roles are often poorly defined and overlapping.

Estimating Workforce Supply and Demand

- The standardized workforce data trended over time that are required to make accurate predictions of workforce supply and demand are not available.

Shortage of Geriatric MH/SU Providers

- The workforce prepared to care for geriatric MH/SU is inadequate in sheer numbers, with the growth of the population threatening to exacerbate this.

Recruiting Geriatric MH/SU Providers

- Across all health professions, relatively few opportunities for specialization in geriatric MH/SU exist. There is little support or mentorship available for those who do pursue specialization.
- Financial incentives are not in place to encourage geriatric MH/SU providers to enter and stay in this field.

Inadequate Preparation of the Geriatric MH/SU Workforce

- Professional training in geriatric MH/SU is inconsistent and not well documented because national standards and requirements in these areas are minimal and vague. MH/SU specialists have little required training in geriatrics; geriatric specialists have little components without considering the others will not solve the workforce crisis at hand.

Training general health care professionals and DCWs is pivotal to improving the workforce because they are the most likely personnel to come into contact with older adults with MH/SU conditions. The extent to which training and education are provided for these groups is not well documented. Relatively few standards are in place to ensure that formal

required training in MH/SU; and most general providers do not have extensive requirements in either area.

Training the Geriatric MH/SU Workforce

- Many professions have made progress on geriatric MH/SU competency development and workforce development, though these efforts are often done in silos where their dissemination and impact are not easily measured.
- Innovations in geriatric MH/SU workforce development are often vulnerable to grant cuts, and many promising programs end without adequate documentation or evaluation to assist future development.

Strengthening the Role of Direct Care Workers (DCWs) in Geriatric MH/SU Care

- Complex factors, including poor working conditions, low wages, lack of training, and limited opportunities for advancement, deter the development of a stable DCW workforce.
- DCWs have the most contact with older adult patients, yet do not have adequate training in geriatrics or MH/SU, and virtually never receive training in both.

Empowering Older Adults and Their Families

- There is a growing emphasis on peer support and self-care, including for older adult populations.
- Family members play a major role as caregivers, but receive little support and training for caring for older adults with any medical conditions, including MH/SU conditions.

training programs include competencies in addressing MH/SU conditions in older adults. Also essential to training are skills in cultural competence and interprofessional collaboration to meet the complex needs of older adults. However, the evidence base to determine what modes of training are most effective in geriatric MH/SU is largely insufficient.

WORKFORCE IMPLICATIONS OF MODELS OF GERIATRIC MH/SU CARE

U.S. health care delivery remains in a mode of care with origins in the early 20th century, when health care problems were typically acute and life expectancy was significantly shorter than today. However, an acute care orientation is not appropriate for much of geriatric care. For the older adult, chronic illness is the norm, not the exception—for both mental and physical health conditions.

A persuasive body of evidence, drawn from two decades of research, indicates that two common MH/SU disorders among older adults—depression and at-risk drinking—are most effectively addressed when care is organized to include these essential ingredients: (1) systematic outreach and diagnosis; (2) patient education and self-management support; (3) provider accountability for outcomes; and (4) close follow-up and monitoring to prevent relapse. Moreover, these elements are best obtained when care is patient centered, in a location easily accessed by patients (e.g., in primary care, senior centers, or patients' homes), and coordinated by trained personnel with access to specialty consultation. This is not likely to be achieved, however, without practice redesign and change in Medicare payment rules. There is a fundamental mismatch between older adults' need for coordinated care and Medicare fee-for-service reimbursement, which precludes payment of trained care managers and psychiatry consultation.

The committee concluded, as have many other studies, that the delivery of and payment for health care services to older adults must be reorganized to reflect the chronic nature of MH/SU and other health conditions prevalent in the 21st-century geriatric population. The workforce implications are daunting. Registered nurses are particularly well suited to coordinate MH/SU and physical health care, but they need additional training to serve in this capacity. Primary care providers, such as physicians, advanced practice registered nurses, and physician assistants have not been trained in collaborative care and do not work in a practice or system supportive of comanagement, colocation, screening, and outcome monitoring required by these models.

Frontline workers within the aging provider network agencies may be a potential source of care managers. However, they will require intensive training in evidence-based program treatment as they are likely to have limited knowledge of MH/SU. Moreover, training alone will not ensure the intended outcome of effectively meeting the MH/SU needs of older adults. Adequate supervision and coaching support of staff are also essential.

Finally, research on effective delivery of MH/SU care for certain older populations is urgently needed, especially for individuals residing in nursing homes and other residential settings, prisoners, rurally isolated elders, and older adults with serious mental illnesses.

RECOMMENDATIONS

There is a conspicuous lack of national attention either to preparing the health care workforce to care for older adults who have MH/SU conditions or to ensuring sufficient numbers of personnel for the rapidly growing elderly population. Many federal agencies, particularly within HHS, influence the makeup, competence, and capacity of the health care workforce to deliver MH/SU services to older adults. Yet, federal responsibility appears to be diffused across various agencies, bureaus, and departments. Moreover, the efforts of these agencies are minimal, lack specific focus on geriatric MH/SU, and, in some cases, are being discontinued. The Agency for Healthcare Research and Quality (AHRQ), for example, has initiated a noteworthy interagency effort—the Academy for Integrating Mental Health and Primary Care—to coordinate the collection, analysis, synthesis, and dissemination of research on integrating MH/SU services in primary care. But the program is underfunded.

The Centers for Medicare & Medicaid Services (CMS) has substantial potential to influence the delivery of geriatric MH/SU services. At present, Medicare and Medicaid reimbursement rules act to deter rather than to facilitate access to effective and efficient geriatric MH/SU services. The agency has numerous projects under way to evaluate new approaches—including payment reform—to improving the quality and effectiveness of services provided to Medicare and Medicaid beneficiaries. These innovation efforts may lead to MH/SU workforce improvements if eventually implemented on a wide scale.

The Health Resources and Services Administration (HRSA) is the central HHS agency tasked with promoting the production and training of key health personnel, but none of its geriatric training programs require exposure to MH/SU conditions.

Several institutes at the National Institutes of Health have missions related to aging and mental health or substance use, but none focus on geriatric MH/SU. The National Institute of Mental Health (NIMH), for example, has funded important research to inform the effective delivery of MH/SU services to older adults, but NIMH is scaling back support for interventions and services research in favor of research in basic translational neuroscience.

SAMHSA is the federal government's lead agency charged with directing services and resources to people with MH/SU conditions, yet it has consistently devoted only a small fraction of its budget to older adults. It is particularly disconcerting that the agency is reducing its activities related to geriatric MH/SU, including the elimination of the Older Adults Targeted Capacity Expansion grants program.

BOX S-4
Recommendations

RECOMMENDATION 1: Congress should direct the Secretary of Health and Human Services (HHS) to designate a responsible entity for coordinating federal efforts to develop and strengthen the nation's geriatric mental health and substance use (MH/SU) workforce.

- The committee urges Congress to fund the already authorized National Health Care Workforce Commission to serve in this capacity. In the absence of congressional action, the Secretary of HHS should act as soon as possible to designate an alternative body.
- The coordinating body should have the following priorities with respect to the geriatric MH/SU workforce:
  - Identification, development, and refinement of methods for improving recruitment and retention of geriatric MH/SU personnel, including ways to build a workforce that reflects the increasingly diverse older adult population.
  - Promotion and support of widescale implementation of evidence-based models of geriatric MH/SU care that effectively deploy personnel.
  - Identification, development, and refinement of model curricula and curriculum development tools in geriatric MH/SU, including effective models of training for integrated rehabilitation, health promotion, health care, and social services for older adults with serious mental illness.
  - Identification, development, and refinement of core competencies in geriatric MH/SU for the entire spectrum of personnel who care for older adults, including direct care workers,

Box S-4 presents the committee's recommendations. Congress and the HHS Secretary must act to establish a locus of responsibility for geriatric MH/SU, to invigorate investment in the human capital that is the geriatric MH/SU workforce, to catalyze basic system redesign to allow for effective deployment of geriatric MH/SU personnel, and to stimulate essential research to inform the education and training of personnel and workforce planning itself.

peer support specialists, primary care physicians, nurses (at all levels), physician assistants, substance use counselors, social workers, psychologists, rehabilitation counselors, and marriage and family therapists.

- o Evaluation and dissemination of all of the above.

RECOMMENDATION 2: The Secretary of HHS should ensure that its agencies—including the Administration on Aging (AoA), Agency for Healthcare Research and Quality (AHRQ), Centers for Medicare & Medicaid Services (CMS), Health Resources and Services Administration (HRSA), National Institute of Mental Health (NIMH), National Institute on Drug Abuse (NIDA), and Substance Abuse and Mental Health Services Administration (SAMHSA)—assume responsibility for building the capacity and facilitating the deployment of the MH/SU workforce for older Americans:

- CMS
    - o CMS should evaluate alternative methods for funding primary care and other personnel who provide evidence-based models of care to older adults with MH/SU conditions. This should include reimbursing care managers as well as the psychiatrists and other mental health specialists providing supervision of their work.
    - o CMS should evaluate alternative payment methods to encourage effective deployment of the workforce to provide integrated primary care, chronic disease self-management, and health promotion for older adults receiving care in community mental health centers and other specialty mental health settings.
    - o CMS should explore approaches and strategies for improving care delivery to older adults with MH/SU conditions through its contracts with quality-improvement organizations.

continued

BOX S-4 Continued

- CMS should enforce and monitor implementation of the Pre-Admission Screening and Resident Review (PASRR) and Minimum Data Set (MDS) nursing home requirements regarding residents' mental health. The agency should also ensure that PASRR and MDS mental health assessments inform residents' care plans and that nursing home personnel implement the care plans accordingly.

- HRSA
  - The HRSA Administrator should ensure that the National Center for Health Care Workforce Analysis devotes sufficient attention to geriatric MH/SU with guidance from the national coordinating body described below.
  - The HRSA Administrator should ensure that the Geriatric Academic Career Awards career development grants include awards to geriatric MH/SU specialists if they commit to working with older adults in acute or long-term care settings.
  - The HRSA Administrator should ensure that the Geriatric Education Centers and the Comprehensive Geriatric Education Program institutional awards fund programs that train individuals in geriatric MH/SU care.
- NIMH
  - The Director of NIMH should ensure that the institute conducts research on methods for increasing the capacity of the mental health workforce to provide competent and effective care for older adults who reside in the community or in nursing homes or other congregate residential settings.
- SAMHSA
  - The SAMHSA Administrator should ensure that the agency devotes sufficient attention to the capacity of the behavioral health workforce to provide both geriatric mental health and geriatric substance use services.
  - The SAMHSA Administrator should ensure that the agency restores funding of the Older Adult Mental Health Targeted Capacity Expansion Grant program.
  - The SAMHSA Administrator should require states that receive MH/SU block grants to document and to report how the funds are used to support local capacity to serve older adults.

RECOMMENDATION 3: Organizations responsible for accreditation, certification, and professional examination, as well as state licensing boards, should modify their standards, curriculum requirements, and credentialing procedures to require professional competence

in geriatric MH/SU for all levels of personnel that care for the diversity of older adults.

- These efforts should include requirements for recredentialing and professional development for already licensed and certified personnel.

RECOMMENDATION 4: Congress should appropriate funds for the Patient Protection and Affordable Care Act (ACA) workforce provisions that authorize training, scholarship, and loan forgiveness for individuals who work with or are preparing to work with older adults who have MH/SU conditions. This funding should be targeted to programs with curricula in geriatric MH/SU and directed specifically to the following types of workers who make a commitment to caring for older adults who have MH/SU conditions:

- Psychiatrists, psychologists, psychiatric nurses, social workers, MH/SU counselors, and other specialists who require skills and knowledge of both geriatrics and MH/SU.
- Primary care providers, including geriatricians and other physicians, registered nurses (RNs), advance practice registered nurses (APRNs), and physician assistants.
- Potential care managers for older adults who have MH/SU conditions, including RNs, APRNs, social workers, physician assistants, and others.
- Faculty in medicine, nursing, social work, psychology, substance use counseling, and other specialties.
- Direct care workers and other frontline employees in home health agencies, nursing homes, and assisted living facilities (including personal care attendants not employed by an agency).
- Family caregivers of older adults with MH/SU conditions.

RECOMMENDATION 5: HHS should direct a responsible entity (as described above) to develop and coordinate implementation of a data collection and reporting strategy for geriatric MH/SU workforce planning. Data collection and reporting should include the following:

- Prevalence data for *Diagnostic and Statistical Manual of Mental Disorders* (DSM)-defined disorders and other MH/SU conditions, including data on comorbidity of these conditions. Representative data on the following subgroups are essential:
  - Age within the 65+ population (65-74, 75-84, and 85 and older)

continued

BOX S-4 Continued

- Gender
- Race and ethnicity (including non-English speakers)
- Veteran status
- Living situation (private household, public housing or senior housing facility, group home, assisted living or other residential care facility, and nursing home)
- Coexisting physical health conditions
- Coexisting cognitive and functional impairments
- Geographic area

- Use of MH/SU services for the above subgroups.
- Comprehensive and comparable information on the full range of geriatric MH/SU personnel with sufficient detail to assess the workforce supply by race and ethnicity; language skills; geographic location and distribution; qualifications, training, and certification; areas of practice; and hours spent in the care of older adults.

1

Introduction

Abstract: *This chapter presents the objectives, scope, and context for this report and describes the approach that the Institute of Medicine (IOM) Committee on the Mental Health Workforce for Geriatric Populations used to undertake the study. The committee's charge was twofold: first, to determine the mental health and substance use (MH/SU) needs of the 65-and-older population and, second, to develop recommendations for ensuring a competent and sufficient workforce to meet these needs. This study was undertaken during a period characterized by considerable uncertainty regarding the future organization and financing of the U.S. health care system, dramatic change in the makeup of the older population, and great concern about the capacity of the nation's MH/SU workforce to meet the needs of older adults. Federal responsibility for geriatric MH/SU is diffused among numerous U.S. Department of Health and Human Services agencies, and the agencies' attention to these concerns is minimal and dwindling.*

The aging of America has and will continue to have profound consequences for the nation's economy and society for years to come. The U.S. Census Bureau projects that the number of adults age 65 and older will increase from 40.3 million to 72.1 million between 2010 and 2030 (Vincent and Velkoff, 2010). During the same period, the ethnic, racial, and cultural makeup of the older adult population will become more diverse than ever (Cummings et al., 2011; Vincent and Velkoff, 2010). The impact on the demand for and cost of health care will be unprecedented. In 2008, the Institute of Medicine (IOM) issued a report, *Retooling for an Aging America: Building the Health Care Workforce*, which highlighted the urgency of expanding and strengthening the geriatric health care workforce to meet the demands of our rapidly aging and changing population (IOM, 2008). The following year, because of similar concerns about geriatric mental health and substance use (MH/SU) needs, Congress mandated that the IOM undertake a complementary study focusing on the geriatric MH/SU workforce needs of the nation (U.S. Congress, House of Representatives, 2009). Thus, in response to the congressional mandate, the IOM entered into a contract with the Office of the Assistant Secretary for Planning and Evaluation in the U.S. Department of Health and Human Services (HHS) in September 2010. The IOM Committee on the Mental Health Workforce for Geriatric Populations was appointed in early 2011 to carry out the charge. The 16-member committee included experts in geriatric psychiatry, substance use, social work, psychology, and nursing; direct care workers; and those with specialties in epidemiology, workforce development, labor economics, long-term care, health care delivery and financing, and health care disparities.[1] Brief biographies of the committee members are provided in Appendix E.

STUDY SCOPE

The charge to the committee was essentially twofold: first, to assess the current and projected MH/SU needs of adults age 65 and older and, second, to recommend how the nation should prepare the MH/SU workforce to meet these needs (Box 1-1). The committee was also asked to address the unique needs of important subgroups in the older adult population, including individuals of diverse ethnic backgrounds, veterans with posttraumatic stress disorder, and persons living with chronic disease. The study sponsor asked the committee to define the MH/SU workforce broadly (Frank, 2011). The committee focused on the full spectrum of workers who are engaged in the diagnosis, treatment, care, and management of MH/SU conditions in older adults—ranging from personnel who may have minimal education to specialty physicians with the most advanced psychiatric and neurological training. This includes

[1]An additional committee member with expertise in the consumer perspective was also appointed, but had to step down from the committee due to illness.

BOX 1-1
Charge to the IOM Committee on the Mental Health Workforce for Geriatric Populations

At the request of the U.S. Department of Health and Human Services Office of the Assistant Secretary for Planning and Evaluation, the Institute of Medicine (IOM) will convene an ad hoc committee to determine the mental and behavioral health care needs of the target population—the population of Americans who are over age 65 years—and then make policy and research recommendations for meeting those needs through a competent and well-trained mental health workforce, especially in light of the projected doubling of the aged population by 2030.

The committee will

- Provide a systematic and trend analysis of the current and projected mental and behavioral health care needs of the target population.
- Within the target population, consider the special needs of growing ethnic populations, of veterans with posttraumatic stress disorder, and of persons with chronic disease.
- Weigh the impact of improved diagnostic techniques, of addressing mental health issues as part of effective chronic disease management, and of the implementation of the federal mental health parity law on meeting the mental health needs of the target population.

When making recommendations, the committee will consider forces that shape the health care workforce, such as education, training, modes of practice, and the financing of public and private programs.

- MH/SU specialists such as general psychiatrists, psychologists, social workers, psychiatric nurses, and substance use counselors who may provide services to patients or clients of any age;
- primary care providers, such as general internists, family medicine practitioners, advanced practice registered nurses, and physician assistants who may provide services to patients of any age (but may have daily contact with older adults who have MH/SU conditions);
- primary care providers with specialized training in the care of older adults, such as geriatricians and geriatric nurses (excludes MH/SU specialists);

- MH/SU providers with specialized training in the care of older adults, such as geriatric psychiatrists, gerontological nurses, geropsychologists, and gerontological social workers;
- direct care workers who, with minimal training, are employed to provide supportive services either in facilities or in the home;
- peer support providers who, with special training, teach peers the skills and behaviors to self-manage their mental illness; and
- informal caregivers such as family members, friends, and volunteer community members with the potential to identify and support older adults who may need MH/SU services.

In its early deliberations, the committee worked on refining its charge and workplan for the study. During the first committee meeting, the study sponsor made five suggestions that helped the committee focus its work: (1) concentrate on the MH/SU conditions that are most prevalent among older adults and for which there are sufficient data for study (Box 1-2); (2) exclude the principal diagnoses of cognitive impairment

BOX 1-2
Geriatric Mental Health and Substance Use Conditions Addressed in This Report

Older adults with the following conditions are the focus of this report. See Chapter 2 for definitions of each condition and related epidemiological data and analysis.

DSM-IV-TR Mental Disorders

- Adjustment disorder
- Anxiety disorders (including posttraumatic stress disorder)
- Bipolar disorder
- Depressive disorders
- Personality disorders
- Schizophrenia
- Substance-related disorders (including alcohol dependence and abuse, drug dependence and abuse)

Other Conditions

- Anxiety symptoms
- At-risk drinking or drug use
- Behavioral and psychiatric symptoms of dementia
- Complicated grief
- Fear of falling
- Hoarding
- Minor depression (depressive symptoms)
- Severe domestic squalor
- Severe self-neglect
- Suicidal ideation, plans, or attempts

(e.g., Alzheimer's disease and other dementias), intellectual disability, and autism spectrum disorder, but include the behavioral and psychiatric symptoms of dementia; (3) do not explore the effectiveness of individual therapeutic interventions (e.g., prescription medications, specific approaches to psychotherapy); (4) exclude tobacco use as a substance use condition; and (5) exclude workforce issues related to caregivers' needs. The sponsor also recommended that the committee limit its inquiry into diagnostic techniques to the question of how the workforce can most effectively identify older adults who need MH/SU services.

METHODS OF THE STUDY

The committee deliberated during four in-person meetings and numerous teleconferences between March 2011 and April 2012. In June 2011, the committee held a public workshop to learn the perspectives of selected stakeholders, including consumers, families, and caregivers; providers who care for older adults in various settings; researchers who have studied the effectiveness of different models of care; and policy makers. Appendix B contains the workshop agenda.

As the subsequent chapters will make clear, data are very limited describing older adults with MH/SU conditions, the workforce that serves them, or the private and public programs that support them. The study committee and staff consulted with many representatives of public- and private-sector organizations to obtain information about relevant programs and policies. Staff from HHS agencies (Administration on Aging, Centers for Medicare & Medicaid Services, Health Resources and Services Administration, National Institute of Mental Health, Substance Abuse and Mental Health Services Administration, and others) and the Veterans Health Administration offered critical insights and program data. The professional organizations listed in Box 1-3 provided information on training and education, requirements for program accreditation, licensing and certification, and trends in the size and makeup of the workforce.

Terminology

This report uses the term "geriatric MH/SU workforce" to refer to the full range of personnel providing services to older adults with MH/SU conditions. The term "older adult" refers to individuals age 65 and older.

Many terms and labels are used to describe mental health conditions and problems related to abuse or misuse of substances. This report uses the term "mental health condition" to describe mental disorders defined

BOX 1-3
Nongovernmental Organizations That Provided Workforce Information to the IOM Committee

- American Association for Geriatric Psychiatry
- American Association of Colleges of Pharmacy
- American Association of Physician Assistants
- American Counseling Association
- American Geriatrics Society
- American Mental Health Counselors Association
- American Occupational Therapy Association
- American Psychiatric Nurses Association
- American Psychological Association
- ARCH National Respite Network
- Council for Social Work Education
- Direct Care Alliance
- National Alliance for Caregiving
- National Association of Social Workers

in the *Diagnostic and Statistical Manual of Mental Disorders* (DSM-IV-TR)[2] as well as the range of symptoms and syndromes that result in significant emotional distress, functional disability, and reduced quality of life in older adults. The term "substance use conditions" refers to abuse, misuse, or dependence on alcohol and drugs (both illicit drugs and prescription and nonprescription medications).

CONTEXT FOR THIS REPORT

A Health Care System in Transition

As this report goes to press, the degree of uncertainty about the future of the U.S. health care delivery system is unprecedented. The nation awaits the outcome of a U.S. Supreme Court decision regarding the constitutionality of the Patient Protection and Affordable Care Act.[3] The outcome has substantial implications for older adults with MH/SU conditions because the Act contains numerous provisions related to the

[2]DSM, or DSM-IV-TR, refers to the *Diagnostic and Statistical Manual of Mental Disorders*. During the course of this study, the Fourth Edition-Text Revision (DSM-IV-TR) was in use. A fifth edition is expected in 2013 (American Psychiatric Association, 2012).

[3]Public Law 111-148.

health care workforce, the delivery and integration of MH/SU services, and the organization and financing of Medicare and Medicaid MH/SU services. In addition, as Box 1-4 describes, recent legislation mandating parity in insurance coverage of physical and mental health conditions will be implemented during the next few years.

The backdrop for these events is a dramatic shift in the age makeup of the U.S. population. Numerous expert reports have stressed the urgency of preparing the nation's health care workforce for the "silver tsunami" of the aging baby boomer population (IOM, 1978, 2008). Along with the sheer growth in numbers of Medicare beneficiaries will be a corresponding rise in demand for health care services. Many of the older adults seeking physical health care services in primary care settings, hospitals, and elsewhere will have coexisting MH/SU conditions. Considerable evidence shows that older adults with MH/SU conditions are among the most costly Medicare beneficiaries (Alecxih et al., 2010; Cummings and Kropf, 2011; MedPAC, 2011). Older adults have complex and multiple health care problems. When these medical conditions are accompanied by a mental health or substance use diagnosis, the older patient is likely to use more costly services and suffer poorer outcomes. If the nation is to confront the growing burden of Medicare costs, it must develop ways to maximize the productive capacity of the geriatric MH/SU workforce. Many reports have also described the inadequate supply of MH/SU personnel (Hogan, 2003; Hoge et al., 2007; IOM, 2006; Jeste et al., 1999). The U.S. health care delivery system has always focused more on physical health than mental health (IOM, 2006). This stems from numerous factors, including long-held societal biases against MH/SU conditions, limitations on health coverage of MH/SU conditions, federal statutes that require states to assume primary responsibility for adults under age 65 with serious mental illness, and the widespread carve-out of MH/SU coverage and service delivery into systems separate from the rest of health care.

Perhaps, as a consequence, MH/SU health care delivery is inadequate and of poor quality for most older adults. Many MH/SU conditions are neither detected nor diagnosed properly in older adults. Because MH/SU problems rarely occur apart from physical health problems, care coordination is integral to good health outcomes (Lin et al., 2003, 2011; Noel et al., 2004). Evidence-based, effective treatments and models exist for coordinating MH/SU care. Moreover, there is growing evidence suggesting that effective identification and treatment of MH/SU conditions may be central to reducing the costs and improving the effectiveness of the Medicare program (Unützer et al., 2008).

BOX 1-4
Parity for Coverage of Geriatric Mental Health/Substance Use (MH/SU) Services

In 2008, two landmark bills mandating parity in health insurance coverage of MH/SU services became law: (1) the Medicare Improvements for Patients and Providers Act of 2008 (Public Law 110-275) and (2) the Paul Wellstone and Pete Domenici Mental Health Parity and Addiction Equity Act of 2008 (Public Law 110-343). The following describes both mandates and briefly considers the possible implications for the geriatric MH/SU workforce:

- **Medicare Improvements for Patients and Providers Act (MIPPA).** Since the creation of the Medicare program, the Medicare coinsurance rate for outpatient mental health services has been much higher than the rate for most other outpatient health care services (i.e., 50 percent vs. 20 percent). MIPPA equalizes the outpatient Medicare coinsurance rates, thus creating "parity" in the coverage of mental health and physical health care. The reduction in the coinsurance rate from 50 to 20 percent is being phased in over a 5-year period starting in 2010.
- **Mental Health Parity and Addiction Equity Act.** This law mandated parity in the coverage of physical and MH/SU conditions by employer-sponsored group health plans with more than 50 insured employees.[a] The health plans are not required to provide MH/SU benefits but, if they do, the benefits must be no more

Changing Face of the Older Population

The older adult age cohort is not only growing rapidly, but the age distribution within the cohort is changing, as is the racial and ethnic makeup of the population (Vincent and Velkoff, 2010). Census projections indicate that, from 2003 to 2030, the proportion of older adults who are white (non-Hispanic) will decline from 83 percent to 72 percent (Table 1-1).

The increasing proportion of older adults who are racial/ethnic minorities will demand a workforce that is prepared to work with diverse populations. In particular, the rapid growth of Hispanic and Asian populations will necessitate increased linguistic competence from the workforce. *Black*, *Hispanic*, and *Asian* are deceptively simple categorizations for the many nationalities, languages, and subcultures represented in these groups. Preparing a culturally and linguistically competent workforce restrictive then the plan's medical and surgical benefits. Thus the deductibles, copays, coinsurance, out-of-pocket maximums, and treatment limitations (including day or visit limits and medical management tools) for MH/SU and physical health conditions must be the same.

Workforce Implications

Little evidence suggests that either parity mandate will have much impact on the geriatric MH/SU workforce. Parity could potentially increase demand for the services of MH/SU providers. However, it is unlikely the increased demand will be large enough to motivate more providers to provide geriatric MH/SU services. In fact, the Congressional Budget Office has predicted that parity will have minimal impact on costs.

Most importantly, parity does *not* affect what MH/SU services are covered by Medicare or which providers can be reimbursed for providing MH/SU care to older adults. As a result, even after full phase-in of parity, the evidence-based innovations in MH/SU care delivery (described in Chapter 4) will continue to be unreimbursable under the Medicare program.

[a]The Patient Protection and Affordable Care Act (ACA) extends the mandate to other types of private health insurance plans.
SOURCES: Congressional Budget Office, 2008; Garfield et al., 2011; MedPAC, 2010; Sarata, 2011.

that reflects the diversity of the wider population will be an important challenge for the coming decades.

Figure 1-1 shows the age distribution of the projected older population through 2050. Currently, persons ages 65 to 69 make up the largest proportion of the older population. However, as the oldest of the baby boomers age, the age distribution will shift, with an increasing percentage of the older population being over 80 years old. Because the "oldest-old" typically require more frequent and more intense care than the "young-old," the changing age distribution of the older population has many implications for the health care workforce.

The Health Care Workforce

This examination of the MH/SU workforce for geriatric populations occurs within the context of the nation's health care workforce at large, the

TABLE 1-1
U.S. Census Projection of the Racial and Ethnic Makeup of the Older Adult Population, by Percentage, 2003 and 2030

Race/Ethnicity	Percentage of Population Ages 65 and Older	
	2003	2030
Non-Hispanic white	83	72
Black	8	10
Hispanic	6	11
Asian	3	5

NOTE: Percentages may not total 100 because of rounding.
SOURCE: Drayer et al., 2005.

workforce that specializes in the care of older adults, and the workforce trained broadly to provide services to individuals with MH/SU conditions. There are numerous and substantive concerns about the workforce as a whole, as well as its specialty sectors. Understanding these concerns is critical to grasping the enormous obstacles to building a strong workforce that can meet the MH/SU needs of the growing geriatric population.

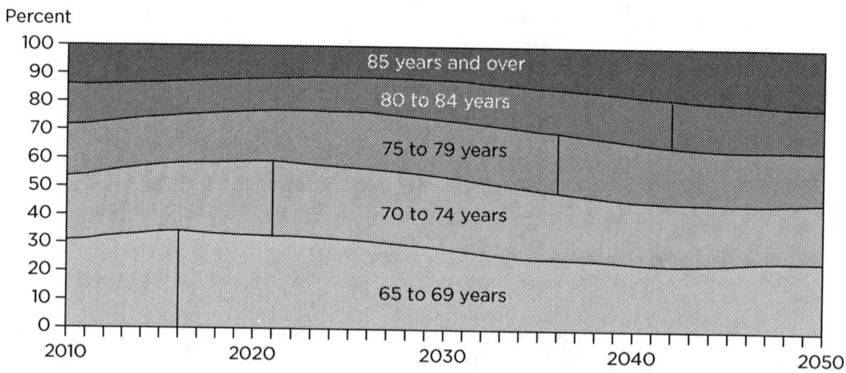

FIGURE 1-1
Distribution of the projected older population by age for the United States, 2010-2050.

NOTE: The vertical line indicates the year that each age group is the largest proportion of the older population.

SOURCE: Vincent and Velkoff, 2010.

Concerns About the Overall Health Care Workforce

In *Crossing the Quality Chasm: A New Health System for the 21st Century*, the IOM called for major changes in health care workforce development, training, and education (IOM, 2001). It highlighted, among other problems, the critical challenges in recruitment and retention, which have been most visible in the field of nursing and the inadequate preparation of the workforce as a whole to function in interdisciplinary teams and to implement evidence-based practices. A subsequent IOM report, *Health Professions Education: A Bridge to Quality*, added to this list of concerns the lack of preparedness among the workforce to address shifts in the nation's patient population, analyze and address problems in health care quality, and use informatics to support the provision and quality of care (IOM, 2003). A myriad of other issues have been identified by other experts, including the limited attention given to preparing and supporting the direct care, largely nondegreed workforce (Hewitt et al., 2008) or the self-care and peer support roles of individuals and family members (Brown and Wituk, 2010; Mowbray et al., 1997).

Improvements in health care workforce development have been impeded by a range of factors, including conservative professional hierarchies that govern health professions education and facilitate a very gradual pace of reform; a dense and inconsistent patchwork of laws, regulations, agencies, and accreditation processes that are slow to adapt and change; continuing education approaches that have minimal effect on clinical practice or health care outcomes; and the absence of methods for ensuring the ongoing competence of practitioners (IOM, 2001).

Concerns About the Workforce for Geriatric Populations

The state of the nation's workforce that is specifically trained to care for older adults was captured recently and comprehensively in *Retooling for an Aging America: Building the Health Care Workforce* (IOM, 2008). As Chapter 3 will describe, the available statistics are sobering. They document how few individuals choose to specialize in geriatrics in any sector of health care, and the frequency with which such individuals decide to let their credentials in geriatric specialties lapse. Among the geriatric specialists that remain in this field, there is marked maldistribution, with few working in rural areas even though older adults are overrepresented in rural areas and are less healthy than their urban counterparts.

For members of the general workforce, professional education provides little training related to the assessment and treatment of older adults and little exposure to geriatric populations. Whatever is provided tends to occur late in the sequence of educational experiences, minimizing its potential to influence interest in specialization. Factors cited as impediments to increasing training regarding geriatric care include the lack of faculty trained in geriatrics, the lack of funds, competition for time in program curricula, the stigma associated with older adults and their care, and financial disincentives to geriatric practice.

Concerns About the General MH/SU Workforce

Challenges confronting the MH/SU workforce were highlighted in detail in a number of reports released over the past decade, including *Improving the Quality of Health Care for Mental and Substance-Use Conditions* (IOM, 2006); *Strengthening Professional Identity: Challenges of the Addiction Treatment Workforce* (Whittier, 2006); and *An Action Plan for Behavioral Health Workforce Development* (Hoge et al., 2007). These reports captured the enormous complexity of the behavioral health workforce with its numerous professions, variation in educational approaches, and varied workforce type, including professionals, direct care workers, persons in recovery, and family members. Data on this workforce have not been collected routinely or in a uniform manner, making it difficult to understand its composition and relevant trends. However, the information available highlighted the striking lack of racial and cultural diversity, particularly at the professional level, and the serious workforce shortages. The latter have been acute, especially in rural and frontier areas of the country and for the field of addictions.

Training in the screening, assessment, and treatment of substance use disorders is typically minimal in all but addiction-specific professional programs despite the prevalence of substance use conditions among those receiving mental health care (see Appendix C). Similarly, there has been a noted dearth of practitioners trained in meeting not only the needs of older adults, but children and youth as well. Many professionals have struggled to understand and incorporate recovery-oriented approaches to care, but the behavioral health disciplines, in general, have had difficulty blending their drive to professionalize their discipline with the growing focus on recovery and peer support. Furthermore, it has been a challenge educating and engaging the MH/SU workforce in evidence-based practices, such as the use of medications to treat addictions. Innovative efforts to address the myriad of workforce problems in behavioral health have tended to be short-lived with little evaluation of their impact or dissemination nationally.

FEDERAL INFLUENCE ON THE GERIATRIC MH/SU WORKFORCE

Many federal policies influence the makeup, competence, and capacity of the health care workforce to deliver MH/SU services to older adults.

Many federal agencies, particularly within HHS, have the authority to catalyze activities to strengthen the geriatric MH/SU workforce and to improve the quality of services they provide. Yet federal responsibility appears to be diffused across various agencies, bureaus, and departments. No one entity within HHS is taking the lead. As Table 1-2 suggests, HHS agencies' attention to the older adult population with geriatric MH/SU conditions has been minimal and is clearly declining.

ORGANIZATION OF THE REPORT

Chapter Objectives

This introductory chapter has described the background, charge to the committee, scope, methods, and context for this report.

Chapter 2, "Assessing the Service Needs of Older Adults with Mental Health and Substance Use Conditions," presents prevalence and use data and considers the impact of population trends, particularly the aging of the baby boomer cohort and growing population diversity, on the makeup of the older population and future needs for MH/SU services.

Chapter 3, "The Geriatric Mental Health and Substance Use Workforce," describes the spectrum of personnel who serve older adults with MH/SU conditions and assesses the capacity and competence of the workforce to meet the needs of this population.

Chapter 4, "Workforce Implications of Models of Care for Older Adults with Mental Health and Substance Use Conditions," describes nine evidence-based MH/SU interventions for older adults, the implications of the models for developing the workforce, and the barriers to implementation.

Chapter 5, "In Whose Hands? Recommendations for Strengthening the Mental Health and Substance Use Workforce for Older Americans," presents the committee's findings and recommendations.

TABLE 1-2
Selected Department of Health and Human Services (HHS) Agencies with the Potential to Strengthen the Geriatric MH/SU Workforce

Key Focus/ Agency	Emphasis on Mental Health and Substance Abuse (MH/SU) Services and Workforces
FINANCING	
Centers for Medicare & Medicaid Services (CMS)	
—Medicare and Medicaid programs	• Medicare—40 million adults age 65+ were Medicare beneficiaries in 2011. Medicare payment rules are the principal driver of (1) which providers and other types of personnel can be reimbursed for providing MH/SU services to older adults, (2) how the geriatric MH/SU workforce is organized to provide services, and (3) the types of services that are provided. o Supports quality-improvement organizations (QIOs), private organizations charged with improving the quality of health care for Medicare beneficiaries. • Medicaid—nearly 10 percent of Medicare beneficiaries over age 64 have dual Medicaid and Medicare coverage. A significant proportion has serious mental illness (SMI). Medicaid is the principal payer of nursing home care for older adults with MH/SU conditions. Thus, the Medicaid program o oversees the implementation the Preadmission Screening and Resident Review Program (PASRR), which requires MH screening and treatment follow-up for nursing home residents. o oversees the implementation of the Minimum Data Set (MDS), a mandatory data collection and screening instrument for assessing nursing home patients' physical and mental health status. • Medicaid also administers two programs that serve older adults with MH/SU conditions: o Home- and community-based waivers for individuals who would otherwise require care

	in a nursing home or other institutional setting (about 30 percent of all long-term care Medicaid spending). o The "Money Follows the Person" rebalancing demonstration program, which helps state Medicaid programs support the use of home- and community-based services in lieu of nursing homes or other institutional services (including for older adults with SMI who are transitioning out of institutions into the community). • The CMS Center for Medicare and Medicaid Innovation (CMMI) sponsors several large-scale initiatives to develop and assess ways to improve the quality, effectiveness, and efficiency of the Medicare and Medicaid programs. These include Accountable Care Organizations (ACOs), Bundled Payments for Care Improvement, the Comprehensive Primary Care Initiative, the Health Care Innovation Challenge, State Demonstrations to Integrate Care for Dual Eligibles, the Medicaid Emergency Psychiatric Demonstration, and others.
RESEARCH	
Agency for Healthcare Research and Quality (AHRQ)	
—Center for Primary Care, Prevention, and Clinical Partnerships	No specific focus on geriatric MH/SU. • Spearheading the creation of an Academy for Integrating Mental Health and Primary Care to serve as a national coordinating center and clearinghouse for the collection, analysis, synthesis, and dissemination of research on integrating MH/SU services in primary care.
—Effective Health Care Program	No specific focus on geriatric MH/SU. • Funds clinical effectiveness research on a broad range of topics related to the needs of the Medicare, Medicaid, and State Children's Health Insurance Programs.

continued

TABLE 1-2 Continued

Key Focus/ Agency	Emphasis on Mental Health and Substance Abuse (MH/SU) Services and Workforces
Centers for Disease Control and Prevention (CDC)	Administers or supports several programs and research related to geriatric MH/SU. • The Healthy Aging Research Network sponsors, translates, and disseminates research on programs and policies to facilitate healthy aging including the Program to Encourage Active and Rewarding Lives for Seniors (PEARLS), one of the first studies to demonstrate the feasibility of collaborating with community service organizations to identify and effectively treat depressed, homebound older adults primarily with counseling rather than prescription drugs. • The National Center for Health Statistics, a CDC division, conducts numerous population-based surveys that collect epidemiologic and use data related to geriatric MH/SU (including the Behavioral Risk Factor Surveillance Survey, the National Health Interview Survey, and others).
National Institutes of Health (NIH)	
—National Institute on Mental Health (NIMH)	
○ NIMH Geriatrics Research Branch	Diminishing focus on research related to effective delivery of geriatric MH/SU services. Access to new funding for the Advanced Centers for Interventions and Services Research has been eliminated. • Supports research, training, and resource development related to the etiology and pathophysiology of late-life mental disorders. • Has also funded research on telehealth, online curricula development, and collaborative care.
○ NIMH Services Research and Clinical Epidemiology	• Supports two programs related to service delivery in MH/SU although neither program focuses on older adults. The Primary Care Research Program supports studies that examine what types of MH/SU care can be integrated into the primary care setting. The Systems Research Program supports studies on organization and coordination of MH/SU care settings, including schools, community organizations, and criminal justice facilities.

—National Institute on Aging (NIA)	• Supports research on Alzheimer's disease and other diseases that cause dementia. • Supports epidemiological research on depression and other mental health conditions as well as research on nursing home populations.
—National Institute on Alcohol Abuse and Alcoholism (NIAAA)[a]	Funds research on alcohol abuse, alcoholism, and health effects of alcohol with some focus on adults age 60 and older.
—National Institute on Drug Abuse (NIDA)[a]	Principal focus is on biomedical neuroscience, but funds some extramural research on epidemiology, services, and prevention, including research on drug abuse in the older adult population.
RESOURCES AND SERVICES	
Administration on Aging (AoA)	Provides nonmedical services to help older adults maintain health and independence and supports research on related topics. • Administers the National Aging Network, a national service infrastructure that funds state-level organizations that provide home- and community-based services (including the Aging and Disability Resource Center and the National Family Caregiver Support Program). • Has supported research and dissemination of evidence on several community-based, MH/SU screening and interventions for older adults, including Healthy IDEAS, PEARLS, HomeMEDS, ElderVention, and the Brief Intervention and Treatment for Elders.

continued

TABLE 1-2 Continued

Key Focus/ Agency	Emphasis on Mental Health and Substance Abuse (MH/SU) Services and Workforces
Health Resources and Services Administration (HRSA)	

—Bureau of Health Professions	MH/SU content is not required in geriatric training programs.
	• Administers several grant programs open to geriatric MH/SU professionals, including
	  o Comprehensive Geriatric Education Program
	  o Geriatric Academic Career Awards
	  o Geriatric Education Center Program
	  o Geriatric Training Program for Physicians, Dentists, and Behavioral and Mental Health Professions
	• From 2007 to 2010, the above programs provided training and education in mental health (88 percent) and substance use (22 percent) to 93,616 individuals. Participants represented a wide range of disciplines, including nursing (24 percent), medicine (15 percent), social work (12 percent), and others (49 percent).

—National Health Service Corps	No emphasis on geriatric MH/SU workforce. • Provides loan repayment and scholarships to providers in exchange for service commitment in underserved areas (primarily to a nonelderly population). • More than 3,000 MH specialists (psychiatrists, psychologists, licensed clinical social workers, psychiatric nurse specialists, marriage and family therapists, and licensed professional counselors) have participated in the corps.
—Bureau of Primary Health Care	No emphasis on geriatric MH/SU workforce. • Provides financial support to community health centers providing primary care to underserved persons; patient population is primarily nonelderly (less than 7 percent is age 65 and older). • Participating health centers must provide or arrange for MH and SU services; about two-thirds of the centers provide mental health services onsite.

Substance Abuse and Mental Health Services Administration (SAMHSA)	Once a priority population, older adults are no longer a focus of SAMHSA activities. Starting in 2013, the agency will not fund any grant programs dedicated specifically to geriatric MH/SU.
	• Notable programs related to older adults:
	  ○ Older Adults Targeted Capacity Expansion (TCE) Grants—a service grant program that directed resources to older adults from 2002 to 2011; 29 programs received grants. Included a Technical Assistance Center.
	  ○ Enhancing Older Adult Behavioral Health currently funds five of the former TCE grantees. This 18-month initiative focuses on suicide prevention and prescription drug misuse/abuse among older adults.

[a] NIH is assessing a possible merger of NIDA and NIAAA into a combined Substance Abuse/Addictions Institute (as recommended by the NIH Scientific Management Review Board in 2010).

SOURCES: AoA, 2011a,b,c; Ciechanowski et al., 2004; Davis et al., 2012; HRSA Bureau of Health Professions, 2011; Medicaid.gov, 2012; Miller, 2011; NIAAA, 2010, 2011; NIDA, 2011; NIH, 2010, 2011; NIMH, 2011a,b,c; SAMHSA, 2006, 2011a,b,c; SCAN Foundation, 2011.

REFERENCES

Alecxih, L., S. Shen, I. Chan, D. Taylor, and J. Drabek. 2010. *Individuals living in the community with chronic conditions and functional limitations: A closer look.* http://www.lewin.com/content/publications/ChartBookChronicConditions.pdf (accessed January 19, 2012).

American Psychiatric Association. 2012. *DSM-IV-TR.* http://www.dsm5.org/Pages/Default.aspx (accessed June 1, 2012).

AoA (Administration on Aging). 2011a. *About AoA.* http://www.aoa.gov/AoARoot/About/index.aspx (accessed November 13, 2011).

———. 2011b. *Behavioral health.* http://www.aoa.gov/AoARoot/AoA_Programs/HPW/Behavioral/index.aspx (accessed November 15, 2011).

———. 2011c. *National aging network.* http://www.aoa.gov/AoARoot/AoA_Programs/OAA/Aging_Network/Index.aspx (accessed April 14, 2011).

Brown, L. D., and S. Wituk, eds. 2010. *Mental health self-help: Consumer and family initiatives.* New York: Springer.

Ciechanowski, P., E. Wagner, K. Schmaling, S. Schwartz, B. Williams, P. Diehr, J. Kulzer, S. Gray, C. Collier, and J. LoGerfo. 2004. Community-integrated home-based depression treatment in older adults: A randomized controlled trial. *JAMA* 291(13):1569-1577.

Congressional Budget Office. 2008. *Cost estimate H.R. 6331: Medicare Improvements for Patients and Providers Act of 2008, enacted as P.L. 110-275 on July 15, 2008.*

Cummings, M. R., V. A. Hernandez, M. Rockeymoore, M. M. Shepard, and K. Sager. 2011. *The Latino age wave: What changing ethnic demographics mean for the future of aging in the United States.* http://www.atlanticphilanthropies.org/sites/default/files/uploads/HIP_LatinoAgeWave_FullReport_Web.pdf (accessed September 6, 2011).

Cummings, S. M., and N. P. Kropf. 2011. Aging with a severe mental illness: Challenges and treatments. *Journal of Gerontological Social Work* 54(2):175-188.

Davis, P. A., C. Binder, J. Hahn, P. C. Morgan, J. Mulvey, and S. R. Talaga. 2012. *CRS report: Medicare primer* (accessed January 27, 2012).

Drayer, R. A., B. H. Mulsant, E. J. Lenze, B. L. Rollman, M. A. Dew, K. Kelleher, J. F. Karp, A. Begley, H. C. Schulberg, and C. F. Reynolds. 2005. Somatic symptoms of depression in elderly patients with medical comorbidities. *International Journal of Geriatric Psychiatry* 20(10):973-982.

Frank, R. 2011. Testimony to the IOM Committee on the Mental Health Workforce for Geriatric Populations. Washington, DC. March 8.

Garfield, R. L., S. H. Zuvekas, J. R. Lave, and J. M. Donohue. 2011. The impact of national health care reform on adults with severe mental disorders. *American Journal of Psychiatry* 168(5):486-494.

Hewitt, A., S. Larson, S. Edelstein, D. Seavey, M. Hoge, and J. Morris. 2008. *A synthesis of direct service workforce demographics and challenges across intellectual/developmental disabilities, aging, physical disabilities, and behavioral health.* Falls Church, VA: The Lewin Group.

Hogan, M. F. 2003. The President's New Freedom Commission: Recommendations to transform mental health care in America. *Psychiatric Services* 54(11):1467-1474.

Hoge, M. A., J. A. Morris, A. S. Daniels, G. W. Stuart, L. Y. Huey, N. Adams, and Annapolis Coalition on the Behavioral Health Workforce. 2007. *An action plan for behavioral health workforce development: Executive summary.* Washington, DC: SAMHSA.

HRSA Bureau of Health Professions. 2011. *Title VI and Title VIII geriatrics program data on the geriatrics mental and behavioral health and substance abuse workforce.* December (unpublished).

IOM (Institute of Medicine). 1978. *Aging and medical education.* Washington, DC: National Academy Press.

———. 2001. *Crossing the quality chasm: A new health system for the 21st century.* Washington, DC: National Academy Press.

———. 2003. *Health professions education: A bridge to quality.* Washington, DC: The National Academies Press.

———. 2006. *Improving the quality of health care for mental and substance-use conditions.* Washington, DC: The National Academies Press.

———. 2008. *Retooling for an aging America: Building the health care workforce.* Washington, DC: The National Academies Press.

Jeste, D. V., G. S. Alexopoulos, S. J. Bartels, J. L. Cummings, J. J. Gallo, G. L. Gottlieb, M. C. Halpain, B. W. Palmer, T. L. Patterson, C. F. Reynolds, and B. D. Lebowitz. 1999. Consensus statement on the upcoming crisis in geriatric mental health—research agenda for the next 2 decades. *Archives of General Psychiatry* 56(9):848-853.

Lin, E. H. B., W. Katon, M. Von Korff, L. Q. Tang, J. W. Williams, K. Kroenke, E. Hunkeler, L. Harpole, M. Hegel, P. Arean, M. Hoffing, R. Della Penna, C. Langston, J. Unützer, and IMPACT Investigators. 2003. Effect of improving depression care on pain and functional outcomes among older adults with arthritis—a randomized controlled trial. *JAMA* 290(18):2428-2434.

Lin, W.-C., J. Zhang, G. Y. Leung, and R. E. Clark. 2011. Chronic physical conditions in older adults with mental illness and/or substance use disorders. *Journal of the American Geriatrics Society* 59(10):1913-1921.

Medicaid.gov. 2012. *Money follows the person (MFP).* http://www.medicaid.gov/Medicaid-CHIP-Program-Information/By-Topics/Long-Term-Services-and-Support/Balancing/Money-Follows-the-Person.html (accessed April 11, 2012).

MedPAC (Medicare Payment Advisory Commission). 2010. *Report to the Congress: Medicare payment policy.* Washington, DC: MedPAC.

———. 2011. *Coordinating care for dual-eligible beneficiaries.* Washington, DC: MedPAC.

Miller, B. 2011. *The AHRQ academy for integrating mental health and primary care.* http://prezi.com/pdwleusvlceo/the-ahrq-academy-for-integrating-mental-health-and-primary-care/ (accessed November 13, 2011).

Mowbray, C. T., D. P. Moxley, C. A. Jasper, and L. L. Howell, eds. 1997. *Consumers as providers in psychiatric rehabilitation.* Columbia, MD: International Association for Psychosocial Rehabilitation Services.

NIAAA (National Institute on Alcohol Abuse and Alcoholism). 2010. *Scientific management review board vote on merger.* http://pubs.niaaa.nih.gov/publications/Newsletter/Fall2010/article05.htm (accessed November 13, 2011).

———. 2011. *Fy 2012 congressional budget justification.* Bethesda, MD: Department of Health and Human Services.

NIDA (National Institute on Drug Abuse). 2011. *Fiscal year 2012 budget information: Congressional justification for National Institute on Drug Abuse.* http://drugabuse.gov/Funding/Budget12.html (accessed November 13, 2011).

NIH (National Institutes of Health). 2010. *Scientific review board: Report on substance use, abuse and addiction research at NIH.* Bethesda, MD: Department of Health and Human Services.

———. 2011. *NIH budget request FY2012.* Bethesda, MD: Department of Health and Human Services.

NIMH (National Institute of Mental Health). 2011a. *Geriatrics Research Branch.* http://www.nimh.nih.gov/about/organization/datr/geriatrics-research-branch/index.shtml (accessed November 13, 2011).

———. 2011b. *Primary Care Research Program.* http://www.nimh.nih.gov/about/organization/dsir/services-research-and-epidemiology-branch/primary-care-research-program.shtml (accessed November 13, 2011).

———. 2011c. *Systems Research Program.* http://www.nimh.nih.gov/about/organization/dsir/services-research-and-epidemiology-branch/systems-research-program.shtml (accessed November 13, 2011).

Noel, P. H., J. W. Williams, J. Unützer, J. Worchel, S. Lee, J. Cornell, W. Katon, and L. H. Harpole. 2004. Depression and comorbid illness in elderly primary care patients: Impact on multiple domains of health status and well-being. *Annals of Family Medicine* 2(6):555-562.

SAMHSA (Substance Abuse and Mental Health Services Administration). 2006. *Strategic plan: FY 2006-FY 2011.* Rockville, MD: SAMHSA.

———. 2011a. *FY 2011 grant request for application (RFA): Grants to enhance older adult behavioral health services (short title: Older adult TCE).* http://www.samhsa.gov/grants/2011/sm_11_009.aspx (accessed November 13, 2011).

———. 2011b. *Leading change: A plan for SAMHSA's role and actions 2011-2014.* Rockville, MD: SAMHSA.

———. 2011c. *Request for applications (RFA) No. Sm-11-009.* http://www.samhsa.gov/grants/2011/sm_11_009.aspx (accessed November 13, 2011).

Sarata, A. K. 2011. *Mental health parity and the Patient Protection and Affordable Care Act.* Washington, DC: Congressional Research Service.

SCAN Foundation. 2011. *Long-term care fundamentals. What is a Medicaid waiver?* Technical Brief Series No. 8. http://www.thescanfoundation.org/sites/scan.lmp03.lucidus.net/files/LTC_Fundamental_8.pdf (accessed September 12, 2011).

Unützer, J., W. J. Katon, M.-Y. Fan, M. C. Schoenbaum, E. H. B. Lin, R. D. DellaPenna, and D. Powers. 2008. Long-term cost effects of collaborative care for late-life depression. *American Journal of Managed Care* 14:95-100.

U.S. Congress, House of Representatives. 2009. Departments of Labor, Health and Human Services, and Education, and related agencies appropriations bill, 2010. *Report of the Committee on Appropriations together with minority views (to accompany H.R. 3293).* Report 111-220.

Vincent, G. K., and V. A. Velkoff. 2010. *The next four decades: The older population in the United States: 2010 to 2050. Current Population Reports,* pp. 25-1138. Washington, DC: U.S. Census Bureau.

Whittier, M. 2006. *Strengthening professional identity: Challenges of the addictions treatment workforce. A framework for discussion.* Rockville, MD: SAMHSA.

2

Assessing the Service Needs of Older Adults with Mental Health and Substance Use Conditions

Abstract: *This chapter analyzes the available information about the prevalence of mental health and substance use (MH/SU) conditions in older adults and identifies the additional information required to plan for a workforce capable of meeting their current and future service needs. The committee estimates that in 2010, at least 5.6 to 8 million older adults had one or more MH/SU conditions. Several million more older adults were probably also affected, but the available data are not adequate to estimate the number. By 2030, expected growth in the older population will increase the number of older people with MH/SU conditions by 80 percent. Many older adults with MH/SU conditions also have physical health conditions and cognitive, functional, and sensory impairments that can complicate the detection, diagnosis, and treatment of their MH/SU conditions and create difficult caregiving situations for their families and professional and other service providers. In 2010, MH/SU conditions were the eighth most costly type of health care conditions for older adults in the United States, but most older adults with these conditions still do not receive the MH/SU services they need.*

An in-depth understanding of the service needs of a target population is integral to analyzing the requirements for a workforce capable of meeting those needs. Thus, the objectives of this chapter are twofold:

first, to describe what is known about the prevalence of mental health and substance use (MH/SU) conditions in older adults and their related service needs, and second, to consider the impact of population trends, particularly the aging of the baby boomer cohort and growing population diversity, on the makeup of the older population and future needs for MH/SU services.

The first two sections of the chapter describe the MH/SU conditions that occur in older adults and present the best available information about the proportion and number of older adults that have one or more of the conditions. The third section provides information about prevalence rates for important subgroups of the older population, including racial and ethnic groups and veterans. Later sections describe the coexisting physical health conditions and cognitive and functional impairments that shape the MH/SU service needs of older adults; review the impact of MH/SU conditions; and discuss the available data on use of MH/SU services by older adults and factors that could affect their future MH/SU service needs. The last section summarizes the chapter findings about the current and future MH/SU service needs of the older population. Unfortunately, much of the information required to analyze their MH/SU service needs and plan for a workforce capable of meeting those needs is not available. Additional information needed for these purposes is discussed.

MH/SU CONDITIONS IN OLDER ADULTS

The Institute of Medicine committee identified 27 MH/SU conditions for attention in this report because of their importance in older adults and their implications for service needs and workforce requirements. Fifteen of the conditions, including two substance use conditions, are defined by explicit criteria in the most recent version of the *Diagnostic and Statistical Manual of Mental Disorders*, Fourth Edition-Text Revision (DSM-IV-TR) (APA, 2000), the accepted source for diagnostic classification of MH/SU conditions in the United States. These conditions are referred to as *mental disorders* in this report. The other 12 conditions are symptoms or clusters of symptoms not classified as mental disorders in DSM-IV-TR. These conditions are referred to as *other MH/SU conditions* in the report.

Two of the 15 DSM-IV-TR mental disorders, bipolar disorder and schizophrenia, constitute the core of a category of mental health conditions usually referred to as *serious mental illness* (SMI). SMI is often defined to include severe forms of other DSM-IV-TR mental disorders, such as major depression, but it does not include substance use conditions.

Box 2-1 describes each of the 27 MH/SU conditions identified by the committee, focusing primarily on symptoms. Descriptions of the 15 DSM-IV-TR mental disorders are taken from the DSM-IV-TR manual. Descriptions of the 12 other MH/SU conditions are compiled from published reports. As discussed later in the chapter, substantial numbers of older adults have more than one of the 27 conditions.

The DSM-IV-TR does not provide diagnostic criteria specifically for older adults, and clinicians and researchers have noted that some of the criteria for DSM-IV-TR mental disorders include symptoms that are expressed less often in older adults than younger people with the conditions. Several studies have shown, for example, that older adults with DSM-IV-TR depressive disorders are significantly less likely than younger people with these disorders to exhibit the depressed mood and sadness that are the first listed criteria for the disorders (Gallo et al., 1994, 1999). Likewise, older adults with bipolar disorder are somewhat less likely to exhibit the manic symptoms that are required criteria for the disorder (Coryell et al., 2009; Depp and Jeste, 2004; Hirschfeld and Vornik, 2004).

Diagnostic criteria for DSM mental disorders are established with the publication of the most recent version of the manual, but clinicians, researchers, and others continue to debate the criteria for existing disorders and whether additional MH/SU conditions should be included as disorders in the next version of the manual. The forthcoming DSM-5, scheduled for publication in 2013, will include criteria for diagnosing some new mental disorders, eliminate some disorders, and revise the criteria for many other disorders. It is likely, for example, that hoarding, one of the other MH/SU conditions identified by the IOM committee as important for older adults, will be included as a mental disorder in the DSM-5 (APA, 2010). Thus, the designation of which MH/SU conditions are defined as DSM mental disorders, although set for years at a time, is also changeable.

The committee's decision to identify both DSM-IV-TR mental disorders and other MH/SU conditions for special attention in this report reflects the report's focus on the service needs of older adults and workforce requirements and competencies to meet those needs. As described in Box 2-1, both DSM-IV-TR mental disorders and other MH/SU conditions result in significant emotional distress, functional disability, and reduced quality of life for the person. In addition, at least four types of age-related factors can cause, complicate, and exacerbate MH/SU conditions. The four factors are physiological effects of normal aging; changes in life circumstances that frequently occur in old age; coexisting physical health conditions that are common in older adults; and cognitive, functional, and sensory impairments that affect substantial numbers of older adults, especially those age 75 and older. In the presence of these age-related factors, MH/SU conditions that do not meet the criteria for a DSM-IV-TR mental disorder can result in pressing and sustained needs for MH/SU services.

BOX 2-1
Symptoms of MH/SU Conditions Identified as Important for Older Adults

DSM-IV-TR Category Depressive Disorders

1. **Major Depressive Disorder** is a DSM-IV-TR mental disorder characterized by one or more Major Depressive Episodes. Major Depressive Disorder and Major Depressive Episode (described below) are often referred to as *major depression*.

2. **Major Depressive Episode** is a period of at least 2 weeks in which the person has five or more of nine symptoms nearly every day, including at least one of the first two: (1) depressed mood that lasts most of the day, as indicated by either subjective report (e.g., the person feels sad or empty) or observations of others (e.g., the person appears tearful); or (2) markedly diminished interest or pleasure in all or nearly all activities that lasts most of the day. The seven additional symptoms are (3) significant weight loss when not dieting, weight gain, or decrease or increase in appetite; (4) insomnia or hypersomnia; (5) psychomotor agitation or retardation; (6) fatigue or loss of energy; (7) feelings of worthlessness or excessive or inappropriate guilt; (8) diminished ability to think or concentrate, or indecisiveness; and (9) recurrent thoughts of death (not just fear of dying), recurrent suicidal ideation, a suicide plan, or a suicide attempt (APA, 2000).

3. **Dysthymic Disorder** is a DSM-IV-TR mental disorder characterized by at least 2 years of depressed mood that lasts most of the day for more days than not, accompanied by at least two of the following additional symptoms: poor appetite or overeating, insomnia or hypersomnia, low energy or fatigue, low self-esteem, poor concentration or difficulty making decisions, and feelings of hopelessness. In the 2-year period, any symptom-free intervals must last no longer than 2 months (APA, 2000).

DSM-IV-TR Bipolar Disorders

4. **DSM-IV-TR Bipolar Disorders I and II.** Bipolar I Disorder is a mental disorder characterized by one or more Manic Episodes or Mixed Episodes (described below), often accompanied by a history of major depressive episodes (APA, 2000). Bipolar II Disorder is a mental disorder characterized by one or more major depressive episodes accompanied by at least one Hypomanic

Episode (APA, 2000). Bipolar I and II disorders are usually referred to as bipolar disorder.

A *Manic Episode* is a period of at least 1 week in which the person has an abnormally and persistently elevated, expansive, or irritable mood. The mood disturbance must be accompanied by at least three of the following symptoms: inflated self-esteem or grandiosity, decreased need for sleep, more talkative than usual or pressured speech, flight of ideas, distractibility, increased goal-directed activities or psychomotor agitation, and excessive involvement in pleasurable activities with a high potential for painful outcomes (e.g., buying sprees, sexual indiscretions, or foolish business investments) (APA, 2000).

A *Mixed Episode* is a period of at least 1 week in which the criteria for both a manic episode and a major depressive episode are met nearly every day. The person has rapidly alternating moods (sadness, irritability, euphoria) often accompanied by agitation, insomnia, appetite dysregulation, psychosis, and suicidal thinking (APA, 2000).

DSM-IV-TR Anxiety Disorders

5. **Panic Disorder** is a DSM-IV-TR mental disorder characterized by recurrent unexpected panic attacks followed by at least 1 month of persistent concern about having another panic attack, worry about the consequences of an attack, or a significant change in behavior to avoid panic attacks. A panic attack is a discrete period in which the person experiences sudden intense apprehension, fear, or terror in the absence of real danger. It must be accompanied by at least 4 of 13 additional symptoms: palpitations, pounding heart, or accelerated heart rate; sweating; trembling or shaking; sensations of shortness of breath or smothering; feelings of choking; chest pain or discomfort; nausea or abdominal distress; feeling dizzy, unsteady, lightheaded or faint; feelings of unreality or being detached from oneself; fear of losing control or going crazy; fear of dying; numbness or tingling sensations; and chills or hot flashes. Panic disorder can occur with or without agoraphobia (APA, 2000).

6. **Agoraphobia Without Panic** is a DSM-IV-TR mental disorder characterized by anxiety about, or avoidance of, places or situations in which escape might be difficult or embarrassing or help might not be available in the event of a panic attack or panic-like symptoms. The person must not have a history of panic attacks.

continued

BOX 2-1 Continued

Agoraphobic fears typically involve specific situations, such as being outside the home alone; being in a crowd; standing in a line; being on a bridge; or traveling in a bus, train, or car (APA, 2000).

7. **Social Phobia** is a DSM-IV-TR mental disorder characterized by clinically significant anxiety provoked by exposure to certain types of social or performance situations in which embarrassment may occur. The person usually tries to avoid the feared situation. The fear and/or avoidance must interfere significantly with the person's normal routine, occupational functioning, or social activities or relationships (APA, 2000).

8. **Obsessive-Compulsive Disorder** is a DSM-IV-TR mental disorder characterized by recurrent obsessions and/or compulsions. Obsessions are persistent ideas, thoughts, impulses, or images that are experienced as intrusive and inappropriate and cause anxiety or distress. Examples are repeated thoughts about contamination, repeated doubts, a need to have things in a particular order, aggressive or horrific impulses, and sexual imagery. Compulsions are repetitive behaviors (e.g., hand washing, ordering, checking) or mental acts (e.g., counting and repeating words silently), the goal of which is to prevent or reduce anxiety or distress. The compulsion is usually intended to reduce distress related to the obsession or to prevent a dreaded event or situation (APA, 2000).

9. **Generalized Anxiety Disorder** is a DSM-IV-TR mental disorder characterized by persistent, excessive anxiety and worry that occurs most days for at least 6 months. The intensity, duration, or frequency of these symptoms is far out of proportion to the likelihood or impact of the feared event. The symptoms are accompanied by at least three of six additional symptoms: restlessness or feeling keyed up or on edge, being easily fatigued, difficulty concentrating, irritability, muscle tension, and disturbed sleep. The person may not realize the anxiety and worry are excessive but is distressed by constant worry, difficulty controlling the worry, and related impairments in important areas of functioning (APA, 2000).

10. **Posttraumatic Stress Disorder (PTSD)** is a DSM-IV-TR mental disorder characterized by symptoms that develop after exposure to an extremely traumatic event involving either (1) direct personal experience of threatened death, serious injury, or other threat

to one's physical integrity; or (2) witnessing an event involving death, injury, or a threat to the physical integrity of another person, or learning about unexpected or violent death, serious harm, or threat of death or injury to a family member or other close associate. The person's response to the event must involve intense fear, helplessness, or horror, and the symptoms must last more than 1 month and include persistent reexperiencing of the traumatic event, avoidance of stimuli associated with the trauma, numbing of general responsiveness, and persistent arousal (e.g., rapid heart rate). Traumatic events experienced directly include military combat, violent personal assault, being kidnapped, being taken hostage, terrorist attack, torture, incarceration as a prisoner of war or in a concentration camp, natural or manmade disasters, severe automobile accidents, or diagnosis of a life-threatening illness. The disorder may be especially severe or long-lasting when the stressor is of human design (e.g., torture or rape) (APA, 2000).

DSM-IV-TR Schizophrenia and Other Psychotic Disorders

11. **Schizophrenia** is a DSM-IV-TR mental disorder that lasts for at least 6 months, including at least 1 month during which the person has two or more of the following: positive symptoms (delusions, hallucinations, disorganized speech, and grossly disorganized or catatonic behavior), and/or negative symptoms (restrictions in the range and intensity of emotional expression, the fluency and productivity of thought and speech, and the initiation of goal-directed behavior). For a significant portion of the time after onset of the disorder, the person's functioning in one or more major areas, such as work, interpersonal relations, and self-care, must be markedly below his or her prior functioning (APA, 2000).

    In 2000, an international panel recommended two new classifications: late-onset schizophrenia, with onset after age 45, and very-late-onset schizophrenia, with onset after age 60 (Howard et al., 2000). DSM-IV-TR criteria do not list these classifications, but the DSM-IV-TR manual discusses late-onset schizophrenia (APA, 2000), and a late-onset specification code can be added to identify the conditions.

DSM-IV-TR Substance-Related Disorders Substance Dependence and Substance Abuse are defined similarly for alcohol and other substances (described below). A person with a DSM-IV-TR diagnosis of

continued

BOX 2-1 Continued

Substance Dependence cannot also have a DSM-IV-TR diagnosis of Substance Abuse.

12. **Alcohol Dependence and Alcohol Abuse** are DSM-IV-TR mental disorders that meet the requirements for substance dependence and abuse defined with respect to alcohol.

13. **Drug Dependence and Drug Abuse** are DSM-IV-TR mental disorders that meet the requirements for substance dependence and abuse defined with respect to illicit drugs and prescribed or over-the-counter drugs used for nonmedical purposes, including amphetamines, cannabis, cocaine, hallucinogens, inhalants, opioids, sedatives, hypnotics, and antianxiety drugs (APA, 2000).

    Substance Dependence is a cluster of symptoms indicating the person continues to use the substance despite significant substance-related impairment or distress. The pattern of repeated self-administration must result in three or more of seven symptoms in three categories: tolerance, withdrawal, and compulsive drug-taking behavior (APA, 2000).

    Substance Abuse is a maladaptive pattern of substance use leading to clinically significant impairment or distress as manifested by one (or more) of the following, occurring within a 12-month period: (1) failure to fulfill major role obligations; (2) recurrent substance use in situations in which it is physically hazardous; (3) recurrent substance-related legal problems; and (4) continued use despite recurrent social or interpersonal problems caused or exacerbated by the substance use (APA, 2000).

DSM-IV-TR Adjustment Disorders

14. **Adjustment Disorder** is a DSM-IV-TR mental disorder characterized by a psychological or behavioral response to an identifiable stressor that results in clinically significant emotional or behavioral symptoms. The symptoms must occur within 3 months of the onset of the stressor and resolve within 6 months after the stressor is resolved. The person must have marked distress that is in excess of what would be expected given the nature of the stressor or significant impairment in social or occupational functioning (APA, 2000).

DSM-IV-TR Personality Disorders

15. **Personality Disorders** are DSM-IV-TR mental disorders characterized by an enduring pattern of inner experience and behavior that deviates markedly from the expectations of the person's culture, is pervasive and inflexible, and leads to distress or impairment. The onset of the disorder can be traced back to adolescence or early adulthood. The 10 personality disorders are paranoid, schizoid, schizotypal, antisocial, borderline, histrionic, narcissistic, avoidant, dependent, and obsessive-compulsive personality disorder (APA, 2000).

MH/SU Conditions That Are Not DSM-IV-TR Disorders

16. **Depressive Symptoms** is a term to describe symptoms, such as depressed mood and feelings of worthlessness and guilt, that do not meet the criteria for a diagnosis of a DSM-IV-TR depressive disorder, usually because of insufficient duration, number, or severity. Other terms for such symptoms are subsyndromal depression, subthreshold depression, subclinical depression, and minor depression (Blazer, 2003; Lavretsky and Kumar, 2002; Lyness et al., 2009).
17. **Anxiety Symptoms** is a term to describe symptoms, such as excessive nervousness, worry, and fear or avoidance of anxiety-causing situations that do not meet the criteria for a DSM-IV-TR diagnosis of an anxiety disorder, usually because of insufficient number or severity. Other terms for such symptoms are subsyndromal anxiety and subthreshold anxiety (Grenier et al., 2011; Lenze and Wetherell, 2011).
18. **At-Risk Drinking** is a term to describe alcohol-related symptoms that do not meet the criteria for a DSM-IV-TR diagnosis of alcohol dependence or abuse, usually because of insufficient number or severity. Symptoms of at-risk drinking include having more than a specified number of drinks (usually 2 per day); binge drinking, and exhibiting any of the symptoms of alcohol dependence or abuse (e.g., tolerance, withdrawal, compulsive alcohol use behaviors, failure to fulfill major role obligations, and recurrent alcohol-related legal, social, or interpersonal problems). Other terms for such symptoms are subsyndromal alcohol dependence, subthreshold alcohol dependence, alcohol misuse, and problem

continued

BOX 2-1 Continued

drinking (APA, 2000; Berks and McCormick, 2008; Blazer and Wu, 2009a, 2011; Blow and Barry, 2002; Merrick et al., 2008).

19. **At-Risk Drug Use** is a term to describe drug-related symptoms that do not meet the criteria for a DSM-IV-TR diagnosis of drug dependence or abuse, usually because of insufficient number or severity. Symptoms of at-risk drug use include drug overdoses and any of the symptoms of drug dependence and abuse (e.g., tolerance, withdrawal, compulsive drug use behaviors, failure to fulfill major role obligations, and recurrent drug-related legal, social, or interpersonal problems). Other terms for such symptoms are subthreshold drug dependence, at-risk use of psychoactive drugs, and extra-medical drug use (Blazer and Wu, 2009b,c; Degenhardt et al., 2007; Wu and Blazer, 2011).

20. **Suicidal Ideation** is a term to describe serious thoughts about suicide and death. It is sometimes subdivided into active suicidal ideation (e.g., thinking about taking one's own life) and passive suicidal ideation or passive death ideation (e.g., feeling that life is not worth living and wishing one were dead) (Bartels et al., 2002; Beck et al., 1979; Paykel et al., 1974; Raue et al., 2007).

21. **Suicide Plans and Attempts** are terms to describe plans and behaviors to kill oneself. Suicide plans can include selecting a time when one will be alone and therefore able to kill oneself, selecting a means for killing oneself, and obtaining the means for killing oneself. Suicide attempts are active behaviors to end one's life.

    Suicidal ideation, suicide plans, and suicide attempts are included as one of the nine symptoms of a DSM-IV-TR major depressive episode (APA, 2000).

22. **Behavioral and Psychiatric Symptoms Associated with Dementia** is a term to describe noncognitive symptoms of diseases and conditions that cause dementia. Such symptoms include delusions, hallucinations, agitation, verbal aggression; physical aggression, anxiety, apathy, depression, dysphoria, irritability, elation, euphoria, aberrant motor behavior, appetite and eating disorders, sleep disorders; inappropriate sexual behavior; and unsafe wandering. Other terms for such symptoms are neuropsychiatric symptoms of dementia and behavioral and psychological symptoms of dementia (Chan et al., 2003; Cohen-Mansfield et al., 1989; Cummings et al., 1994; Jeste and Finkel, 2000; Lyketsos

et al., 2000; McNeese et al., 2009; Smith and Buckwalter, 2005; Teri et al., 1992).

DSM-IV-TR defines diagnostic criteria for several dementia-related mental disorders, and coding specifications for behavioral and psychiatric symptoms can be added to these disorders, but behavioral and psychiatric symptoms associated with dementia are not classified as DSM-IV-TR mental disorders.

23. **Hoarding** is a term to describe symptoms, such as the accumulation of a large volume of paper, newspapers, containers, food, books, trash, and other materials that clutter living areas to the extent that they cannot be used for their intended purposes. Severe hoarding can create health and safety hazards for the person and others living in the same home, building, or community. The person is often unaware of the problem, but it may result in a referral or complaint to a public health, adult protective services, or case management agency. Another term for these symptoms is compulsive hoarding (Ayers et al., 2010; Frost et al., 2000; Kim et al., 2001; Pertusa et al., 2008).

24. **Severe Domestic Squalor** is a term to describe a living situation, often from the perspective of a public health or adult protective services worker who is responding to a referral or complaint. The living situation is said to be filthy; cluttered with dirt, garbage, and rubbish; and infested with vermin, excrement, and decomposing food. Visitors experience disgust and revulsion, and the smell is sometimes said to be unbearable to all except the occupant, who often refuses help to clean the living situation (Snowdon and Halliday, 2011; Snowdon et al., 2007).

25. **Severe Self-Neglect** is a term used to describe health-related symptoms, such as malnutrition, dehydration, untreated medical conditions, and hazardous living conditions, that result from a person's failure to provide for his or her own needs. The National Center on Elder Abuse says that self-neglect "generally manifests itself in an older person as a refusal or failure to provide himself/herself with adequate food, water, clothing, shelter, personal hygiene, medication (when indicated), and safety precautions" (NCEA, 2011). Severity of self-neglect is usually defined in the domains of personal hygiene, cleanliness, health needs, household and environmental hazards, and home safety (Dong et al., 2010; Kelly et al., 2008).

continued

BOX 2-1 Continued

The DSM-IV-TR category Problems Related to Abuse or Neglect includes seven mental disorders related to abuse and neglect, but not self-neglect (APA, 2000).

26. **Fear of Falling** is a term used to describe persistent, often exaggerated, concerns about falling that occur in adults who have or have not fallen. The symptoms can result in loss of confidence in ability to perform daily activities, activity restriction, changes in posture and gait, future falls, avoidance of feared activities and environments, loss of mobility, and loss of independence (Delbaere et al., 2010; Jorstad et al., 2005; Murphy et al., 2003; Oh-Park et al., 2011; Yardley and Smith, 2002).

The following examples illustrate the impact of interactions among the four age-related factors noted earlier and MH/SU conditions in older adults:

1. Age-related changes in the metabolism of alcohol and drugs, including prescription drugs, can cause or exacerbate DSM-IV-TR and other alcohol and drug use conditions and increase an older person's risk of dangerous overdoses. This can happen even to people who have used alcohol and drugs at the same dose and frequency for many years without serious negative effects (Blow and Barry, 2002; Dowling et al., 2008; Wu and Blazer, 2011).
2. Losses that occur frequently in old age, such as the death of a spouse, partner, close relative, or friend, can trigger emotional responses that cause or exacerbate DSM-IV-TR depressive disorders and depressive symptoms (Alexopoulos, 2005; Zisook and Shuchter, 1991) and lead to severe, debilitating symptoms, such as those seen in complicated grief (Kersting et al., 2011). In a person with significant loss, differentiating major depression and grief is often difficult.
3. Acute and chronic physical health conditions that are common in older adults and medications to treat the conditions can cause and exacerbate DSM-IV-TR mental disorders and other MH/SU conditions and worsen their impact on the person (Blow and Barry, 2002; Jeste et al., 2005; Schultz, 2011).

27. **Complicated Grief** is a term used to describe symptoms associated with bereavement that are intense and go beyond the usual and culturally expected response to a death. These symptoms include disbelief and/or anger and bitterness about the death; severe, recurrent, and painful feelings of intense longing for the deceased; preoccupation with thoughts of the deceased, often involving intrusive images and thoughts; avoidance of situations and activities that remind one of the death; and neglect of necessary adaptive activities (Horowitz et al., 1997; Shear et al., 2005).

4. Cognitive, functional, and sensory impairments can complicate the detection and diagnosis of DSM-IV-TR mental disorders and other MH/SU conditions and reduce an older person's ability to comply with recommended treatments, including health-related behaviors and medications prescribed for the person's MH/SU and physical health conditions (Cohen, 1996; Schultz, 2011; Wolitzky-Taylor et al., 2010).

The complex interactions among MH/SU conditions and these age-related factors, especially coexisting physical health conditions and cognitive, functional, and sensory impairments, have been described by many geriatric mental health professionals and researchers as a key or defining characteristic of the field (Alexopoulos, 2005; Blazer et al., 2004; Borson et al., 2001; Bruce et al., 1994; Bryant et al., 2009; Cohen, 1996; Flint, 2002; Katz, 1996; Knight, 2004; Lyness et al., 2006; Reynolds et al., 2002). The adverse consequences of these interactions work both ways (Bryant et al., 2009; Wolitzky-Taylor et al., 2010). In the case of an older person with depression, for example, physical health conditions and cognitive and functional impairments can worsen the person's depression and, conversely, depression can worsen the person's physical health and cognitive and functional impairments (Blazer, 2003).

People of any age can experience physiological changes, losses, physical health conditions and cognitive, functional, and sensory impairments that may cause, complicate, and exacerbate MH/SU conditions. These factors are, however, more prominent and pervasive in older people (Bartels, 2004; Kilbourne et al., 2005).

At worst, interactions among mental disorders, other MH/SU conditions, and age-related factors can result in what has been described as a "spiral" or "cascade" of decline in physical, cognitive, and psychological health (Blazer, 2000; Bruce et al., 1994; Bryant et al., 2008). In such situations, even a highly skilled clinician can have difficulty disentangling the components of the problem and deciding what to do first to reverse the decline.

Because of their coexisting physical health conditions, older adults with MH/SU conditions are frequently seen in medical care settings, such as primary care offices, hospitals, and emergency departments. Likewise, because of their coexisting physical health conditions and cognitive and functional impairments, older adults with MH/SU conditions may be receiving nursing and nonmedical personal care services at home or in a residential care setting, such as a nursing home or assisted living facility. In all these settings, the interactions of MH/SU conditions and age-related physiological changes, losses, physical health conditions, and cognitive and functional impairments can create difficult caregiving situations. Health care professionals and service providers who work with older adults at home or in general medical care, nursing home, and other residential care settings may not expect or recognize the MH/SU conditions, understand their implications for the person's physical health and cognitive and functional status, or know how to respond.

In the same way, specialty MH/SU service providers, especially those who do not have geriatric training, may not recognize physical health conditions or cognitive, functional, or sensory impairments in the older adults for whom they provide services. They may not understand the complex interactions among these coexisting conditions and the person's MH/SU condition or know how to adapt usual treatments and services to accommodate the coexisting conditions. As a result, treatable physical health conditions may not be treated, and medications that can seriously worsen the person's physical health and cognitive and functional status may be unknowingly prescribed (Druss and Walker, 2011).

PREVALENCE OF MH/SU CONDITIONS IN OLDER ADULTS

To analyze the service needs of older adults with DSM-IV-TR mental disorders and other MH/SU conditions and then plan for the workforce required to meet the needs, it is necessary to know how many older adults have the conditions. As noted earlier, some older adults have more than one MH/SU condition. For planning purposes, it is necessary to know how many people have each condition, for example, how many have depressive disorders and how many have alcohol dependence or abuse, as well as how many have two or more conditions, for example, how many have both depressive disorders and alcohol dependence or abuse. The latter information is required to determine the total number of people who need MH/SU services, whether for only one or more than one condition.

To estimate the number of older adults who have any of the 27 MH/SU conditions identified by the committee and how many have more than one such condition, the committee gathered available information from published research conducted in population-based samples in the United States. To fill gaps, unpublished data were obtained whenever possible, but many gaps remain.

To ensure that all older adults with MH/SU conditions were included in its estimates and, at the same time, avoid double counting, the committee used a U.S. Census Bureau classification system that divides the population into two categories: (1) people living in *housing units*, including houses, apartments, mobile homes, and single rooms occupied as separate living quarters, and (2) people living in *group quarters*, including nursing homes, prisons and jails, psychiatric hospitals, residential treatment centers, and homeless shelters (Census Bureau, 2010a). People categorized as *living in housing units* are referred to in this report as *people living in the community* or *community-living people*.

The 2010 Census found there were 40.3 million adults age 65 and older in the United States (Census Bureau, 2011a). Of the 40.3 million older adults, about 38.8 million (96 percent) were living in the community, and 1.5 million (4 percent) were living in group quarters settings (Census Bureau, 2010b). These U.S. Census figures are used in this section to develop population estimates of the number of older adults who had each of the identified MH/SU conditions and the number who had one or more of the conditions in 2010.

Some older adults with MH/SU conditions developed the conditions after age 65, and some grew older with conditions they had for many years. Both groups are included in the estimates presented in this section. Likewise, many older adults have MH/SU conditions that have not been recognized, and as a result, they do not have formal diagnoses of the conditions. The information presented in this section does not rely on formal diagnoses, and the estimates provided in the section include people with diagnosed and undiagnosed conditions.

The U.S. Census Bureau classification system used by the committee categorizes people who live in assisted living, senior housing, and other public housing facilities as people living in the community and does not distinguish them from people who live in single-family housing.

Although use of this classification system is important for placing the committee's estimates in the context of U.S. Census figures for the number of older adults in the country and avoiding double counting, classifying people who live in assisted living, senior housing, and other public housing facilities in a different category from people living in nursing homes is not ideal for characterizing MH/SU conditions in older adults. In fact, the proportion of older adults in these non–nursing home, residential facilities who have MH/SU conditions is closer to the proportion of nursing home residents with the conditions than it is to the proportion of other community-living older adults with the conditions (Gruber-Baldini et al., 2004; Rabins et al., 1996; Rosenblatt et al., 2004; Watson et al., 2003). Available information about the proportions of assisted living, senior housing, and public housing facility residents that have MH/SU conditions and implications for their service needs and related workforce requirements are discussed later in the chapter. For purposes of estimating the proportion and number of older adults with MH/SU conditions, however, residents of non–nursing home, residential facilities are included with other community-living older adults in this section.

In the following discussion, available information about the proportion and number of older adults that have particular MS/SU conditions identified by the committee is presented in four tables. Particular conditions are included in each table based on two factors: (1) whether the available information about the particular MH/SU condition pertains to older people who live in the community (Tables 2-1 and 2-2), in group quarters settings (Table 2-4), or both (Table 2-3); and (2) whether the available information about the prevalence of the particular MH/SU condition can be combined with prevalence information for other MH/SU conditions without double counting (Tables 2-1, 2-3, and 2-4) or not (Table 2-2). Table 2-5 shows the totals for the proportion and number of older adults who had MH/SU conditions for which adequate data are available.

Prevalence of MH/SU Conditions in Community-Living Older Adults

Information about the prevalence of some of the 27 identified conditions in community-living older adults is available from large-scale surveys of MH/SU conditions that have been conducted in nationally representative, population-based samples in the United States (see Box 2-2). These surveys used structured interviews based primarily on DSM-IV-TR diagnostic criteria to identify people with particular MH/SU conditions. The exact wording and number of questions about each condition and the decision rules used to identify people who do or do not have the condition vary from one survey to another, and most of the surveys were conducted a decade ago. Despite these caveats, the surveys provide useful

BOX 2-2
Selected Population-Based Surveys of Mental Health and Substance Use Conditions in Nationally Representative Samples of Community-Living Adults in the United States

Collaborative Psychiatric Epidemiological Studies (CPES). The CPES is a group of three related surveys (below) funded by the National Institute of Mental Health. The three surveys were conducted independently, but used a common sampling process that allows for analyses of pooled data as if they were from a single, nationally representative sample (Heeringa et al., 2004). The samples included people living in the community and excluded people living in prisons, jails, nursing homes, and long-term medical or dependent care facilities, and military personnel living on a military base. The surveys used a structured interview, a modified version of the World Mental Health Composite International Diagnostic Interview (Kessler and Ustun, 2004), administered in person by a research interviewer. The combined sample for the three surveys was 20,013 people, including 2,584 adults age 65 and older.

- **National Comorbidity Survey-Replication (NCS-R).** The NCS-R was conducted from 2001 to 2002 in a sample of 9,282 English-speaking people, including 1,461 adults age 65 and older.
- **National Latino and Asian American Study (NLAAS).** The NLAAS was conducted in 2002-2003 in a sample of 4,649 Latinos (i.e., Mexicans, Puerto Ricans, Cubans, and other Latinos) and Asians (i.e., Chinese, Filipinos, Vietnamese, and other Asians), including 701 adults age 65 and older. Ethnicity was self-defined and classified according to U.S. Census categories. Interviews were conducted in English, Spanish, Tagalog, Vietnamese, or Mandarin.
- **National Study of American Life (NSAL).** The NSAL was conducted in 2001-2003 in a sample of 6,082 English-speaking African Americans, Afro-Caribbeans, and non-Hispanic whites, including 422 adults age 65 and older.

National Epidemiological Survey of Alcohol and Related Conditions Wave 1 (NESARC 1). The NESARC 1 was funded by the National Institute on Alcohol Abuse and Alcoholism (NIAAA) and conducted from 2001 to 2002 in a sample of 43,093 English-speaking people, including 8,205 adults age 65 and older. The

continued

BOX 2-2 Continued

sample included people living in the community and noninstitutional group quarters, such as boarding houses, rooming houses, nontransient hotels, motels, shelters, and group homes; it excluded people in prisons, jails, and nursing homes (Grant and Dawson, 2006). The survey used a structured interview, the "Alcohol Use Disorder and Associated Disabilities Interview Schedule—DSM-IV version" (Grant et al., 2001) that was administered in person by a lay interviewer.

National Epidemiological Survey of Alcohol and Related Conditions Wave 2 (NESARC 2). The NESARC 2 was funded by NIAAA and was conducted from 2004 to 2005. The sample included 34,653 of the initial 43,093 NESARC 1 respondents (NIAAA, 2010), including 7,177 adults age 65 and older. Of the 8,440 Wave 1 respondents of all ages who were not interviewed in Wave 2, 3,114 were not eligible because they were institutionalized, mentally or physically impaired, on active duty in the armed forces, deceased, or deported, and 5,306 refused or could not be located. The survey used the same structured interview and in-person administration procedure that was used for the NESARC 1 survey.

National Survey of Drug Use and Health (NSDUH). The NSDUH is funded by the Substance Abuse and Mental Health Services Administration and is conducted annually. The 2010 sample was 68,487 people, including 2,517 adults age 65 and older (CBHSQ, 2011n). The sample includes residents of households and noninstitutional group quarters, such as shelters, halfway houses, and rooming houses, and civilians living on military bases, and excludes homeless people who do not use shelters, military personnel on active duty, and residents of prisons, jails, nursing homes, mental institutions, and long-term hospitals. The survey used a structured interview and was conducted in person by a lay interviewer, but most of the questions were administered with a computer-assisted self-interviewing technology to provide a highly confidential mode of response.

information about the proportion and number of older adults who have the conditions. Data on adults age 65 and older that were not included in published reports from the surveys were generated for the committee by the Center for Multicultural Mental Health Research and the Substance Abuse and Mental Health Services Administration (SAMHSA).

The surveys described in Box 2-2 and some of the other sources used in this section provide information about the proportion of people who had particular MH/SU conditions in the previous month, the previous 12 months, or at any time in the person's life. For purposes of analyzing current and relatively sustained service needs, the committee decided to use 12-month prevalence rates whenever possible.

Prevalence of 10 MH/SU Conditions in Community-Living Older Adults

Table 2-1 shows 12-month prevalence rates and the estimated number of older adults with any of 10 MH/SU conditions for which data are available from three surveys, the Collaborative Psychiatric Epidemiologic Studies (CPES), National Epidemiological Survey of Alcohol and Related Conditions Wave 1 (NESARC 1), and National Epidemiological Survey of Alcohol and Related Conditions Wave 2 (NESARC 2) (see Box 2-2). The 10 conditions are all DSM-IV-TR mental disorders. The middle column shows the range of rates from the three surveys for each condition, one or more conditions, only one, two or more, and three or more conditions. The third column shows the range of estimates for the number of adults age 65 and older who had the condition(s) in 2010, calculated by multiplying the rates in the middle column by 38.8 million, the 2010 Census figure for the number of community-living adults age 65 and older.

As shown in Table 2-1, 6.8 to 10.2 percent of community-living adults age 65 and older had one or more of the conditions included in the table. Given the differences in the surveys, this range and the ranges for specific conditions are reassuringly small.

Using the 2010 Census figure for the community-living population age 65 and older, the 6.8 to 10.2 percent range indicates that in 2010, 2.6 million to 4 million community-living older adults had one or more of the 10 MH/SU conditions. Among those people, 800,000 to 900,000 people had two or more conditions, and 200,000 to 300,000 people had three or more conditions.

The conditions with the highest prevalence are depressive disorders, including major depressive episode and dysthymic disorder. In 2010, 3 to 4.5 percent of community-living older adults, about 1.2 million to 1.8 million people, had these conditions. The condition with the next highest prevalence is social phobia, which affected 0.9 to 2.6 percent of community-living older adults, about 400,000 to 1 million people in 2010.

TABLE 2-1
12-Month Prevalence Rates and Estimated Number of Community-Living Adults Age 65 and Older with 10 MH/SU Conditions

Mental Health or Substance Use Condition	Prevalence Rate[a] (%)	Estimated Number of Older Adults in 2010[b] (Millions)
Mental health conditions		
Depressive disorders	3.0-4.5	1.2-1.8
Major depressive episode(s)	3.0-4.3	1.2-1.7
Dysthymic disorder	0.6-1.6	0.2-0.6
Panic disorder	0.8-1.1	0.3-0.4
Agoraphobia without panic	[c]-0.3	[d]-0.1
Social phobia	0.9-2.6	0.4-1.0
Generalized anxiety disorder	1.1-2.1	0.4-0.8
Posttraumatic stress disorder (PTSD)[c]	0.6-2.6	0.2-1.0
Substance use conditions		
Alcohol dependence or abuse	[d]-1.9	[e]-0.7
Drug dependence or abuse	[d]-0.2	[e]-0.1
Summary figures		
One or more of the conditions	6.8-10.2	2.6-4.0
One of the conditions	4.8-7.8	1.8-3.0
Two or more of the conditions	2.0-2.4	0.8-0.9
Three or more of the conditions	0.5-0.8	0.2-0.3

[a] Prevalence rate is the range of rates from the Collaborative Psychiatric Epidemiological Studies (CPES), National Epidemiological Survey of Alcohol and Related Conditions Wave 1 (NESARC 1), and National Epidemiological Survey of Alcohol and Related Conditions Wave 2 (NESARC 2).

[b] The estimated number of older adults was calculated by multiplying the prevalence rates (middle column) by 38.8 million.

[c] The NESARC 1 survey did not measure PTSD; thus, the figures for PTSD represent data from only two of the surveys, the CPES and NESARC 2.

[d] The lowest prevalence rate from the three surveys is less than 0.2 percent.

[e] The lowest number of people with the condition from the three surveys is less than 50,000.

SOURCE: Center for Multicultural Mental Health Research, 2011.

The range of rates for alcohol dependence or abuse indicates that up to 700,000 community-living older adults had this condition in 2010. Data from the National Survey on Drug Use and Health (NSDUH) (see Box 2-2) support the high end of the range, showing that 780,000 older adults had alcohol dependence or abuse in 2010 (CBHSQ, 2011m).

The rates for drug dependence or abuse are smaller, up to 0.2 percent of community-living older adults, or about 78,000 people in 2010. The comparable figure from the NSDUH is even smaller, about 22,000 people in 2010 (CBHSQ, 2011m).

Posttraumatic stress disorder (PTSD) had the widest range of rates, 0.6 to 2.6 percent, and number of older adults affected, 200,000 to 1 million (see Box 2-3). PTSD is known to occur in veterans as a result of combat-related trauma. Many other kinds of traumatic events can also lead to PTSD, and available data show that older women, who are rarely veterans, are somewhat more likely than older men to have PTSD (Pietrzak et al., 2012). Moreover, older men, including older veterans who experienced combat-related trauma, can develop PTSD as a result of other traumatic events (Cook et al., 2005; Pietrzak et al., 2012; Schnurr et al., 2002).

For people with preexisting PTSD, various trajectories have been shown to occur with aging, including symptom stability, worsening, improvement, and fluctuation (Lapp et al., 2011). The onset and progression of dementia sometimes can trigger and exacerbate symptoms in older adults with PTSD, resulting in frightening situations for spouses and other family members (Johnston, 2000; Mittal et al., 2001).

Prevalence of Nine Additional MH/SU Conditions in Community-Living Older Adults

In addition to the 10 MH/SU conditions included in Table 2-1, the committee found data to support estimates of the prevalence of 10 of the remaining MH/SU conditions identified as important for older adults. These data come from a wider array of sources, including any one of the surveys shown in Box 2-2; other population-based surveys conducted in community samples using comprehensive, structured interviews; population-based surveys conducted in national samples using only one or a few questions to identify such people; and Medicare claims.

Table 2-2 shows the 12-month prevalence rates and estimated number of older adults who have 9 of the 10 conditions. Rates for the tenth condition, behavioral and psychiatric symptoms associated with dementia, are not included in Table 2-2 because the only available population-based data for this condition come from a survey that included both community-living older adults and nursing home residents, whereas the data for the other nine conditions come from studies that include only community-

BOX 2-3
Posttraumatic Stress Disorder (PTSD) in Older Adults

Data from the National Epidemiological Survey of Alcohol and Related Conditions Wave 2 (NESARC 2) indicate that 2.4 percent of community-living older adults in the United States have PTSD. The 2.4 percent figure represents current prevalence, as assessed at the time of the interview, based on DSM-IV-TR criteria, including the requirement that exposure to the traumatic event must precede development of the condition. The current prevalence of PTSD was higher for people age 65-74 than for those age 75 and older (2.7 percent vs. 2.0 percent, respectively). It was also higher for Hispanic/Latinos age 65 and older (4.3 percent) than for whites (2.3 percent) and African Americans (2.0 percent) in that age group.

NESARC 2 survey data also indicate that current prevalence of PTSD is higher in community-living adults under age 65 than in those age 65 and older. The data show that 4.2 percent of adults age 55-64 had PTSD, compared with 2.4 percent of those age 65 and older. The reasons for this difference are not known, but plausible explanations include cohort effects related to exposure, for example, to military service; earlier mortality in those with PTSD; underreporting of symptoms by older adults; and underrecognition of PTSD symptoms that may manifest differently in older adults (Lapp et al., 2011; Owens et al., 2005; van Zelst et al., 2003a,b).

After exposure to a traumatic event, older and younger adults generally experience similar risk of developing PTSD (Acierno et al., 2002; Chung et al., 2004; Kohn et al., 2005). Factors associated with susceptibility for PTSD are also similar across age groups. These factors include female gender, childhood adversity, low self-efficacy, lack of social support, and personality traits, such as neuroticism (Acierno et al., 2002; Lapp et al., 2011; Ozer et al., 2003; van Zelst et al., 2003b).

In the United States, research on PTSD in older adults has focused most on older combat veterans and prisoners of war (Dirkzwager

living older adults. Prevalence rates for behavioral and psychiatric symptoms associated with dementia are discussed later in this section.

The middle column of Table 2-2 shows the prevalence rate or range of rates for each of the nine conditions. The third column shows the figure or range of figures for the number of adults age 65 and older who had the condition in 2010, calculated by multiplying the rate(s) in the et al., 2001; Port et al., 2001). One study found that World War II veterans who experienced moderate-to-heavy combat were 13 times as likely to have PTSD 45 years later compared with noncombat veterans (Spiro et al., 1994).

Some studies have focused on PTSD in Holocaust survivors (Trappler et al., 2007; Yehuda et al., 2009). Other studies have documented PTSD in people exposed to other traumatic life events, such as sexual and criminal assault, disasters, life-threatening illness, accidents (including falls), and unexpected loss of a loved one (Chung et al., 2009; Spitzer et al., 2008).

Comorbid mental health and substance use conditions, including depression, anxiety disorders, and alcohol and drug use disorders, are common in older adults with PTSD (Brady, 1997; Jacobsen et al., 2001; Lapp et al., 2011; Spitzer et al., 2008). High levels of coexisting physical health conditions, especially heart disease and ulcers, are also common in such people (Pietrzak et al., 2012; Schnurr et al., 2000).

Several studies conducted in large samples of veterans have found that veterans with PTSD are twice as likely as those without PTSD to develop dementia (Qureshi et al., 2010; Yaffe et al., 2010). Questions have been raised about the mechanism for this association (Borson, 2010; Pittman, 2010). Despite these questions, numerous case studies have documented that dementia can result in the emergence or exacerbation of PTSD symptoms in some older adults (Cook et al., 2003; Dallam et al., 2011; Johnston, 2000; Mittal et al., 2001; van Achterberg et al., 2001). Older veterans with PTSD and dementia may become extremely agitated, paranoid, and physically combative, occasionally attacking their spouse or, conversely, attempting to protect their spouse from other, imagined attackers.

SOURCE: K. M. Bohnert, Health Services Research and Development Service, Department of Veterans Affairs, Ann Arbor, MI, text provided to the IOM committee, January 10, 2012.

middle column by 38.8 million, the U.S. Census figure for the number of community-living adults age 65 and older in 2010.

The proportions of community-living older adults who have any of the nine conditions included in Table 2-2 range from less than 0.2 percent to 11.1 percent. Because the data come from unrelated studies, it is not possible to determine the proportion that has one or more of the conditions.

TABLE 2-2
12-Month Prevalence Rates and Estimated Number of Adults Age 65 and Older with Nine Additional MH/SU Conditions

Mental Health or Substance Use Condition	Prevalence Rate[a] (%)	Estimated Number of Older Adults in 2010[b] (Millions)
Mental health conditions		
Bipolar disorder	[c]-0.2	[d]-0.1
Schizophrenia	0.2-0.8	0.1-0.3
Obsessive-compulsive disorder	0.8	0.3
Depressive symptoms	1.1-11.1	0.4-4.3
Anxiety symptoms	4.3	1.7
Suicidal ideation	0.5-1.7	0.2-0.7
Suicide plans and attempts	[c]	[d]
Substance use conditions		
At-risk drinking	5.2	2.0
At-risk drug use	0.9	0.4

[a] Prevalence rate is the rate or range of rates from the cited sources.
[b] The number of people was calculated by multiplying the percentages in the middle column by 38.8 million.
[c] The prevalence rate is less than 0.2 percent.
[d] The number of people with the condition is less than 50,000.
SOURCES: Blazer and Wu, 2011; Blazer et al., 1987; CBHSQ, 2011i, 2012c; Center for Multicultural Mental Health Research, 2011; Gum et al., 2009; Harris and Cooper, 2006; Hybels et al., 2009; Jeste et al., 1999; Kessler et al., 2005; Steffens et al., 2000; Weissman et al., 1988; Wolitzky-Taylor et al., 2010; Wu et al., 2006.

Three of the MH/SU conditions in Table 2-2 are DSM-IV-TR mental disorders: bipolar disorder, schizophrenia, and obsessive-compulsive disorder (OCD). They are not included in Table 2-1 with other DSM-IV-TR disorders because information about their prevalence is not available from all three surveys used to create Table 2-1. In fact, relatively little information is available about the proportion of community-living older adults who have any of the three disorders. The limited information reflects the difficulty of measuring these disorders in population-based surveys. Some researchers and clinicians question whether the prevalence of mental disorders in general, and the three disorders in particular, is identified accurately by the structured interviews used in the large-scale, population-based surveys conducted to date. For bipolar disorder, schizophrenia, and OCD, they question whether the surveys have found and interviewed representative samples of older adults with the disorders and whether valid prevalence rates can be generated from the relatively small numbers of older survey respondents that have the disorders (Alegria et al., 2007; Cohen et al., 2000; Depp and Jeste, 2004; Gum et al., 2009; Nelson and Rice, 1997; Palmer et al., 1999; Wu et al., 2006).

One of the few population-based sources of information about the proportion of older adults who have any of the three disorders is the Epidemiologic Catchment Area (ECA) survey that was conducted in five U.S. communities in the early 1980s. It used a structured interview based primarily on diagnostic criteria from the previous version of the DSM, DSM-III. ECA data show that the 12-month prevalence rate for bipolar disorder was 0.1 percent in older adults (Weissman et al., 1988). Another U.S. survey that provides population-based prevalence data on bipolar disorder, the NCS-R (see Box 2-2), found that 0.2 percent of older adults had the disorder (Gum et al., 2009). These rates suggest that 39,000 to 78,000 community-living older adults (rounded to 100,000 in the table) may have had bipolar disorder in 2010.

ECA data show that the 12-month prevalence rate for schizophrenia was 0.2 percent in community-living adults age 65 and older (Jeste et al., 1999). A comprehensive analysis of findings from the National Comorbidity Survey-Replication (NCS-R) (see Box 2-2), that included clinical evaluations of a subsample of NCS-R subjects, found a 12-month prevalence rate of 0.2 percent for a somewhat broader group of disorders composed of schizophrenia, schizophreniform disorder, schizoaffective disorder, delusional disorder, and other psychoses (Kessler et al., 2005). Another analysis based on Medicare claims found a 0.8 percent prevalence rate for schizophrenia in Medicare beneficiaries age 65 and older (Wu et al., 2006). The figures from these three studies suggest that in 2010, 78,000 to 300,000 older adults may have had schizophrenia.

The ECA survey is the only population-based source of U.S. data on the 12-month prevalence rate for OCD. The ECA found that 0.8 percent of community-living older adults had this condition (Wolitzky-Taylor et al., 2010), suggesting that about 300,000 older adults may have had OCD in 2010. A follow-up study showed, however, that only 19 percent of ECA subjects who met the criteria for OCD at the time of the survey still met the criteria 1 year later, and the stability of the survey-based diagnosis was particularly low for older adults (Nelson and Rice, 1997). Thus, the 0.8 percent prevalence rate and the associated estimate of the number of older adults with OCD in 2010 are uncertain.

The committee believes that the prevalence rates presented above for bipolar disorder, schizophrenia, and OCD likely underestimate the true rates of these conditions in community-living older adults, but other data are not available from U.S. population-based surveys. Accurate information about the proportion and number of older adults who have these conditions is essential for evaluating the MH/SU service needs of older adults because the conditions are frequently severe, and people with the conditions often require specialty mental health services. As noted earlier, bipolar disorder and schizophrenia are core conditions in the category usually referred to as serious mental illness (SMI), a category of conditions associated with especially high mental health service needs. More accurate and up-to-date information about these conditions is needed to plan for a workforce capable of providing appropriate mental health services for older adults with SMI.

In addition to prevalence rates for the three DSM-IV-TR mental disorders, Table 2-2 shows prevalence rates for six other MH/SU conditions. The 5.2 percent rate for at-risk drinking represents the proportion of community-living adults age 65 and older with *subsyndromal alcohol dependence,* defined as self-reported alcohol use that meets one or two of the seven DSM-IV-TR criteria for alcohol dependence, but not the three or more criteria required for a DSM-IV-TR diagnosis of the disorder (Blazer and Wu, 2011). Using the 2010 U.S. Census figure for the population age 65 and older, the 5.2 percent rate suggests that in 2010, about 2 million community-living older adults had subsyndromal alcohol dependence.

Prevalence rates for at-risk drinking from other studies vary, depending on how the condition is defined and measured. The 2010 Behavioral Risk Factors Surveillance System (BRFSS) survey found that 3.8 percent of community-living adults age 65 and older (about 1.5 million people) reported *binge drinking,* defined as having four or more alcoholic drinks for women and five or more for men on at least one occasion in the previous month (Kanny et al., 2012). Compared with adults age 18-64, older adults who reported binge drinking had a significantly higher average number of drinks per occasion (5.5 drinks for those age 65 and older versus 4.1-4.7 drinks for those age 18-64). The 2010 NSDUH found that 7.6 percent of community-living older adults (about 2.9 million people) reported *binge drinking* (CBHSQ, 2011k,l). One-fifth of these people (about 600,000) reported *heavy drinking,* defined as having five or more drinks per occasion on five or more days in the previous month.

The 4.3 percent prevalence rate for anxiety symptoms represents the proportion of community-living older adults with symptoms that do not meet the DSM-IV-TR criteria for a diagnosis of an anxiety disorder (about 1.7 million people in 2010). To be included in the 4.3 percent rate, individuals with anxiety symptoms also had to have substantial associated functional impairment. Other studies that did not require this high level of functional impairment have found higher rates of anxiety symptoms. One study found, for example, that 19 percent of a population-based sample of about 3,000 community-living Medicare beneficiaries ages 70-79 reported having at least one of three anxiety symptoms: feeling fearful, nervous or shaky inside, or tense and keyed up (Mehta et al., 2003). Some of these people may have had diagnosable DSM-IV-TR anxiety disorders, such as generalized anxiety disorder or major depression with anxiety, but it is not possible to determine the proportion that did.

The range of prevalence rates for depressive symptoms, 1.1 to 11.1 percent, comes from four population-based studies intended to measure depressive symptoms that did not meet the DSM-IV-TR diagnostic criteria for a depressive disorder. One study found that 11 percent of a national random sample of 137,000 community-living Medicare beneficiaries age 65 and older reported feeling "depressed or sad much of the time over the previous year" (Harris and Cooper, 2006). Two population-based studies of older adults in five North Carolina counties found that 4 and 11.1 percent, respectively, had depressive symptoms (Blazer et al., 1987; Hybels et al., 2009). A fourth study conducted in Cache County, Utah, found that only 1.1 percent of older adults had depressive symptoms (Steffens et al., 2000). This range of rates, 1.1 to 11.1 percent, suggests that 430,000 to 4.3 million older adults may have had depressive symptoms in 2010.

The researchers who conducted the Cache County study note that the relatively low rate of depressive symptoms in their study, 1.1 percent, could reflect characteristics of the sample that predict reduced risk for the condition, such as low rates of cardiovascular disease and cancer and high rates of social and religious involvement. They note alternatively that the low rate of depressive symptoms could reflect reluctance of the older adults in their sample to report "minor mental health problems" (Steffens et al., 2000).

The 0.9 percent prevalence rate for at-risk drug use in Table 2-2 comes from the 2010 NSDUH and represents the proportion of community-living adults age 65 and older who reported nonmedical use of prescription psychotherapeutic drugs in the previous year. The 0.9 percent rate indicates that about 350,000 older adults reported nonmedical use of such drugs (CBHSQ, 2011g,h). Nearly half of these people reported nonmedical use of prescription pain relievers (CBHSQ, 2011i,j).

In 2010, 1.7 percent of older adults (about 650,000 people) reported use of any illicit drugs, including 1 percent (nearly 400,000 people) who reported using marijuana (CBHSQ, 2011c,d,e,f). The proportion of older adults who reported using other illicit drugs in 2010 is not given because of small numbers, but combined NSDUH data for 2005 and 2006 indicate that 0.7 percent of community-living adults age 65 and older reported using marijuana in the previous year, and less than 0.1 percent reported using cocaine, heroin, hallucinogens, or inhalants (Blazer and Wu, 2009b). Whether all older adults who use any illicit drug would be considered to have at-risk drug use is unclear, however.

Many of the figures for the nine conditions shown in Table 2-2 come from unrelated studies; thus it is not possible to determine how many older adults have more than one of the conditions. Likewise, it is not possible to determine how many older adults that have one or more of the conditions shown in Table 2-2 also have one or more of the conditions shown in Table 2-1. This information about comorbidity is required to estimate the total number of older adults who needs MH/SU services.

Prevalence of Behavioral and Psychiatric Symptoms Associated with Dementia

Table 2-3 shows prevalence rates and the estimated number of older adults that had behavioral and psychiatric symptoms associated with dementia in a one-month period. The rates come from the Aging, Demographics, and Memory Study (ADAMS), a study conducted in a stratified random sample of adults age 71 and older, drawn from the national, population-based samples used for the 2000 and 2002 Health and Retirement Study surveys (Okura et al., 2010; Plassman et al., 2007). Unlike the other data sources used to develop the figures shown in Tables 2-1 and 2-2, the ADAMS sample included nursing home residents, and the figures in Table 2-3 pertain to both community-living people and nursing home residents. The table shows the proportions of ADAMS subjects with normal cognition and dementia who had each of the symptoms, one or more symptoms, one or two symptoms, and three or more symptoms.

As shown, 57.2 percent of the older adults with dementia had one or more symptoms in the previous month, including 30.5 percent who had one or two symptoms and 26.7 percent who had three or more symptoms. The most common behavioral and psychiatric symptoms in older adults with dementia were depression or dysphoria (depressed mood) (28 percent), apathy or indifference (22.9 percent), agitation or aggression (22.5 percent), and delusions (18.2 percent) (Okura et al., 2010). Older adults with normal cognition, including older adults with MH/SU conditions but no dementia, were much less likely than those with dementia to have any of the symptoms.

ADAMS is the only U.S. study conducted to date that has measured these behavioral and psychiatric symptoms in a nationally representative sample of community-living older adults and nursing home residents, but

TABLE 2-3
Proportion of Community-Living Adults and Nursing Home Residents Age 71 and Older with Normal Cognition or Dementia Who Had Associated Behavioral and Psychiatric Symptoms in the Previous Month[a]

Symptom[b]	Older Adults with Normal Cognition n = 303 (%)	Older Adults with Dementia n = 299 (%)
Delusions	0.6	18.2
Hallucinations	0.0	14.7
Agitation/aggression	3.6	22.5
Depression/dysphoria	11.9	28.0
Anxiety	6.5	15.2
Irritability or lability	5.9	13.4
Disinhibition	0.5	11.2
Elation/euphoria	1.5	1.6
Apathy/indifference	3.0	22.9
Aberrant motor behavior	0.0	16.5
Summary figures		
One or more symptoms	17.7	57.2
One or two symptoms	13.3	30.5
Three or more symptoms	4.3	26.7

[a] The data are weighted to adjust for the study's complex sampling design.

[b] The behavioral and psychiatric symptoms measured in the Aging, Demographics and Memory Study come from the 10-item version of the Neuropsychiatric Inventory (Cummings et al., 1994).

SOURCE: T. Okura, Bajikoen Clinic, Geriatrics Section, Tokyo, Japan, unpublished data from the Aging, Demographics, and Memory Study provided to the IOM committee, September 14, 2011.

three other studies have measured behavioral and psychiatric symptoms associated with dementia in population-based samples at the county or local level (Chan et al., 2003; Lyketsos et al., 2000, 2002). The samples for these studies included adults age 65 and older, thus supplementing the ADAMS data on adults age 71 and older. Each of the studies found somewhat higher prevalence rates, ranging from 61 to 75 percent, for older adults with dementia and associated behavioral and psychiatric symptoms, suggesting that the 57.2 percent figure from ADAMS may be conservative.

Estimates of the total number of adults age 65 and older who have dementia range from 3.9 million to 5.1 million people (see calculations below).[1] Combining these figures and the 57.2 percent rate for older adults with dementia and associated behavioral and psychiatric symptoms indicates that in 2010, 2.2 to 2.9 million older adults had such symptoms in the previous month.

Many researchers and clinicians believe that nearly all people with dementia will have behavioral and psychiatric symptoms at some time in the frequently long course of their illness (Gauthier et al., 2010; Lyketsos et al., 2011; McKeith and Cummings, 2005). Dementia-related behavioral and psychiatric symptoms often change over time as the person's dementia worsens. Thus, the services and workforce competencies required to meet the needs of older adults with behavioral and psychiatric symptoms associated with dementia also change over time.

MH/SU Conditions for Which Population-Based Prevalence Data Are Not Available

The committee did not find population-based data to support estimates of the proportion or number of community-living older adults who have 7 of the 27 identified MH/SU conditions. The seven conditions include two DSM-IV-TR mental disorders (adjustment disorder and personality disorders) and five other MH/SU conditions (hoarding, severe

---

[1]U.S Census data show there were 25.7 million people age 71 and older in 2010, and ADAMS data indicate that 13.9 percent of people in that age group (about 3.6 million people) had dementia. U.S. Census data also show there were 14.5 million people ages 65-70 in 2010. No national data are available on the number of people ages 65-70 who have dementia, but two sources indicate that 2 percent of people in that age group, or about 290,000 people, have Alzheimer's disease (Brookmeyer et al., 1998; Hebert et al., 2003). Combining these figures indicates that about 3.9 million people age 65 and older had dementia in 2010. Other data from the U.S. Centers for Medicare & Medicaid Services show that in 2008, 12.6 percent of Medicare fee-for-service beneficiaries had Medicare claims with a diagnostic code for Alzheimer's disease or another dementia (CMS, 2011). Combining the 12.6 percent rate and the U.S. Census figure for the population age 65 and older in 2010, 40.3 million people, indicates that about 5.1 million people age 65 and older had dementia in 2010.

domestic squalor, severe self-neglect, fear of falling, and complicated grief).

Although older adults with adjustment disorder are seen with some frequency in clinical settings (Casey and Bailey, 2011; Lantz, 2008), no U.S. population-based data were found for the proportion or number of community-living adults age 65 and older who have this condition. One Swiss study found that 2.3 percent of community-living older adults had an adjustment disorder (Maercker et al., 2008).

Personality disorders were measured in the NESARC 1 and 2 surveys (see Box 2-2). The Wave 1 survey found that many community-living adults age 65 and older had one or more of seven DSM-IV-TR personality disorders; for example, 1.8 percent of older adults (about 700,000 people in 2010) had *lifetime* paranoid personality disorder, and 5.2 percent (about 2 million people in 2010) had *lifetime* obsessive-compulsive personality disorder (Grant et al., 2004). The committee did not find published data on the 12-month prevalence of the seven personality disorders. Moreover, a reanalysis of the NESARC 1 data on personality disorders in adults of all ages concluded that the published rates for lifetime prevalence were too high for each disorder because they included people who did not meet the DSM-IV-TR-required level of distress, impairment, or dysfunction associated with each of the criteria for each disorder (Trull et al., 2010). The NESARC 2 survey measured three DSM-IV-TR personality disorders that were not included in the NESARC 1 survey (Sansone and Sansone, 2011), but the committee did not find published data on 12-month prevalence of these disorders.

An analysis of findings from the Baltimore site of the Epidemiologic Catchment Area survey found that 6.6 percent of adults age 55 and older had personality disorders (Cohen et al., 1994). The disorders were diagnosed in a psychiatric evaluation using diagnostic criteria from the previous version of the DSM, DSM III. Half of those diagnosed with any personality disorder had obsessive-compulsive personality disorder. The researchers note that older adults with personality disorders are likely to express more severe symptoms of the disorder when they are experiencing stress-related situations such as serious illness, prolonged ill health, or the death of a spouse, other relative, or close friend.

The available data on three other MH/SU conditions—hoarding, severe domestic squalor, and severe self-neglect—come from case reports and administrative records of public health departments and aging and adult protective services agencies. For example:

- Massachusetts public health officers who responded to a survey about formal complaints of hoarding received by their departments identified 471 complaints received from 1992 to 1997, sug-

gesting a 5-year rate of 0.3 complaints per 1,000 people living in the areas served by the departments (Frost et al., 2000).
- Case records from a psychiatry agency in Sydney, Australia, showed that 173 older adults were referred to the agency for moderate or severe domestic squalor from 2000 to 2009, suggesting a 1-year rate of 0.7 referrals per 1,000 people in the agency's service area (Snowdon and Halliday, 2011). No U.S. data were found on severe domestic squalor.
- Ombudsman records for New Haven, Connecticut, showed that 92 of 2,161 community-living older adults followed for 9 years (4.3 percent) had confirmed self-neglect, indicating a weighted rate of 7 cases per 1,000 person-years (Abrams et al., 2002).
- Administrative records from the Texas Adult Protective Services Division show that self-neglect by adults age 65 and older accounted for 40 percent of the 61,380 referrals for adult abuse and neglect received by the agency in 1997 (Pavlik et al., 2001).

These findings cannot be used to estimate the population-based prevalence of the three conditions because the findings only represent reported cases. Clearly, however, they have important implications for workforce competencies in public health departments and aging and adult protective services agencies.

The committee did not find population-based data on the prevalence of fear of falling, but studies conducted in convenience samples suggest that substantial proportions of older adults have this condition (Lach, 2005; Murphy et al., 2003; Oh-Park et al., 2011). A study of more than 500 community-living adults age 70 and older in New York City found, for example, that 31 percent reported fear of falling at baseline, and 45 percent of those who did not report fear of falling at baseline developed the condition in the next 2 to 5 years (Oh-Park et al., 2011).

No U.S. population-based studies of complicated grief were found. Studies conducted in Europe show that, depending on how complicated grief is defined, 0.9 to 9 percent of bereaved older adults had the condition (Forstmeier and Maercker, 2007; Kersting et al., 2011).

Prevalence of MH/SU Conditions in Older Adults Living in Group Quarters Settings

With the exception of the figures presented earlier on behavioral and psychiatric symptoms associated with dementia, the figures presented thus far in this section have been for community-living older adults. To estimate the total proportion and number of older adults with MH/SU conditions, older adults living in group quarters settings must be added.

As noted earlier, the 2010 Census found that 1.5 million adults age 65 and older, about 4 percent of the 40.3 million older adults in the United States, were living in group quarters settings (Census Bureau, 2010b). Of the 1.5 million older adults, 82 percent were living in nursing homes; 2 percent were living in prisons, jails, or other adult correctional facilities; and about 3 percent were homeless or living in homeless shelters or other transitional housing (Census Bureau, 2010d). The remaining 13 percent (fewer than 200,000 people) were in other group quarters settings, such as psychiatric hospitals, residential treatment centers, inpatient hospice facilities, and religious group residences. As discussed earlier, for purposes of this analysis of the proportion and number of older adults with MH/SU conditions, older adults living in assisted living, senior housing, and public housing facilities are included in the community-living population.

Prevalence of MH/SU Conditions in Older Nursing Home Residents

Table 2-4 shows the proportion and number of older adults living in nursing homes in April 2009 who had depression, anxiety disorders, bipolar disorder, or schizophrenia and the proportion and number that had one or more of these conditions. The data come from residents' Minimum Data Set (MDS) assessments and reflect diagnoses noted in their nursing home medical records. The diagnoses can be primary or secondary.

TABLE 2-4
Prevalence and Estimated Number of Nursing Home Residents Age 65 and Older with Selected Mental Health Conditions, 2009

Condition	Prevalence Rate (%)	Number of Residents with the Condition
Mental health conditions		
Depression	49.6	590,834
Anxiety disorders	16.1	192,071
Bipolar disorder	2.8	33,416
Schizophrenia	3.6	42,521
Summary figures		
One or more conditions	56.8	675,622

SOURCE: Shaping Long-Term Care in America Project and Brown University, data provided to the IOM committee, November 2011.

As shown in Table 2-4, MDS data indicate that 56.8 percent of nursing residents age 65 and older (675,622 people) had at least one of the four conditions. Depression was the most prevalent condition, affecting nearly half of all older residents. Sixteen percent of residents age 65 and older had anxiety disorders, and smaller proportions had bipolar disorder and schizophrenia.

Various concerns have been raised about the precision of resident diagnoses based on MDS data. In particular, the committee believes that the 49.6 percent figure for depression in Table 2-4 probably includes both DSM-IV-TR depressive disorders and depressive symptoms that do not meet the criteria for a diagnosis of a DSM-IV-TR depressive disorder. Data on mental health conditions in nursing home residents are available from other sources, but many of these sources are quite old, and the characteristics of nursing home residents, including the proportions that have various mental health conditions, have changed in recent years (see Box 2-4).

The proportion of nursing home residents with mental health conditions will probably continue to change as nursing homes increasingly admit people for short-term, postacute care as opposed to long-term personal care and supervision. From 1999 to 2005, the proportion of long-stay residents among new admissions to nursing homes decreased from 39 to 25 percent, and the proportion of people with dementia among new admissions decreased from 24 to 18 percent (Fullerton et al., 2009). These trends reflect higher Medicare payments for postacute nursing home care as well as ongoing government and private initiatives to discourage nursing home placement from the community and encourage discharges of nursing home residents to assisted living, other residential care facilities, and home. In the same period during which admissions of long-stay residents and people with dementia decreased, however, the proportion of all residents and new residents with depression increased substantially (see Box 2-4). Thus, the likely direction of future changes in the proportion of nursing home residents with particular mental health conditions is uncertain.

In addition to the four mental health conditions shown in Table 2-4, many nursing home residents have behavioral symptoms. National data from residents' MDS assessments show that in 2010, 28 percent of residents of all ages had such symptoms (AHCA, 2010). Many of these residents are individuals with dementia who are included in Table 2-3, and some are residents with mental health conditions who are included in Table 2-4. Thus, for purposes of this analysis of the proportion and number of older adults with MH/SU conditions, these individuals are already counted. The implications of such symptoms for residents' service needs and related workforce requirements are discussed later in this report.

Small proportions of older nursing home residents have other MH/SU

BOX 2-4
Changing Prevalence of Mental Health Conditions in Nursing Home Residents

The proportion of nursing home residents age 65 and older with depression has increased greatly, at least since 1999. One study of residents age 65 and older in more than 5,000 nursing homes in eight states found that among those who had been in the facility for at least 90 days, the proportion with depression increased from 34 percent in 1999 to 45 percent in 2003 and 52 percent in 2007 (Gaboda et al., 2011).

Among people newly admitted to nursing homes, the proportion with depression has also increased. From 1999 to 2005, the proportion of new admissions of all ages with depression increased from 11 to 16 percent (Fullerton et al., 2009). During the same period, the proportion of new residents with bipolar disorder and schizophrenia remained the same, while the proportion of new admissions with anxiety disorders decreased from 3 to 2 percent.

New nursing home admissions with mental health conditions are more likely than other new admissions to stay in the nursing home for at least 90 days (Grabowski et al., 2009). In 2005, about half of all new admissions age 65 and older with bipolar disorder or schizophrenia who survived at least 90 days were still living in the nursing home at that time (Aschbrenner et al., 2011). The greater likelihood that new admissions with these conditions are staying in the nursing home for at least 90 days means that the overall prevalence of the conditions is probably also increasing.

conditions. The 2004 National Nursing Home Survey found, for example, that 1 percent of residents age 65 and older had alcohol dependence or abuse (Seitz et al., 2010).

Prevalence of MH/SU Conditions in Older Inmates in Adult Correctional Facilities

In 2010, 29,000 adults age 65 and older were inmates in adult correctional facilities, including federal and state prisons and local jails (Census Bureau, 2010d). Due to changes in prison sentencing and release policies enacted three decades ago, the number of older inmates is increasing rapidly. In the 4 years from 2007 to 2010, the number of older inmates in federal prisons increased by 67 percent, compared with a 0.7 percent increase in the prison population as a whole (Human Rights Watch, 2012).

One study conducted in 2004 found that 36 to 52 percent of inmates age 55 and older in adult correctional facilities had mental health conditions, based on documentation of a recent diagnosis, recent mental health treatment, or symptoms that met the DSM-IV-TR diagnostic criteria for conditions, such as major depressive episode, mania, and psychosis (James and Glaze, 2006). Data from the Iowa prison system for the years 1996-2001 show that 23 percent of inmates age 55 and older had mental health conditions and 71 percent had a history of substance dependence or abuse, primarily involving alcohol (Arndt et al., 2002). The committee did not find comparable data on the proportion and number of inmates age 65 and older who have MH/SU conditions, but the proportions for inmates age 55 and older cited above suggest that 23 to 71 percent of older inmates (6,670 to 20,600 people) may have had such conditions in 2010.

Prevalence of MH/SU Conditions in Homeless Older Adults

National data on the number of homeless people come from a survey conducted on 1 day each year. In 2010, 649,917 people were found to be homeless on the designated day, including 403,308 people who were in a homeless shelter and 239,759 people who were unsheltered (HUD, 2011). The survey report does not show how many of these people were age 65 and older, but 26 percent had SMI and 35 percent had chronic substance abuse. From October 2009 to September 2010, about 44,000 adults age 62 and older spent at least one night in an emergency shelter or transitional housing (HUD, 2011), but the committee did not find information about how many of these people had MH/SU conditions.

Prevalence of MH/SU Conditions in Older Adults in Other Group Quarters Settings

Psychiatric hospitals are categorized as group quarters settings in the U.S. Census Bureau's classification system. In 2008, 4 percent of the 180,496 people in state psychiatric hospitals were age 65 and older (about 7,200 people) (SAMHSA, 2009). The average length of stay in these hospitals was 131 days for people of all ages, but comparable information is not available for older adults.

The committee did not find information about the number of older adults in private psychiatric hospitals or their average length of stay. The committee also did not find information about the number of older adults with MH/SU conditions in other group quarters settings. It is likely that all older adults in private psychiatric hospitals and substantial proportions of older adults in other group quarters settings have MH/SU conditions.

Comorbid MH/SU Conditions

As noted earlier, some older adults with MH/SU conditions have more than one such condition. Some have both a mental health condition, such as a depressive disorder, and a substance use condition, such as alcohol dependence. In addition, some older adults have more than one mental health condition, for example, a depressive disorder and generalized anxiety disorder, and some have more than one substance use condition, for example, alcohol dependence and nonmedical use of prescription drugs.

To estimate the proportion and number of older adults that have MH/SU conditions and avoid double counting, it is necessary to account for comorbidity. Some information about comorbidity is available from the large-scale, population-based surveys described in Box 2-2. This information is frequently reported for younger people but rarely reported for older adults, often because small numbers make the data for older adults unreliable. The figures on comorbidity presented below come from studies selected to illustrate the extent of comorbidity in the older population. The studies used clinical, research, or registry-based samples.

- In a sample of 1,801 primary care patients age 60 and older who had major depression or dysthmia, 11 percent also had PTSD and 15 percent also had panic disorder (Hegel et al., 2005).
- In a sample of 182 research subjects age 60 and older who had major depression or depressive symptoms, 23 percent also had an anxiety disorder, including 9 percent that had panic disorder and 7 percent that had social phobia (Lenze et al., 2000).
- In a sample of 2,240 primary care patients age 65 and older, 28 percent had major depression and 12 percent of those individuals also had suicidal ideation; 21 percent of the full sample had both major depression and an anxiety disorder, and 18 percent of those individuals also had suicidal ideation (Bartels et al., 2002).
- In a sample of 76 research subjects age 60 and older who had dysthymic disorder, 31 percent also had personality disorders, including 17 percent who had obsessive-compulsive personality disorder (Devanand et al., 2000).
- In a research sample of 1,552 adults age 53 to 100 who had consumed any alcohol in the previous 5 years, 29 percent had depressive symptoms, and of those individuals 33 percent screened positive for alcohol abuse or misuse (Rodriguez et al., 2010).

- In a registry-based sample of about 15,000 veterans age 60 and older who had bipolar disorder, 9 percent also had substance abuse, 5 percent also had PTSD, and 10 percent also had other anxiety disorders (Sajatovic et al., 2006).
- In a small research sample of 18 adults age 60 and older who had a hoarding condition, 28 percent also had major depressive disorder; 22 percent also had dysthymia; 16 percent also had OCD; 5 percent also had social phobia; and 5 percent also had general anxiety disorder (Ayers et al., 2010).

Because the samples for these studies are not population based, the findings cannot be used to determine average comorbidity figures for the older population. They do, however, portray the complex mix of comorbid MH/SU conditions that occur in some older adults and shape their service needs and related workforce requirements.

Committee Estimates of the Proportion and Number of Older Adults with MH/SU Conditions in 2010

This section has presented information the committee was able to obtain about the proportion and number of older adults who have MH/SU conditions. Many gaps remain in the information that would be required to create a comprehensive picture of these conditions in older adults that could, in turn, be used to analyze their service needs and plan for a workforce capable of meeting those needs. The difficulties confronted by the committee in obtaining even the information presented thus far in the chapter would likely also confront others, including policy makers, administrators, and educators, who require comprehensive information to understand and address service needs. Moreover, the information presented in the chapter pertains only to national-level prevalence, whereas many policy makers, administrators, and educators need state- or local-level information, some of which would probably be even more difficult to obtain.

Table 2-5 shows the estimated number of adults age 65 and older with MH/SU conditions for which the committee found both population-based prevalence data and comorbidity information sufficient to avoid double counting. Most of the figures come from Tables 2-1, 2-3, and 2-4, shown earlier. Figures from Table 2-2 on bipolar disorder and schizophrenia are also included because the committee assumes that most community-dwelling older adults with these conditions do not have other conditions shown in Table 2-1 and therefore are not already included in the numbers shown in Table 2-5.

As shown in Table 2-5, an estimated 5.6 million to 8 million older

TABLE 2-5
Estimated Number of Adults Age 65 and Older with MH/SU Conditions in 2010

MH/SU Condition	Estimated Number of Older Adults with the Conditions (Millions)
Community-living adults	
One or more of 10 conditions[a]	2.6-4.0
Bipolar disorder[b]	[c]-0.1
Schizophrenia[b]	0.1-0.3
Nursing home residents	
One or more of four conditions[d]	0.7
Community-living adults and nursing home residents	
Behavioral and psychiatric symptoms associated with dementia[e]	2.2-2.9
Totals	5.6-8.0

[a] Estimated number of community-living people with one or more of the 10 conditions included in Table 2-1, i.e., depressive disorders, major depressive episode, dysthymic disorder, panic disorder, agoraphobia without panic, social phobia, generalized anxiety disorder, posttraumatic stress disorder, alcohol dependence or abuse, and drug dependence or abuse.
[b] Estimated number of community-living people with the disorder (see Table 2-2).
[c] The estimated number of people with the disorder is less than 50,000.
[d] Estimated number of nursing home residents with one or more of the four conditions included in Table 2-4.
[e] Estimated number of community-living people and nursing home residents with one or more of the behavioral and psychiatric symptoms associated with dementia (see Table 2-3).

adults had one or more of the MH/SU conditions included in the table. These figures represent 14 to 20 percent of the population age 65 and older in 2010.

The conditions with the highest prevalence are behavioral and psychiatric symptoms associated with dementia and depressive disorders. As shown in Table 2-5, an estimated 2.2 million to 2.9 million community-living older adults and nursing home residents have behavioral and psychiatric symptoms associated with dementia. Combining the number of community-living older adults with depressive disorders from Table 2-1 (1.2 million to 1.8 million people) and the number of older nursing home residents with depression from Table 2-4 (590,000 residents) indicates that 1.8 million to 2.4 million older adults had this condition in 2010, with the caveat discussed earlier that some of the nursing home residents may have depressive symptoms rather than a DSM-IV-TR depressive disorder.

The figures in Table 2-5 represent only 13 of the 27 MH/SU conditions identified by the committee. Data presented earlier about three of the remaining conditions—depressive symptoms, anxiety symptoms, and at-risk drinking—suggest that several million older adults may have each condition. Adding older adults with these conditions to Table 2-5 would greatly increase the estimated totals. The ranges for the three conditions are wide. For example, the range for depressive symptoms is 430,000 to 4.3 million people. More importantly for estimating the proportion and number of older adults with MH/SU conditions, no information is available to account for comorbidity, and it is unclear is how many older adults who have one of the three conditions also have two or three of the conditions. Likewise, it is unclear how many older adults with one or more of the three conditions also have other conditions that are included in Table 2-5 and are, therefore, already included in the totals.

The figures for four other conditions—suicidal ideation, suicide plans and attempts, OCD, and at-risk drug use—are smaller. Nevertheless, adding older adults with each of these conditions to Table 2-5 would increase the estimated totals by about 2 million people. Again, however, no information is available to account for comorbidity.

Adding older adults with the remaining seven conditions for which sufficient population-based prevalence data were not found—adjustment disorders, personality disorders, hoarding, severe domestic squalor, severe self-neglect, fear of falling, and complicated grief—would probably increase the estimated totals. On the other hand, some, and perhaps many, older adults who have these conditions may also have one or more of the other conditions included in Table 2-5 and therefore, may already be included in the totals.

Gaps in the information needed to analyze MH/SU service needs and related workforce requirements exist across different categories of conditions and settings. In general, more prevalence and comorbidity information is available for DSM-IV-TR mental disorders than for other MH/SU conditions. Still, the available information about two DSM-IV-TR disorders, adjustment disorder and personality disorders, is not sufficient to allow for inclusion of these conditions in the committee's estimated totals. The available prevalence data for some DSM-IV-TR disorders are quite old, and as noted earlier, the committee believes the data for bipolar disorder in community-living older adults probably underestimate its true prevalence.

With the exception of nursing home residents, more prevalence and comorbidity information is available for older adults living in the community than in group quarters settings. The number of older adults in non–nursing home group quarters settings, such as adult correctional facilities and homeless shelters, is small in comparison with the numbers in the community and nursing homes. As a result, even if large proportions of older adults in these settings have MH/SU conditions, the numbers would probably be too small to change the committee's estimated totals. For purposes of analyzing service needs and workforce requirements, however, it is important to know how many older adults in non–nursing home group quarters settings have MH/SU conditions. The same is true for hoarding, severe domestic squalor, and severe self-neglect, where the number of people with the conditions is relatively small, but the implications of the conditions for workforce requirements in public health departments and aging and adult protective services agencies are significant.

Committee Estimates of the Proportion and Number of Older Adults with SMI in 2010

The estimated proportion and number of people with SMI depend on how SMI is defined. In general, the term is intended to identify very serious mental health conditions that create a high need for mental health services. Over the years, other terms have been used, such as *severe mental illness* and *severe and persistent mental illness*. Regardless of the specific term, however, people with the identified conditions generally have been accorded high priority for publicly funded mental health services (Goldman and Grob, 2006).

As noted earlier, schizophrenia and bipolar disorder are included in all definitions of SMI. Severe forms of other mental disorders, such as major depression, are sometimes also included, but substance use conditions are not included.

In 1993, people with *serious mental illness* were defined in federal regulations as people "age 18 and older, who currently or at any time in the past year, have had a diagnosable mental, behavioral, or emotional disorder of sufficient duration to meet diagnostic criteria specified within DSM-III-R, that has resulted in functional impairment that substantially interferes with or limits one or more major life activities" (SAMHSA, 1993). The regulations also stated that, "In the case of adults, this most seriously mentally ill population is largely composed of persons with schizophrenia and major mood disorders." Substance use conditions were explicitly excluded. Fiscal year 1993 federal appropriations legislation used a different term, *severe mental illness*, and specified "disorders with psychotic symptoms such as schizophrenia, schizoaffective disorder, manic depressive disorder, autism, as well as severe forms of other disorders such as major depression, panic disorder, and obsessive compulsive disorder" (Narrow et al., 2000).

In 2006, SAMHSA convened an expert panel to recommend ways to estimate the prevalence of SMI in people of all ages. Based on the panel's recommendations, SAMHSA developed a detailed methodology for use with data from the National Survey on Drug Use and Health (NSDUH), including follow-up telephone interviews conducted by a mental health clinician with a subsample of NSDUH respondents (CBHSQ, 2012b). Using that methodology, data from the 2010 NSDUH show that 1.4 percent of community-dwelling adults age 65 and older, about 535,000 people, had SMI (CBHSQ, 2012d).

The 535,000 figure does not include nursing home residents or older adults living in certain other group quarters settings, and the SAMHSA methodology has not been applied to these people. As shown earlier, about 76,000 nursing home residents had bipolar disorder and schizophrenia in 2009 (see Table 2-4). It is not clear whether all these individuals would be found to have SMI based on the SAMHSA methodology or how many additional nursing home residents and other older adults who are homeless or living in adult correctional facilities, psychiatric hospitals, or other residential treatment facilities would be found to have SMI based on the methodology. At a minimum, combining the 535,000 community-living older adults identified as having SMI based on the SAMHSA methodology and the 76,000 nursing home residents with bipolar disorder and schizophrenia indicates that at least 611,000 older adults (about 1.5 percent of the older population) had SMI in 2010.

Definitions of SMI have not been developed specifically for older adults. In fact, with some notable exceptions (see, e.g., Bartels, 2004, 2011), SMI research and analyses to date have focused almost entirely on people under age 65.

In considering how to define SMI for this report, the IOM committee wanted to identify older adults with very serious mental health conditions that create not only high need for mental health services, but also high priority for workforce training and competencies. While acknowledging the extensive conceptual work and research conducted to develop the SAMHSA methodology, the committee was uncertain about whether this methodology adequately identifies older adults with SMI. The committee considered whether SMI in older adults should ideally be defined more in terms of functional impairment and less in terms of particular mental health conditions, but a methodology for estimating the proportion and number of older adults with SMI defined in this way has not been developed.

To estimate the prevalence of SMI in older adults using information obtained for this report, the committee decided to focus on four mental health conditions: schizophrenia, schizoaffective disorder, bipolar disorder, and treatment-refractory major depression. No population-based data are available on the prevalence of treatment-refractory major depression, so data on major depressive episode are used as a substitute in developing the estimate. The committee's estimate is based on the following figures presented earlier in this chapter:

- the range of figures for major depressive episode in community-living older adults: 1.2 million to 1.7 million people (see Table 2-1);
- the figure for *nonaffective psychoses*, including schizophrenia, schizophreniform disorder, schizoaffective disorder, delusional disorder, and other psychosis in community-living older adults: 78,000 people (Kessler et al., 2005);
- the range of figures for bipolar disorder in community-living older adults: 39,000 to 78,000 people (see Table 2-2); and
- the number of nursing home residents with schizophrenia and bipolar disorder: 76,000 (see Table 2-4).

Combining the figures above indicates that 1.4 million to 1.9 million older adults, 3 to 4.8 percent of the older population, had SMI in 2010. Using a range of these figures and the SAMHSA figures noted earlier, the committee estimates that in 2010, 611,000 to 1.9 million older adults (1.5 to 4.8 percent of the older population) had SMI.

A study of MH/SU conditions in older adults in Massachusetts (Clark et al., 2009) provides state-level information about the prevalence of SMI, defined in the study as schizophrenia and paranoid disorders, bipolar disorder, and major depression (see Table 2-6). The study sample includes all older Medicare and Medicaid beneficiaries in the state as of January 1, 2005, with the exception of Medicare managed care enrollees. People with MH/SU conditions were identified by the presence of a code for the condition as either a primary or secondary diagnosis on at least one Medicare or Medicaid claim during the year. Medicare managed care enrollees were excluded because Medicare claims are not submitted for them. People were counted as living in long-term care (LTC) if they were in a nursing home or hospital for a combined total of 120 days or longer during 2005.

As shown in Table 2-6, 5.4 percent of older Medicare and Medicaid beneficiaries had SMI in 2005, including 1.1 percent who had schizophrenia and paranoid disorders, 1.1 percent who had bipolar disorder, and 3.2 percent who had major depression. Among those with SMI, the data indicate that

TABLE 2-6
Number and Proportion of Massachusetts Medicare and Medicaid Beneficiaries Age 65 and Older with Serious Mental Illness, Other Mental Illness, and No Mental Illness by Age, Gender, Place of Residence, Insurance, and Coexisting Dementia, 2005, N = 679,182[a]

Characteristics	Mental Health Status					
	Serious Mental Illness (SMI)	Serious Mental Illness (SMI) Conditions			Other Mental Illness	No Mental Illness
		Schizophrenia and Paranoid Disorders	Bipolar Disorder	Major Depression		
Number	36,686	7,174	7,780	21,732	90,462	552,034
	5.4%	1.1%	1.1%	3.2%	13%	81%
Age						
65-74	15,161	2,971	3,406	8,784	32,484	275,003
	41%	41%	44%	40%	36%	50%
75-84	14,126	2,649	3,039	8,438	36,232	200,792
	39%	37%	39%	39%	40%	36%
85+	7,399	1,554	1,335	4,510	21,746	76,239
	20%	22%	17%	21%	24%	14%
Gender						
Male	11,074	2,166	2,514	6,394	27,754	235,812
	30%	30%	32%	29%	31%	43%

Female	25,612	5,008	5,266	15,338	62,708	316,222
	70%	70%	68%	71%	69%	57%
Residence						
Community	32,492	5,798	6,962	19,372	85,913	550,068
	89%	81%	89%	91%	95%	99.6%
Long-term care	4,194	1,376	818	2,000	4,549	1,966
	11%	19%	11%	9%	5%	0.4%
Insurance						
Medicare only	20,532	2,373	4,721	13,946	64,683	467,011
	56%	33%	61%	64%	72%	85%
Medicaid only	508	*b*	*b*	*b*	738	18,008
	1%	*b*	*b*	*b*	0.8%	3%
Dual eligible	15,646	4,801	3,059	7,786	25,041	67,015
	43%	67%	39%	36%	28%	12%
Dementia	16,632	4,421	3,611	8,600	30,362	37,309
	45%	62%	46%	40%	34%	7%

[a] Some data taken from R. E. Clark, University of Massachusetts Medical School, unpublished data provided to the IOM committee, November 2011.
[b] Numbers were not reported because of small cell size (<11) in some disease groups for Medicaid-only sample members.
SOURCES: Clark et al., 2009; Lin et al., 2011.

- 89 percent lived in the community, including 81 percent of those with schizophrenia and paranoid disorders, 89 percent of those with bipolar disorder; and 91 percent of those with major depression;
- 70 percent were women, including 70 percent of those with schizophrenia and paranoid disorders, 68 percent of those with bipolar disorder, and 71 percent of those with major depression;
- 43 percent were dually eligible for Medicare and Medicaid, including 67 percent of those with schizophrenia and paranoid disorders; 39 percent of those with bipolar disorder; and 36 percent of those with major depression; and
- 45 percent had coexisting dementia, including 62 percent of those with schizophrenia and paranoid disorders; 46 percent of those with bipolar disorder; and 36 percent of those with major depression.

There are several caveats with respect to the data from the Massachusetts study. The data represent only one state, and comparable data from other states would undoubtedly differ. In addition, the accuracy of diagnoses based on Medicare and Medicaid claims is uncertain, and the exclusion of Medicare managed care enrollees means that 18 percent of older Medicare beneficiaries in the state are not represented (Lin et al., 2011). Acknowledging these caveats, the data provide state-level information about the proportion, number, and characteristics of this high-priority population that is useful for analyzing their service needs and related workforce requirements. Especially notable are the high proportions of older adults with SMI that were dual eligibles, had coexisting dementia, and were living in the community as opposed to long-term care settings.

PREVALENCE OF MH/SU CONDITIONS IN SIX SUBGROUPS OF THE OLDER POPULATION

The prevalence rates and estimated numbers of older adults with MH/SU conditions discussed in the previous section pertain to the older population as a whole. This section focuses on differences in prevalence rates for six subgroups within that population:

1. Adults ages 65-74, 75-84, and 85 and older
2. Older women and men
3. Racial and ethnic groups
4. Residents of assisted living, senior housing, and public housing facilities
5. Older adults who are dually eligible for Medicare and Medicaid
6. Older veterans

As discussed in the section, differences in prevalence rates and estimated numbers of people with MH/SU conditions in the older population as a whole versus in these subgroups have important implications for service needs and workforce requirements.

Adults Ages 65-74, 75-84, and 85 and Older

Among the 40.3 million adults age 65 and older in 2010, more than half (54 percent) were age 65-74, about 21.7 million people (Census Bureau, 2011b). The 13.1 million adults age 75-84 constituted 32 percent of the older population, and the 5.5 million adults age 85 and older, often referred to as the *oldest-old*, constituted the remaining 14 percent.

National data on prevalence rates and numbers of older adults with MH/SU conditions in the age subgroups 65-74, 75-84, and 85 and older are not easily accessible. Published reports of findings from population-based surveys of MH/SU conditions rarely include information about age subgroups within the older population. Published reports from some of the surveys provide information about "older people" defined as adults age 50 and older or 55 and older, rather than adults age 65 and older. The limited amount of information about age subgroups within the older population in published reports from these surveys is often attributed to small sample sizes, suggesting the need for larger samples. At the same time, since the data exist, at least for the age groups 65 and older, 65-74, and 75 and older, the limited amount of published information probably also reflects decisions about the relative importance of including information about people in older versus younger age groups in published reports of survey findings.

Some survey-based information about the prevalence of MH/SU conditions for adults ages 65 and older, 65-74, and 75 and older can be accessed online, and additional information can be obtained through special analyses conducted by the agency that funded the survey or other researchers who have access to the raw data. Prevalence rates for adults age 65-74 and 75 and older for the MH/SU conditions that were measured in the population-based surveys of MH/SU conditions described in Box 2-2 were provided to the IOM committee by the Center for Multicultural Mental Health Research and SAMHSA. Sample sizes were too small to generate reliable rates for adults age 85 and older.

For the 10 MH/SU conditions measured in each of three surveys (the CPES, NESARC 1, and NESARC 2), prevalence rates were generally higher for the age group 65-74 than the age group 75 and older, although some differences are very small (Center for Multicultural Mental Health Research, 2011). The midpoint of the rates for having one or more of the 10 conditions is 9.5 percent for adults age 65-74 and 6.9 percent for adults age

75 and older. The differences in rates for particular MH/SU conditions are generally smaller, but show the same pattern of higher rates in younger versus older age groups within the older population.

Prevalence rates for substance use conditions measured in the NSDUH and calculated for the age groups 65-69, 70-74, and 75 and older also show this pattern. The 2010 rate for alcohol dependence or abuse in the past year was 2.8 percent for adults age 65-69, 1.8 percent for those age 70-74, and 1.4 percent for those age 75 and older.[2] Likewise, the 2010 rate for binge drinking in the past month was 11 percent for adults age 65-69, 8.6 percent for those age 70-74, and 4 percent for those age 75 and older. The 2009 National Health Interview Survey (NHIS) also found higher rates of binge drinking for adults age 65-74 than for those age 75 and older (NCHS, 2011b).

For drug dependence or abuse in the past year, prevalence rates from the 2010 NSDUH are higher for adults age 65-69 (0.2 percent), decreasing to rates too low to be reported for adults age 70-74 and 75 and older.[2] The 2010 rate for nonmedical use of prescription drugs was 1.3 percent for adults age 65-69, compared to 0.7 percent for adults age 70-74 and 75 and older. Similarly, the 2010 rate for nonmedical use of prescription pain relievers was 0.5 percent for adults age 65-69 compared to 0.4 percent for adults age 70-74 and 75 and older. The few exceptions to the pattern of higher rates in the age group 65-74 than in the age group 75 and older all come from one of the surveys, the CPES (see Box 2-2). CPES data show slightly lower proportions of adults age 65-74 than adults age 75 and older for three conditions: panic disorder, suicidal ideation, and depressive symptoms.

Very little information is available about prevalence rates for MH/SU conditions in the oldest old, with one important exception. For at least the past 60 years, reported suicide rates have been higher for white men age 85 and older than for any other group. Suicide rates for white men age 75-84 have been second highest in the same period (NCHS, 2011a). Rates are lower for older men in other racial and ethnic groups and for women in all age groups.

Prevalence rates for behavioral and psychiatric symptoms associated with dementia are probably higher for the oldest old than for adults ages 65-74 and 75-84. This is because dementia is much more common in adults age 85 and older than in the younger age subgroups (Brookmeyer et al., 1998; Hebert et al., 2003). It is not clear whether adults age 85 and older with dementia are more likely than adults ages 65-74 or 75-84 with dementia to have behavioral and psychiatric symptoms.

[2]Center for Behavioral Health Statistics and Quality, unpublished data from the 2010 National Survey on Drug Use and Health provided to the IOM committee, 2011.

Psychotic symptoms, including hallucinations, delusions, and paranoid ideation, have been found to occur in 7 to 10 percent of adults age 85 and older in population-based Swedish samples (Ostling and Skoog, 2002; Ostling et al., 2007). Similar data are not available from population-based samples in the United States.

Calculations by the committee based on data from the Massachusetts study discussed earlier (Clark et al., 2009) indicate that 7 percent of Medicare and Medicaid beneficiaries age 85 and older had SMI. Another 20.6 percent of those age 85 and older had other mental health conditions, including other depression, anxiety, and other mental illness. Interestingly, the rate for SMI in the oldest old is higher than in those ages 65-74 and 75-84 in the Massachusetts sample (7 percent for those age 85 and older versus 4.7 percent for those age 65-74 and 5.6 percent for those age 75-84). Likewise, the rate for schizophrenia is higher in the oldest old than in the younger age subgroups (1.5 percent of those age 85 and older versus 0.9 percent of those age 65-74 and 1.1 percent of those age 75-84). This pattern of higher rates for the oldest old in comparison with those age 65-74 and 75-84 holds true for each mental health condition measured in the Massachusetts study. It is not clear whether the pattern would also be seen in national, population-based samples if the samples were large enough to support accurate findings for the oldest old.

As discussed later in this chapter, the number of adults age 85 and older is expected to increase from 5.5 million in 2010 to 8.7 million in 2030 (Census Bureau, 2011b). Information about the prevalence of MH/SU conditions in the oldest old is needed to plan for adequate services and workforce competencies to care for this population that also has very high rates of coexisting physical health conditions and cognitive and functional impairments.

Older Women and Men

On average, women live longer than men and, therefore, constitute a larger proportion of the older population. Among the 40.3 million adults age 65 and older in 2010, 22.9 million (57 percent) were women and 17.4 million (43 percent) were men (Census Bureau, 2011a). The difference is greater in older age subgroups. Among the 5.5 million adults age 85 and older in 2010, 3.7 million (67 percent) were women, and 1.8 million (33 percent) were men.

Because of the larger number of women in the older population, one would expect to find larger numbers of older women than older men with mental health conditions, even if the proportion of older women and men with each condition were the same. For most conditions, however, the proportion of older women with the conditions is higher. This is true for 8 of the 10 conditions measured in three population-based surveys of MH/SU conditions described in Box 2-2 (CPES, NESARC 1, and NESARC 2). For example, the midpoint of the prevalence rates from the three surveys for depressive disorders is 4.8 percent for older women and 2.6 percent for older men (Center for Multicultural Mental Health Research, 2011). Likewise, the midpoint of the rates for having one or more of the 10 conditions is 9.8 percent for older women and 6.4 percent for older men.

The two conditions for which these surveys found lower rates for older women than older men are alcohol dependence or abuse, where the midpoint of rates is 0.3 percent for older women and 1.9 percent for older men, and drug dependence or abuse, where the midpoint of the rates is 0.05 percent for older women and 0.11 percent for older men (Center for Multicultural Mental Health Research, 2011). The 2010 National Survey of Drug Use and Health also found lower rates for alcohol dependence or abuse, drug dependence or abuse, or both conditions for older women than men (1.3 percent for older women versus 3.1 percent for older men).[3] Similar patterns have been found in studies of some other MH/SU conditions. Older women are more likely than older men to have depressive and anxiety symptoms that do not meet the criteria for a DSM-IV-TR diagnosis of a depressive or anxiety disorder (Grenier et al., 2011; Judd et al., 1996; Lyness et al., 2009). In contrast, older women are less likely than older men to have at-risk drinking. The 2005 and 2006 NSDUH surveys show, for example, that 3 percent of women age 65 and older reported binge drinking, compared with 15 percent of men in that age group (Blazer and Wu, 2009a).

Only about half of all older adults drink alcohol. In 2010, 47 percent of women age 65 and older and 55 percent of men in that age group reported having any alcoholic drinks in the previous year.[3] Women are more susceptible than men to the physical effects of alcohol throughout their lives, but age-related physiological changes can increase the susceptibility of all older adults to alcohol-related problems (Blow and Barry, 2002; Epstein et al., 2007).

In 2010, 1.4 percent of older women and 2.2 percent of older men reported past-year use of illicit drugs, including marijuana, cocaine, heroin, and prescription psychotherapeutic medications, such as pain relievers and antianxiety medications that are used for nonmedical purposes.[3] Many older adults take prescription psychotherapeutic medications. From 2005 to 2008, 18 percent of older women and men reported taking prescription pain relievers in the past month, and 12 percent of older women and 7 percent of older men reported taking prescription sedatives,

[3]Center for Behavioral Health Statistics and Quality, unpublished data from the 2010 National Survey on Drug Use and Health provided to the IOM committee, 2011.

hypnotics, and antianxiety medications (NCHS, 2011c). These medications are needed and effective for many older adults, but they have high potential for negative side effects, including addiction, overdoses, and impaired physical and cognitive functioning, the likelihood of which is increased by age-related physiological changes (Blow, 1998; Simoni-Wastila, 2000; Simoni-Wastila and Yang, 2006).

Wide exposure to prescription pain relievers, antianxiety medications, and other prescription psychotherapeutic medications creates high risk for misuse, which can range from infrequent, intentional or unintentional use of a higher dose than prescribed to repeated use of high doses, sometimes combined with alcohol and over-the-counter sleeping medications that exacerbate their effects (Blow and Barry, 2002; Epstein et al., 2007; Gleason et al., 1998; Simoni-Wastila and Yang, 2006). Older women are particularly at risk for misuse of antianxiety medications, usually benzodiazepines. Long-term use of these medications is not recommended, especially for older adults (Blow, 1998). Yet longitudinal studies have found that older women were not only more likely than older men to be taking the medications at the beginning of the study, but also more likely to be taking them 1 to 10 years later (Blazer et al., 2000b; Gray et al., 2003). Greater awareness of the risks associated with misuse of these prescription medications is important for older adults, especially older women, and for the physicians and other health care professionals who prescribe the medications. Other health care, residential care, and home- and community-based service providers should also be aware that many older adults use these medications and observant for possible misuse and its negative side effects.

Racial and Ethnic Groups

In 2010, 80 percent of the population age 65 and older was non-Hispanic white; 8 percent was African American; 7 percent was Hispanic/Latino; 3 percent was Asian; and 1 percent was American Indian, Native Alaskan, Native Hawaiian, or Pacific Islander. The remainder was two or more races or ethnicities (Census Bureau, 2011c).

Prevalence rates for MH/SU conditions differ for older adults in various racial and ethnic groups. Table 2-7 shows these differences for community-living adults age 65 and older in four groups, with the Asian and American Indian, Native Alaskan, Native Hawaiian, and Pacific Islander groups combined because of small numbers. The data come from three of the national, population-based surveys of MH/SU conditions described in Box 2-2 (CPES, NESARC 1, and NESARC 2). All the conditions are DSM-IV-TR mental disorders. The figures show the midpoint of

TABLE 2-7
12-Month Prevalence of Selected Mental Disorders in Community-Living Adults Age 65 and Older in the United States in Four Racial and Ethnic Groups

Mental Disorder	Racial or Ethnic Group			
	White (%)	African American (%)	Hispanic/ Latino (%)	Asian/ Native Hawaiian/ Pacific Islander (%)
Mental health disorders				
Depressive disorders	3.8	3.6	6.9	4.0
Major depressive episode	3.5	3.4	6.1	3.5
Dysthymic disorder	1.0	0.7	2.0	0.7
Panic disorder	0.9	0.7	1.8	1.8
Agoraphobia without panic	0.1	0.2	0.3	0.1
Social phobia	1.7	1.7	1.1	1.5
Generalized anxiety disorder	1.5	1.7	1.7	2.5
Posttraumatic stress disorder (PTSD)[a]	1.5	2.3	3.2	1.3
Substance use disorders				
Alcohol dependence or abuse	1.1	1.1	1.2	0.0
Other drug dependence or abuse	0.1	0.1	0.1	0.0

TABLE 2-7 Continued

Mental Disorder	Racial or Ethnic Group			
	White (%)	African American (%)	Hispanic/ Latino (%)	Asian/ Native Hawaiian/ Pacific Islander (%)
Summary figures				
One or more of the disorders	8.0	8.7	11.7	9.0
Two or more of the disorders	2.2	2.1	3.1	1.6
Three or more of the disorders	0.6	0.7	1.2	0.6

[a] The NESARC 1 survey did not measure PTSD; thus, the PTSD figures represent the midpoint of the prevalence rates from only two surveys, the CPES and NESARC 2.
SOURCE: Center for Multicultural Mental Health Research, 2011.

the range of prevalence rates from the three surveys for each disorder and for one or more, two or more, and three or more disorders.

The figures in Table 2-7 suggest that prevalence rates for some disorders and for one or more, two or more, and three or more disorders may be higher for Hispanic/Latinos than for the other three groups. Differences in the midpoints of rates among the groups have not been tested for statistical significance, however.

Until about 10 years ago, little information was available from national, population-based surveys about the prevalence of MH/SU conditions in racial and ethnic groups in the older population. Starting in 2001, several national surveys included large enough numbers of people in various groups to allow for meaningful prevalence estimates. In addition, NESARC conducted interviews in English and Spanish, and the National Latino and Asian American Study conducted interviews in English, Spanish, Tagalog, Vietnamese, and Mandarin, thus allowing people with limited English proficiency to be interviewed in their primary language (Alegria et al., 2007).

Findings from these national, population-based surveys provide valuable information about differences among racial and ethnic groups in prevalence rates for MH/SU conditions. Yet, aggregation of findings for the four major groups shown in Table 2-7 obscures important differences in rates within each of the groups. Some of these differences pertain to subgroups defined specifically by race or ethnicity, for example, Puerto Rican and Mexican American subgroups within the Hispanic/Latino group. Other differences pertain to an array of factors that have been found to be related to the prevalence of MH/SU conditions in older adults in various racial and ethnic groups. These factors include whether the person was born in the United States or elsewhere, and, if born elsewhere, how old the person was at the time of immigration; how long the person has been in the United States; the person's gender, education, and income; perceived financial strain; life events; and region of the country. The following examples come from studies selected to illustrate the interrelationships among these factors and prevalence rates:

- Among older Asian Americans living in the United States, the prevalence of major depression was much higher for Chinese Americans age 65-74 than for Filipino and Vietnamese Americans in that age group. In contrast, prevalence was lower for Chinese Americans age 75 and older than for adults in that age group in the other two Asian subgroups. Likewise, within the Hispanic/Latino group, prevalence of major depression was higher for Cuban Americans and Puerto Ricans age 65-74 than for Mexican Americans in that age group, and much higher for Puerto Ricans age 75 and older than for adults age 75 and older in the other two Hispanic/Latino subgroups (Gonzalez et al., 2010).
- Among older blacks living in the United States, the prevalence of major depressive disorder was much higher for older blacks of Caribbean descent than for African Americans (11 percent versus 3 percent, respectively) (Aranda et al., 2011).
- Among older Asian Americans living in the United States, prevalence of MH/SU conditions was higher for those born in the United States than for those born outside the country. For Asian Americans born outside the United States, prevalence was higher for those who arrived in the country as children than for those who arrived as adolescents or adults (Breslau and Chang, 2006).
- Among older Mexican Americans living in the United States, prevalence of depressive symptoms was higher for those born outside the United States than for those born in the United States, and highest for those who arrived in this country less than 6 years before the survey (Black et al., 1998). Within these three categories (born in the United States, arrived in the United States less

than 6 years before the survey, and arrived in the United States 6 or more years before the survey), prevalence differed for women and men. Among older Mexican Americans who were born in the United States, prevalence of depressive symptoms was 28 percent for women and 17 percent for men. Among those who arrived in the United States 6 or more years before the survey, prevalence was also higher for women than men (35 percent versus 15 percent, respectively). Among those who arrived more recently (less than 6 years before the survey), prevalence was very high for both women and men (57 percent for older Mexican American women and 58 percent for older Mexican American men). Low levels of education, low income, financial stress, recent death of a spouse, and health problems were also associated with higher prevalence of depressive symptoms (Chiriboga et al., 2002).

- Among African Americans age 55 and older, prevalence of any of 13 MH/SU conditions was lower for those living in the south than for those living in other parts of the country (Ford et al., 2007). Prevalence of major depressive disorder was 2.6 percent for those living in the south, compared with 6 percent for those living outside the south (Aranda et al., 2011). The researchers hypothesize that these findings may be due to protective effects of greater religious involvement and the larger family networks of older blacks living in the south.

For policy makers, administrators, and others who have to plan services to meet the needs of older adults with MH/SU conditions, the complex interrelationships among race, ethnicity, and the associated factors illustrated above mean that aggregated information about the prevalence of these conditions in the four or five major racial and ethnic groups is not sufficient. Information about differences within these groups is also required. For the workforce, the need for diversity training and competency as well as access to staff with proficiency in numerous languages is also clear. These implications are relevant now and will affect the availability of appropriate MH/SU services for increasing numbers of older adults as racial and ethnic group populations grow in coming years.

Residents of Assisted Living, Senior Housing, and Public Housing Facilities

Many older adults live in assisted living, senior housing, and public housing facilities. The first National Survey of Residential Care Facilities found that in 2010, there were about 31,100 assisted living and other residential care facilities in the United States (Park-Lee et al., 2011). On any given day in 2010, an average of 730,000 people were living in these facilities, 89 percent of whom (about 650,000 people) were age 65 and older (Caffrey et al., 2012). The facilities included in the survey were licensed or otherwise regulated at the state level and had to provide room and board, at least two meals per day, around-the-clock supervision, and assistance with personal care, such as bathing and dressing, or health-related services, such as medication management. Among the 31,100 facilities, 65 percent had 4 to 25 beds and provided care for about one-fifth of all residents. The remaining 35 percent were larger, with 26 to more than 100 beds, and provided care for four-fifths of all residents.

About 300,000 adults age 65 and older were living in federal government–supported public housing facilities in the period from November 2010 to February 2012 (HUD, 2012), and some of those facilities are designated specifically as senior housing. Older adults also live in public housing facilities run by local housing authorities with federal, state, and local government funding, and some of these facilities are designated specifically as senior housing. Public housing and senior housing facilities vary greatly in the extent to which they provide services that could help older adults with MH/SU conditions, but various public and private organizations have ongoing projects to increase services for older adults in such facilities.

Assisted living, senior housing, and public housing facilities are sometimes referred to as *congregate-living facilities* because their residents live in close proximity. In the context of this report, it is important to note that practical and effective approaches for the detection, diagnosis, treatment, and ongoing management of MH/SU conditions in older adults probably differ in congregate-living facilities versus single-family housing.

Recently published national data show that in 2010, 28 percent of all residents in assisted living and residential care facilities had been told by a physician that they had depression, and 42 percent had been told they had dementia (Caffrey et al., 2012). No other national data are available about the proportion or number of residents of assisted living, senior housing, and public housing facilities who have MH/SU conditions, but findings from three studies suggest that many do. One study of 198 residents age 58-104 in 22 randomly selected assisted living facilities in central Maryland used an expert panel to identify those with mental disorders based on resident records and in-person interviews (Rosenblatt et al., 2004). The study found that 26 percent of the residents had one or more mental disorders, including 19 percent with mood disorders, 13 percent with anxiety disorders, and 12 percent with psychotic disorders. In addition, 68 percent of the residents had dementia, and 14 percent had both dementia and a mental disorder. Among those with dementia, 83 percent had exhibited behavioral and psychiatric symptoms in the previous month.

A second study of 2,078 residents age 65 and older in 193 assisted living and other residential care facilities in four states used various sources of information to identify residents with mental health conditions (Gruber-Baldini et al., 2004):

- 28 percent were found to have any mental or psychiatric illness, based on resident records or the report of an informant, usually a family member.
- 14 percent were found to have depression based on their score on a widely used depression assessment instrument.
- 13 percent were found to have psychosis based on staff report of the presence of hallucinations or delusions in the previous 7 days.
- About half of the 2,078 residents had dementia, and 49 percent of them were found to have one or more of four kinds of behavioral symptoms in the previous week: (1) physically aggressive symptoms, such as hitting, kicking, biting, throwing things, or self-abuse; (2) physically nonaggressive symptoms, such as pacing, restlessness, and inappropriate dressing or undressing; (3) verbal symptoms, such as screaming, constant requests for help, and repeated calling out; and (4) resistance to care, including resistance to taking medications and resistance to help with bathing, dressing, and other activities of daily living. As shown in Table 2-8, large proportions of residents with any mental or psychiatric illness, depression, or psychosis also had one or more of these behavioral symptoms in the previous week.

These data on residents with depression and psychosis who also had behavioral symptoms are surprising because the proportions are higher than the comparable proportions for residents with dementia. The proportions of residents with any mental or psychiatric illness who also had behavioral symptoms are only slightly below the comparable proportions for residents with dementia.

A third study of 945 residents age 60 and older in six public housing facilities designated specifically for seniors used in-person screening tests and structured interviews to identify residents with mental disorders (Rabins et al., 1996):

- 8 percent were found to have mood disorders, including 5.6 percent with major depression, 1.7 percent with dysthymia, and 0.4 percent with bipolar disorder;
- 4.6 percent were found to have psychotic disorders, including 2.1 percent with schizophrenia;

TABLE 2-8
Proportion of Assisted Living and Residential Care Residents with Behavioral Symptoms in the Previous Week, by Mental Health Conditions and Dementia

	Behavioral Symptoms				
Condition	One or More Behavioral Symptoms (%)	Physically Aggressive Symptoms (%)	Physically Nonaggressive Symptoms (%)	Verbal Symptoms (%)	Resistance to Care (%)
Any mental or psychiatric illness	40	17	28	29	15
Depression	77	38	50	61	32
Psychosis	69	30	50	52	31
Dementia	49	19	34	31	17

SOURCE: Gruber-Baldini et al., 2004.

- 2 percent were found to have anxiety disorders, including 0.4 percent with panic disorder and 0.8 percent with generalized anxiety disorder; and
- 4.4 percent were found to have substance use disorders, including 4 percent with alcohol dependence or abuse and 0.5 percent with drug dependence or abuse.

The findings from these three studies are not precisely comparable because they focused on different MH/SU conditions and used different methods to identify residents with the conditions. Likewise, findings from the three studies are not precisely comparable with findings discussed earlier in this chapter on MH/SU conditions in community-living older adults and nursing home residents. On the other hand, some differences in the prevalence of MH/SU conditions among older adults in these settings are obvious. With respect to major depression, which was measured in public housing, assisted living and nursing home residents and community-living people, the proportion of older adults with the condition is lowest in those living in the community; it is progressively higher in public housing residents and assisted living residents, and highest in nursing home residents. For alcohol dependence or abuse, which was measured in public housing– and community-living older adults, the proportion of public housing residents with the condition was higher. Similarly, for psychosis, which was measured in public housing and assisted living residents, the proportion of assisted living residents with the condition was higher.

Two other studies that included both assisted living and nursing home residents found little, if any, difference in the proportion of residents who had behavioral and psychiatric symptoms associated with dementia. One study of 347 adults age 65 and older with dementia in 10 nursing homes and 45 assisted living facilities found that 66 percent of the nursing home residents and 56 percent of the assisted living residents had behavioral symptoms (Boustani et al., 2005). Another study of 1,252 adults age 65 and older with dementia in 40 nursing homes and 166 assisted living facilities found no difference in the proportions that also had behavioral symptoms (Sloane et al., 2005).

Many factors other than an older person's MH/SU conditions affect whether the person will be living in the community, a public housing, senior housing, assisted living facility, or a nursing home. In addition to the person's and family's preferences and whether the person has coexisting physical health conditions, cognitive and functional impairments, and a caregiver at home, these factors include federal, state, and local government policies that affect the number of available beds in various types of congregate-living facilities. Such policies determine, for example, which types of facilities can admit older adults with MH/SU conditions and whether Medicaid or other public funding is available to people with these conditions in the facilities that can admit them. Some states do not allow assisted living facilities to admit people with mental health conditions, and some require a special license or limit the number of people with these conditions that can be admitted (Becker et al., 2002; Polzer, 2011). All states provide Medicaid funding for nursing home care for people who meet the state's financial and functional eligibility criteria, but some states also provide subsidies for low-income assisted living residents (Polzer, 2011). States vary greatly in the amount and types of home- and community-based services they provide (Ng et al., 2010; Reinhard et al., 2011). Differences in state policies suggest that the proportions of older adults with MH/SU conditions in these settings probably differ across states, and available data indicate that is the case (Grabowski et al., 2009; Zimmerman et al., 2011).

Policies and practices of the nursing home and residential care industries also affect whether older adults with MH/SU conditions will be living in the community, public housing, senior housing, an assisted living facility, or a nursing home. As noted earlier, nursing homes are increasingly admitting people who need short-term, postacute care as opposed to long-term personal care and supervision, and the proportion of residents with dementia among all new admissions has decreased (Fullerton et al., 2009). At the same time, the number of beds in assisted living facilities has increased. As the relevant federal, state, and local government policies and industry policies and practices change over time, the proportions of older adults with MH/SU conditions in various settings are also likely to change.

For purposes of planning for services to meet the needs of older adults with MH/SU conditions and structuring a workforce capable of providing those services, the preceding discussion has three important implications. First, it is clear that substantial numbers of older adults with these conditions live in assisted living, public housing, and senior housing facilities. Two of the studies described earlier show that 26 to 28 percent of older assisted living residents had mental health conditions. These figures do not include residents with dementia and associated behavioral symptoms who probably constitute an additional 20 to 25 percent of older residents. The numbers are smaller, but still significant in senior housing and public housing facilities. Planning for services for older adults with MH/SU conditions should include these people explicitly.

Second, as noted earlier, practical and effective approaches for delivering MH/SU services probably differ for people in congregate-living facilities versus people living in single-family housing in the community. In this context, it should be noted that nursing homes are also congregate-living facilities. The needed skills and competencies for staff working with older adults with MH/SU conditions in nursing homes are probably similar in many ways to the needed skills and competencies for staff working with older adults with these conditions in other congregate-living facilities. The combined number of older adults with MH/SU conditions in these settings suggests that the development of workforce skills and competencies that are practical and effective for congregate-living settings is a high priority.

Finally, it is clear that better information is needed about the proportion and number of older adults with MH/SU conditions who live in assisted living, public housing, and senior housing facilities. Research and analyses conducted to date to categorize and identify assisted living and other residential care facilities for the 2010 National Survey of Residential Care Facilities should allow for the identification of these facilities as a distinct type of congregate-living setting in future surveys of MH/SU conditions. Similar research and analyses are needed to allow for the identification of public housing and senior housing facilities as distinct types of congregate-living settings. Because planning for services and related workforce requirements often occurs at the state level, information about the number and proportions of older adults with MH/SU conditions in all types of congregate-living facilities should be available both nationally and by state.

Older Adults Who Are Dually Eligible for Medicare and Medicaid

In 2008, about 6 million adults age 65 and older were dually eligible for Medicare and Medicaid (Clemans-Cope and Waidmann, 2011). National figures on the proportion of dual eligibles who have mental health conditions vary, depending on the source of the data. The most recent available data come from the 2007 Medicare Current Beneficiary Survey, a large-scale survey of a nationally representative sample of Medicare beneficiaries. These 2007 data show that 19.6 percent of dual eligibles age 65 and older had self- or proxy-reported mental illness.[4] An analysis of 2003 data from the same source shows that 20.2 percent of dual eligibles age 65 and older had mental illness (Coughlin et al., 2009), Other analyses show that in the years 2004 through 2006, 26 percent of dual eligibles age 65 and older had one or more mental disorders (MedPAC, 2010) and in 2003, 20 percent of dual eligibles age 65 and older had depression; 2.3 percent had schizophrenia; and 19 percent had other affective and serious mental disorders (Kasper et al., 2010). Finally, an analysis of Medicare, Medicaid, and pharmacy data found that in 2002, 36 percent of dual

[4]T. Coughlin, Urban Institute, personal communication, April 30, 2012.

eligibles age 65 and older had mental disorders, including depressive disorders, bipolar disorder, anxiety disorders, and schizophrenia (Kronick et al., 2009).

Calculations by the committee based on data from the Massachusetts study described earlier in this chapter (Clark et al., 2009) show that in 2005, 38 percent of dual eligibles age 65 and older had SMI or other mental health conditions. Conversely, among older adults with SMI or other mental health conditions, 32 percent were dual eligibles.

Older Veterans

In 2010, there were about 22 million veterans age 18 and older, including about 9 million who were age 65 and older (Census Bureau, 2010c). Not all veterans enroll in the VA health care system, and not all of those who enroll use VA health care services. This section focuses on veterans age 65 and older who enroll in the VA health care system and use VA health care services. The committee's estimates, presented earlier, of the proportion and number of older adults who have MH/SU conditions include all older veterans, but older veterans who use VA health care services are a special population because they are more likely than other older adults to have MH/SU conditions and more likely to have particular conditions that affect their service needs and the workforce competencies required to meet those needs.

In FY 2011, 4 million veterans age 65 and older were enrolled in the VA health care system, and 2.4 million of those veterans used VA health care services. Table 2-9 shows the prevalence rates and number of older veterans who used VA health care services in FY 2011 and had a diagnosis of an MH/SU condition, one or more conditions, only one condition, two or more conditions, and three or more conditions. The figures include veterans who were living in VA nursing homes and VA domiciliary care facilities, but they do not include veterans who were living in non-VA nursing homes and other facilities, even if the VA was paying for their care in the facility.

As shown in the table, 16 percent of older veterans who used VA health care services had a diagnosis of one or more of the MH/SU conditions. About 11 percent had one diagnosed condition; 4.9 percent had two or more diagnosed conditions, and 1.5 percent had three or more diagnosed conditions. These proportions represent older veterans who have had a diagnostic evaluation and received a clinical diagnosis of one or more MH/SU conditions. In this respect, the figures differ from some of the rates and numbers shown earlier in this chapter that are based on research interviews conducted in population-based surveys and include people who have diagnosed and undiagnosed MH/SU conditions. Veter-

TABLE 2-9
Prevalence Rates and Number of Veterans Age 65 and Older Who Used VA Inpatient or Outpatient Health Care Services in FY 2011 and Had Diagnoses of Selected MH/SU Conditions

Mental Health and Substance Use Diagnoses	Prevalence Rate (%)	Number of Older Veterans
Mental health diagnoses		
Major depressive disorder	2.3	52,822
Dysthymia	1.3	31,104
Other mood spectrum disorders	8.1	189,536
Panic disorder	0.3	7,863
Agoraphobia without panic	[a]	[b]
Social phobia	[a]	[b]
Generalized anxiety disorder	1.0	22,267
Posttraumatic stress disorder	4.3	101,181
Schizophrenia	0.7	16,447
Bipolar disorder	0.8	17,650
Other psychoses	0.8	18,674
Substance use diagnoses		
Alcohol dependence or abuse	2.6	59,801
Drug dependence or abuse	0.6	14,458
Summary figures		
One or more of the diagnoses	16.0	372,721
One of the diagnoses	11.1	258,474
Two or more of the diagnoses	4.9	114,247
Three or more of the diagnoses	1.5	33,755

[a] Proportion is less than 0.1 percent.
[b] Number is less than 500.
SOURCE: Department of Veterans Affairs, FY 2011 data provided to the IOM committee, March 22, 2012.

ans who receive diagnoses of MH/SU conditions are usually those who come to VA health care providers with more severe symptoms, including veterans who are seeking treatment because of these symptoms.

The rates and numbers in Table 2-9 provide valuable insights about the prevalence of particular MH/SU conditions in this important population. The conditions with the highest prevalence are other mood disorders and PTSD. *Other mood disorders* are defined as mood or depressive disorders that do not meet the criteria for a DSM-IV-TR diagnosis of major depressive disorder or dysthymia. They include diagnoses of minor depression, affective personality disorder, and depressive disorders that are either superimposed on another mental disorder that is the person's primary diagnosis or cannot be disaggregated from an underlying physical health or substance use condition.

Behavioral and psychiatric symptoms associated with dementia are not included in Table 2-9. VA projections indicate that about 307,000 veterans age 65 and older with dementia would be enrolled in the VA health care system in 2009, and 185,000 of these veterans would use VA health care services (Cooley and Asthana, 2010). No projection is given for the proportion or number of veterans with dementia who would have behavioral and psychiatric symptoms.

In 2006, about 11,000 veterans of all ages lived in VA nursing homes, including about 8,000 veterans age 65 and older (Lemke and Schaefer, 2010). From 1998 to 2006, the proportion of veterans of all ages who lived in VA nursing homes and had depressive disorders, schizophrenia, PTSD, drug use disorders, and dementia increased, and the proportion that had alcohol use disorders decreased. Among new residents age 65 and older, the proportion with PTSD increased from 1998 to 2006, especially among those born between 1918 and 1925, who were mainly World War II veterans.

A study of 9,618 veterans of all ages who lived in VA nursing homes in 2001 found that 19.6 percent had dementia; 15.1 percent had SMI, defined as schizophrenia, bipolar disorder, and other psychoses; and an additional 2.8 percent had both dementia and SMI (McCarthy et al., 2004). Large proportions of these veterans had behavioral symptoms. An analysis of three types of behavioral symptoms (labeled "physically aggressive," "verbally disruptive," and "socially inappropriate") found that very similar proportions of veterans with dementia, SMI, or both conditions had one or more of the three types of behavioral symptoms (68.7 percent, 65.8 percent, and 67.7 percent, respectively).

COEXISTING PHYSICAL HEALTH CONDITIONS AND COGNITIVE IMPAIRMENT

As noted at the beginning of this chapter, many older adults with MH/SU conditions also have one or more physical health conditions, and some have dementia-related cognitive impairment. These coexisting conditions and any medications and other treatments for the conditions can interact with an older person's MH/SU conditions in ways that make it more difficult to detect, diagnose, treat, and manage any of the conditions. Sometimes it is clear that the person's mental health or substance use condition or a treatment for the condition directly caused the physical health condition or cognitive impairment, or vice versa. Research and clinical experience have identified some direct causal relationships. Knowledge about these relationships is an important competency for physicians and other health care and MH/SU professionals who work with older adults because that knowledge may allow them to prevent some conditions or at least to recognize a causal relationship and reduce its negative effects on the person. Often, however, there is no direct causal relationship between a person's mental health or substance use conditions and his or her physical health conditions or cognitive impairment. One condition is not directly causing the other. The conditions simply coexist in the same person. From a workforce perspective, both kinds of situations are important, although probably to a greater or lesser degree for service providers with different responsibilities for detection, diagnosis, treatment, and management of MH/SU conditions in older adults. Although awareness of possible casual relationships is essential for physicians and others who diagnose and prescribe medications for the conditions, awareness that MH/SU conditions, physical health conditions, and cognitive impairment are likely to coexist in older adults is probably most important for direct care workers who often have the first and most frequent opportunities to detect such conditions.

This section presents descriptive information about coexisting MH/SU conditions, physical health conditions, and cognitive impairment in older adults. The text and tables are intended to illustrate the extent of coexisting conditions in settings, such as primary care, home, and community-based care, and hospitals. The information comes from published articles, most of which used the data only to describe the study sample.

Descriptive information about MH/SU conditions, physical health conditions, and cognitive impairment in older adults is usually presented from the perspective that represents the primary interest of particular researchers, clinicians, and others. Those who are primarily interested in MH/SU conditions often describe these conditions as central and refer to the physical health and cognitive conditions as "coexisting." Conversely, researchers, clinicians, and others who are primarily interested in physical health conditions or cognitive impairment often describe these conditions as central and refer to the MH/SU conditions as "coexisting" (Proctor et al., 2003). The same data can be used to study "coexisting" physical health conditions and cognitive impairment in people with depression and "coexisting" depression in people with physical health conditions and cognitive impairment. For many service providers, it may be less important that particular conditions are considered central or "coexisting" than that the conditions are occurring in the same person.

Table 2-10 shows the proportion of 1,801 community-living adults age 60 and older who had major depression or dysthymia and various physical health conditions (Noel et al., 2004). The people were recruited from primary care settings for a study of a model of depression treatment. Information about their physical health conditions was self-reported.

TABLE 2-10
Proportion of Community-Living Primary Care Patients Age 60 and Older with Depressive Disorders and Selected Physical Health Conditions, *N* = 1,801

Physical Health Conditions	Prevalence Rate (%)
Chronic lung disease	23
Hypertension	58
Diabetes	23
Arthritis	56
Loss of hearing or vision	55
Cancer, excluding skin cancer	11
Neurological conditions, e.g., epilepsy, seizures, Parkinson's disease, stroke	8
Heart disease	28
Gastrointestinal disease	21
Urinary tract and prostate disease	39
Chronic pain	57

SOURCE: Noel et al., 2004.

As shown in the table, substantial proportions of older adults with major depression or dysthymia also had one or more of the physical health conditions included in the study. The average number of physical health conditions was 3.8. People with severe cognitive impairment were excluded from the study, but 35 percent of people who were included had mild cognitive impairment in addition to their mental health and physical health conditions (Noel et al., 2004).

Another study of 539 community-living adults age 65 and older who were receiving home health care services found that 13.5 percent had major depression and substantial proportions of those individuals also had physical health conditions, including chronic lung disease (23 percent); diabetes (34 percent); metastatic cancer (4 percent); stroke (22 percent); congestive heart failure (30 percent); and peripheral vascular disease (34 percent) (Bruce et al., 2002). About one-fifth (21 percent) of those with major depression also had cognitive impairment.

Anxiety disorders and anxiety symptoms also coexist with physical health conditions and cognitive impairment (Palmer et al., 1997; Wolitzky-Taylor et al., 2010). A study of 377 community-living adults age 60 and older who were receiving in-home care management services found that 27 percent had clinically significant symptoms of anxiety. Of those with anxiety symptoms, 73 percent had five or more physical health conditions; 67 percent had moderate or severe pain; and 11 percent had cognitive impairment (Richardson et al., 2011).

Many older adults with SMI have coexisting physical health conditions (Bartels, 2004). One study of 8,083 male veterans age 60 and older with SMI found that 41 percent had one or more of 18 physical health conditions, including chronic obstructive pulmonary disease (18 percent); hypertension (36 percent); diabetes (21 percent); arthritis (9 percent); cancer (7 percent); stroke (5 percent); ischemic heart disease (14 percent); congestive heart failure (6 percent); and peripheral vascular disease (5 percent). Seven percent also had alcohol or drug use disorders (Kilbourne et al., 2005).

Older adults hospitalized for mental health conditions often have coexisting physical health conditions (Woo et al., 2003; Zubenko et al., 1997). A study of 195 adults age 60 and older who were hospitalized for major depression found that 75 percent also had one or more physical health conditions, including chronic obstructive pulmonary disease (7 percent), hypertension (59 percent), diabetes (22 percent), arthritis (27 percent), heart disease (25 percent), congestive heart failure (10 percent), thyroid conditions (12 percent), and Parkinson's disease (9 percent) (Proctor et al., 2003). One-quarter of the people had three or more of the conditions. The researchers note that the study sample included only older adults who were discharged from the hospital to home and that older adults discharged to a nursing home probably had more coexisting physical health conditions.

Some older adults hospitalized for physical health conditions also have mental health conditions (Banta et al., 2010; Koenig and George, 1998). A study of 1,007 male veterans of all ages hospitalized for heart disease, cancer, or other medical conditions found that 18 percent had one or more MH/SU conditions, including anxiety disorders (11 percent), depressive disorder (7 percent), alcohol abuse disorder (5 percent), and schizophrenia (0.8 percent) (Booth et al., 1998).

Lastly, a study of 18,939 community-living adults age 65 and older who were enrolled in two Michigan home care programs found high levels of physical and mental health conditions and cognitive impairment (Li and Conwell, 2007). The programs provide personal care, homemaker, and other supportive services to help individuals who are eligible for nursing home placement to remain at home instead. Information about the older adults was obtained in structured in-person interviews conducted by a nurse and social worker in the person's home. Table 2-11 shows only those physical health conditions that were present in 20 percent or more of the people.

As shown in the table, large proportions of the older adults had one or more of the physical health conditions included in the study. The average number of conditions was 5.3. Nearly half of the people (47.6 percent) experienced pain every day, including 25.1 percent with severe daily pain; more than 40 percent had mental disorders; about one-quarter had other mental health symptoms; and 43 percent had cognitive impairment.

The preceding text and tables illustrate the complex array of MH/SU conditions, physical health conditions, and cognitive impairment that service providers may encounter in various care settings. Some of the conditions are causally related, and some simply coexist in the same older person. Analysis of service needs and the workforce competencies required to meet those needs must take into account the high rates of coexisting physical health conditions and cognitive impairment in older adults with MH/SU conditions.

IMPACT OF MH/SU CONDITIONS

MH/SU conditions in older adults are associated with a wide range of negative effects, including emotional distress, functional disability, reduced physical health, increased mortality, suicide, high rates of hospitalization and nursing home placement, and high costs. Much of the published research about these negative effects in older adults pertains to depression, including many studies that compare the negative effects of DSM-IV-TR depressive disorders versus depressive symptoms that do not

TABLE 2-11
Proportion of Community-Living Adults Age 65 and Older with Selected Physical Health Conditions, Mental Health Conditions, and Cognitive Impairment in Two Michigan Home Care Programs, N = 18,939[a]

Physical Health Conditions	Prevalence Rate (%)
Chronic lung disease, including emphysema and asthma	27.0
Hypertension	69.2
Diabetes	32.9
Arthritis	73.3
Stroke	27.0
Coronary artery disease	29.1
Cardiac dysrhythmia	22.2
Congestive heart failure	35.0
Pain	
Moderate daily pain	22.5
Severe daily pain	25.1
Mental disorders	
Depression	32.9
Anxiety	18.8
Schizophrenia	0.6
Other mental health conditions	
Depressive symptoms	24.5
Suicidal ideation in the past 30 days	1.2
Suicide attempts in the past 12 months	0.3
Cognitive impairment	
Mild or moderate cognitive impairment	34.1
Severe cognitive impairment	9.0

[a] Some data derived from L. W. Li, University of Michigan School of Social Work, Ann Arbor, MI, unpublished data provided to the IOM committee, March 12, 2012.
SOURCE: Li and Conwell, 2007.

meet the criteria for a DSM-IV-TR diagnosis of depression. Less research is available about negative effects of the other MH/SU conditions identified by the IOM committee, although many studies address the negative effects of some of these conditions, for example, bipolar disorder and schizophrenia, in people under age 65.

Anecdotal evidence and a relatively small number of studies indicate that families of older adults with MH/SU conditions experience negative effects of the conditions in terms of their own emotional distress, psychological and physical consequences of caregiving, and out-of-pocket costs. These negative effects have been studied extensively in families of older adults with behavioral and psychiatric symptoms associated with dementia. Negative effects on families of people with other MH/SU conditions have been studied less in families of older adults than in families of younger people with the conditions.

This section provides a brief overview of findings from available research on emotional distress and health-related quality of life, mortality, suicide, and costs. Many of the available studies are based on cross-sectional data and therefore cannot demonstrate a causal relationship between MH/SU conditions and negative effects. In addition, as discussed previously, MH/SU conditions, physical health conditions, and cognitive impairment frequently coexist in older adults, and it is difficult to disentangle the relative contributions of these conditions to the negative effects.

Emotional Distress and Health-Related Quality of Life

Many older adults with MH/SU conditions experience severe emotional distress. It has been noted, however, that some older adults are unwilling to report this effect. In addition, some older adults may not experience the emotional effects that are usually associated with an MH/SU condition. For example, as described earlier in this chapter, some older adults who have major depressive disorder do not experience sadness.

Three surveys of nationally representative samples of community-living adults regularly include questions about emotional distress. The BRFSS survey asks, "Now, thinking about your mental health, which includes stress, depression, and problems with emotions, for how many days during the past 30 days was your mental health not good?" In 2006, 6.5 percent of community-living people age 65 and older (about 2.5 million people in 2010) indicated that they experienced these symptoms on 14 or more of the previous 30 days (CDC and National Association of Chronic Disease Directors, 2008).

The NHIS asks how often in the past 30 days the respondent has felt "so sad that nothing could cheer you up"; "nervous"; "restless or fidgety"; "hopeless"; "that everything was an effort"; or "worthless." In 2010, 2.3 percent of community-living people age 65 and older (about 900,000 people) had scores indicating frequent, serious distress (NCHS, 2011d). Using the same questions, the 2010 NSDUH found that 2.1 percent of community-living adults age 65 and older (about 800,000 people) reported frequent, serious distress (CBHSQ, 2012e).

Studies that have used structured assessments of quality of life or health-related quality of life also show that MH/SU conditions, including depressive disorders, depressive symptoms, generalized anxiety disorder, and substance use disorders, are associated with reduced health-related quality of life (Booth et al., 2001; Chachamovich et al., 2008; Porensky et al., 2009; Spitzer et al., 1995). One study of 134 adults age 58-104 with dementia who were living in assisted living facilities found that behavioral and psychiatric symptoms were associated with reduced quality of life (Samus et al., 2005).

Mortality

People of all ages with MH/SU conditions experience higher mortality rates than other people without these conditions. Their higher mortality has been attributed to many factors, including poor compliance with prescribed medical treatments for physical health conditions; toxic effects of medications prescribed for their MH/SU condition; negative health behaviors, such as excessive use of alcohol and drugs, smoking, and inactivity; poor-quality medical care; poverty; lack of health insurance; and lack of coordination in the medical and specialty MH/SU systems (Druss and von Esenwein, 2006).

- A 2006 report of the National Association of State Mental Health Program Directors indicates that people with SMI die 25 years earlier than the general population and that recent state studies show that premature mortality is increasing (Parks et al., 2006).
- An analysis of data from the New Haven ECA site shows that survey participants *age 55 and older* with major depressive disorder were four times more likely than other survey participants to die in a 15-month period (Bruce and Leaf, 1989).
- An analysis of data on public mental health clients in eight states found that they had higher mortality rates and died at a younger age than the general population. Those with major mental illnesses were more likely to die than those with less severe mental illnesses and more likely to die at a younger age (Colton and Manderscheid, 2006).

- An analysis of data on people interviewed for the 1989 NHIS and followed for 17 years found that those with a mental disorder died an average of 8.2 years earlier than other survey participants (Druss et al., 2011).

Suicide

In 2007 (the most recent data available), there were 5,421 suicides among adults age 65 and older, including 4,569 men and 852 women (Xu et al., 2010). Suicide rates for men increased with age from 22.4 per 100,000 men age 65-69 to 41.8 per 100,000 men age 85 and older, the highest rate for any age group (Crosby et al., 2011). Suicide rates for women were lower and decreased from 4.5 per 100,000 women age 65-74 to 3.1 per 100,000 women age 85 and older.

Costs

National figures on the costs of MH/SU conditions in older adults vary depending on which older adults, conditions, services, and payers are included. The 2009 Medical Expenditure Panel Survey (MEPS) found that 7.4 million adults age 65 and older received services for mental disorders (AHRQ, 2009a) at a cost of $17.1 billion (AHRQ, 2009b), making mental disorders the eighth most costly condition for adults age 65 and older in the United States in 2009.

The MEPS includes community-living people and excludes people living in nursing homes, prisons, or jails. Mental disorders are self-reported and include substance use conditions. Survey respondents identify which services they received for the reported conditions. Services included in the $17.1 billion for 2009 are hospital, emergency department, and outpatient services, physician and other medical provider office visits, home health services, other home care services, and prescribed medications. Medical equipment and supplies, ambulance services, eyeglasses, dental care, and over-the-counter medications are not included.

The $17.1 billion figure from MEPS includes expenditures by all payers. In 2009, Medicare paid more than half (52.5 percent) of the cost of services for mental disorders for adults age 65 and older. The remaining 47.5 percent was paid by Medicaid (11.4 percent), private insurance (11.7 percent), out-of-pocket (18.3 percent), and other sources, including the VA, state and local health departments, state programs other than Medicaid, and community and neighborhood clinics (6.1 percent) (AHRQ, 2009c).

Medicare reimbursement data for 2009 provide a different perspective on the costs of MH/SU services for older adults. Table 2-12 shows 2009

Medicare reimbursements for MH/SU services for beneficiaries age 65 and older who were enrolled in fee-for-service Medicare.

As shown in the table, Medicare reimbursements for MH/SU services for older fee-for-service Medicare beneficiaries amounted to $2.4 billion in 2009. Most of the $2.4 billion (93 percent) was for mental health services. The remaining 7 percent was for alcohol use services (4 percent) and drug use services (3 percent). The $2.4 billion total represents 1 percent of Medicare reimbursements for all covered services for Medicare fee-for-service beneficiaries in 2009.

The large gap between the $17.1 billion figure from MEPS and the $2.4 billion figure based on Medicare reimbursement data reflects differences in the people, conditions, services, and payers included in each figure.

- The Medicare reimbursement data pertain to all community-living adults and nursing home residents age 65 and older who were enrolled in fee-for-service Medicare in 2009 but exclude about 9.8 million Medicare beneficiaries (25 percent of all Medicare beneficiaries age 65 and older) who were enrolled in Medicare Advantage health plans (CMS, 2010). In contrast, Medicare Advantage enrollees are included in the MEPS figure.
- The Medicare reimbursement data include services for which an MH/SU condition is listed as the primary diagnosis on the Medicare claim. In contrast, the MEPS survey respondent identifies the services received for MH/SU conditions, and no distinction is made between primary and secondary diagnoses.
- The Medicare reimbursement data include services that are covered by Medicare, including ambulance services and medical equipment, but exclude prescription drugs, which account for $6.4 billion of the Medicare costs included in the MEPS figure. The MEPS figure also includes Medicare copayments and deductibles and nursing home and home care services that are not covered by Medicare.
- The Medicare reimbursement data include only Medicare costs, whereas the MEPS figure includes costs to all payers, including Medicare, Medicaid, private insurance, out-of-pocket, and other payers.

USE OF MH/SU SERVICES BY OLDER ADULTS

The kinds of services required to meet the needs of older adults with MH/SU conditions include detection, diagnosis, treatment, ongoing management, and monitoring. To the extent that older adults receive these kinds of services, the services are provided by a bewildering array of

TABLE 2-12
Medicare Reimbursement for Mental Health and Other Substance Use Services for Fee-for-Service Beneficiaries Age 65 and Older, 2009

MH/SU Service Providers	Medicare Reimbursement ($ Millions)			
	All MH/SU Services	Mental Health Services Only	Alcohol Use Services Only	Drug Use Services Only
All providers	2,440	2,259	108	73
Hospitals	1,558	1,413	85	60
• Community hospitals	1,267	1,136	75	57
o Inpatient care	935	818	63	53
–Specialty MH/SU unit	694	680	8	5
–General unit	241	138	55	48
o Outpatient care	319	306	11	3
–Specialty MH/SU unit	3	3	0	0
–General unit	317	303	11	3

• Psychiatric hospitals	291	278	10	3
o Inpatient care	214	202	9	3
o Outpatient care	77	76	0	0
Nursing homes	174	160	12	2
Home health care	119	117	1	1
Physicians	294	282	7	5
• Psychiatrists	203	200	2	1
• Other physicians	90	81	5	4
Psychologists, nurses, social workers, counselors, other nonphysician MH/SU service providers, and other professionals	245	243	1	0
Laboratories	13	9	1	4
Ambulance services	50	46	2	2

SOURCE: Thomson Reuters, 2011.

organizations and individuals. Chapter 3 describes the geriatric MH/SU workforce, focusing primarily on the education, training, credentials, and competencies of the many types of individual providers who are or could be part of the workforce that provides the services. This section describes the types of organizations and settings that provide or could provide MH/SU services for older adults. It discusses older adults' attitudes and beliefs about using MH/SU services and reviews the available data about their past and current use of these services.

The available information about older adults' use of MH/SU services is not sufficient to support a credible analysis of the number and proportion of older adults that need but do not use MH/SU services. Available data suggest, however, that there is substantial unmet need.

Organizations and Settings That Provide MH/SU Services

From a national perspective, the organizations and settings that provide MH/SU services for older adults can be categorized in various ways. In Box 2-5, these organizations and settings are categorized in six broad types and a catch-all "other" type, based on their primary focus. The categorization also differentiates: (1) *general* medical care, residential, and community social service organizations and settings intended to serve people who do and do not have MH/SU conditions, and (2) *specialty* mental health and substance use organizations and settings intended to serve only people who have MH/SU conditions. From the federal government perspective, the organizations and settings included in Box 2-5 could also be categorized on the basis of the federal agency or agencies with primary administrative responsibility for the services. Alternatively, the organizations and settings could be categorized on the basis of their main sources of funding (Medicare, Medicaid, private insurance, out-of-pocket payments, federal block grants, state funds, and other).

From a state perspective, the organizations and settings listed in Box 2-5 are often categorized differently, with a stated designation of some organizations and settings as part of the "public mental health system." Every state has a State Mental Health Agency (SMHA) that is responsible for the delivery of public mental health services. The public and private organizations and settings operated and/or funded by the SMHA are generally considered to comprise the state's public mental health system. In 2009, SMHAs across the country operated and/or funded nearly 20,000 public and private mental health organizations, settings, and providers, including 212 state psychiatric hospitals, 70 private psychiatric hospitals, 440 general hospitals with a separate psychiatric unit, 59 nursing homes and intermediate care facilities for mental illness (ICF-MI), and 18,847 community mental health centers and providers (SAMHSA, 2009). In

2008, 5 percent of the 6.3 million people of all ages who received SMHA-operated or SMHA-funded mental health services were age 65 and older (about 315,000 people) (SAMHSA, 2009).

States differ considerably in terms of the mental health organizations and settings that are operated or funded by the state's SMHA versus other state agencies, for example, agencies with primary responsibility for Medicaid, criminal justice and corrections, and housing (NRI, 2009). States also differ in terms of whether the SMHA has administrative responsibility for the state's substance use services. In 2009, SMHAs in 27 states had administrative responsibility for substance use services (SAMHSA, 2009). Responsibility for these services was located in another agency in the remaining states.

During the recent financial depression, many states have reduced funding for their SMHA. For FY 2010, 9 to 20 SMHAs reported cuts in state funding for various mental health services, including inpatient long-term care (20 states), inpatient acute care (19 states); clinic services (12 states), and other inpatient and day treatment services (9 states) (CBHSQ, 2012a). Eight to 17 SMHAs reported anticipated cuts in funding for the same services in FY 2011.

States' define the eligibility criteria for services operated or funded through their public mental health system, but all states include services for people with SMI, and states generally prioritize services for people with low income and those who are uninsured or have only Medicaid (Garfield, 2011). National data show that SMHAs operate or fund mental health services for disproportionate numbers of older people in racial and ethnic minority groups. In 2008, the population rates for use of mental health services operated or funded by SMHAs were higher for black, Hispanic/Latino, and Native American people age 65 and older (11.8, 10.6, and 8.6 persons per 1,000 in the population, respectively) than for whites and Asian Americans (6.3 and 4.9 persons per 1,000, respectively) (SAMHSA, 2009). Moreover, in at least some states, the SMHA operates or funds mental health services for a disproportionate number of older people living in rural versus urban areas (Karlin and Norris, 2006). Recent reductions in state funding for SMHAs raise concerns about the current and future capacity of SMHAs to provide mental health services for these vulnerable groups of older adults.

From the perspective of a county or local government, the organizations and settings listed in Box 2-5 might be categorized differently than they are usually categorized from either a national or state perspective. Especially in smaller jurisdictions, these organizations and settings might be thought of less in broad categories and more as unique local agencies that provide various combinations of mental health, substance use, and general medical, residential, and community-based aging and social

BOX 2-5
Types of Organizations and Settings That Provide Some MH/SU Services for Some Older Adults

General medical care organizations and settings. Includes thousands of public and private acute care hospitals; emergency departments; primary medical care settings, such as individual physician offices, group medical practices, ambulatory care clinics, community health centers (CHCs), federally qualified health centers (FQHCs), and rural health centers; and Medicare-certified home health care agencies. The main focus of these organizations and settings is medical and medically related care for physical health conditions. All of these organizations and settings provide care for older adults, and most of them provide some MH/SU services for some older adults.

General residential care organizations and settings. Includes nursing homes; assisted living and other residential care facilities; and congregate-living settings, such as senior housing and public housing facilities. The main focus of these organizations and settings is housing and services ranging from skilled nursing care, rehabilitative services, and extensive assistance with personal care in nursing homes to health-related and supportive services in residential care facilities and congregate-living settings. All of these organizations and settings provide services for older adults, and many of them provide some MH/SU services for some of their older residents.

Aging network agencies and other social service organizations and settings. Includes Area Agencies on Aging (AAAs); senior centers; adult day centers; and many other community agencies that provide health-related and social services, such as personal care, homemaker, and chore services, congregate and home-delivered meals, transportation, information, referrals, and counseling about services and benefits, care management, family caregiver support, and respite care. The main focus of these organizations and settings is supportive services to help individuals remain at home and as functionally independent as possible. Nearly all of the organizations and settings provide services for older adults, and many of them provide some MH/SU services for some older adults.

Specialty mental health organizations and settings. Includes public and private psychiatric hospitals; residential mental health treatment centers; day treatment centers; outpatient mental health clinics; community mental health centers; mental health group homes; individual and group mental health practices that provide psychiatric, psychological, and counseling services; crisis and emergency mental health organizations; lay- and volunteer-led organizations that provide mental health support and self-help services; and specialty managed care organizations that provide mental health services through "carve-out" arrangements with insurers and other payers. All of these organizations and settings provide mental health services, and many of them provide some mental health services for some older adults.

Specialty substance use organizations and settings. Includes public and private residential and outpatient substance use treatment centers, day treatment centers, substance use group homes, crisis and emergency substance use organizations, lay- and volunteer-led organizations that provide substance use support and self-help services, and specialty managed care organizations that provide substance use services through "carve out" arrangements with insurers and other payers. All of these organizations and settings provide substance use services, and some of them provide some substance use services for some older adults.

Veterans Affairs (VA). The VA provides a wide array of medical, mental health, substance use, residential, and home and community-based services for veterans who enroll in the VA health care system. At its medical centers, community-based outpatient centers, and other facilities and through contracts with other organizations, the VA provides all these services for some older veterans with MH/SU conditions.

Other. Includes adult correctional facilities, housing organizations, settings that serve homeless people, adult protective service agencies, public health agencies, and organizations and settings funded by the Indian Health Service.

services, using funding from an array of federal, state, and local government sources, private insurance, and donations from philanthropic organizations and individuals. A local Area Agency on Aging (AAA), for example, might be thought of less as part of a national network of aging services agencies and more as a unique community agency that provides information and referrals, care management, home-delivered meals, and assessments for Medicaid-funded home- and community-based services, using many funding sources in addition to the federal Older Americans Act. In many counties and local jurisdictions, the police department and ambulance service(s) might also be thought of as organizations that provide MH/SU services in crisis and emergency psychiatric situations.

Differences in the way organizations and settings that provide MH/SU services are categorized at the national, state, county, and local government levels make it difficult to create a coherent description of these organizations and settings. More importantly in the context of this report, differences in the way the organizations and settings are categorized at different levels of government make it very difficult to design and implement comprehensive initiatives to address problems in the care of older adults with MH/SU conditions. Such initiatives and the regulatory and financing policies to support them generally target types of organizations and settings that reflect the categories used at the level of government that develops the initiative. Yet, federal government initiatives that target, for example, organizations, settings, and providers that receive Medicare payments and may include training, credentialing, or other workforce requirements will apply to some but not all organizations, settings, and providers that are part of the state-defined public mental health system or the array of community agencies that are considered by local governments to be providing MH/SU services. Likewise, state government initiatives that target organizations, settings, and providers that comprise the state's public mental health system will apply to some, but not all organizations and settings categorized as providing MH/SU services at the federal or local level.

As noted in Box 2-5, the VA provides MH/SU services for veterans enrolled in the VA health care system, which is the largest integrated health care system in the United States. VA health care system integration, which includes common categorizations of types of services, settings, and providers at the national, regional, and local levels as well as an advanced electronic medical record system that is accessible across all levels, greatly facilitates the design and implementation of comprehensive, systemwide initiatives to address medical and medically related conditions, including MH/SU conditions. Box 2-6 describes the VA's systemwide programs to prevent suicide in veterans of all ages. A recent report funded by SAMHSA described these suicide prevention programs as "perhaps the most comprehensive suicide prevention initiative in history" (Suicide Prevention Resource Center and SPAN USA, 2010).

Older Adults' Attitudes and Beliefs About Using MH/SU Services

It is sometimes said that older adults do not use MH/SU services because of stigma associated with the conditions and related services. Their greater tendency to use MH/SU services provided in general medical, residential, and home- and community-based settings versus specialty MH/SU settings is sometimes also attributed to perceived stigma. Available data support the concept that substantial proportions of older adults perceive stigma associated with MH/SU conditions and related services, but the data also identify other attitudes and beliefs, some of which may have an even greater impact on older adults' use of MH/SU services.

One study of more than 600 community-living adults age 60 and older who were receiving health-related and social services from a public long-term care agency assessed their attitudes and beliefs about mental health service use and compared the attitudes and beliefs of those who had depression (either a DSM-IV-TR depressive disorder or depressive symptoms) and those who did not (Morrow-Howell et al., 2008). The study found that more than 90 percent of both groups of older adults said people with mental or emotional problems should seek professional help. Nearly the same proportions said they would seek treatment if they had a mental or emotional problem (89 percent of those who had depression and 94 percent of those who did not). On the other hand, more than 80 percent of both groups said the cost of treatment would be more than they could afford, and only 41 percent said they knew where to obtain treatment. Relatively small proportions said their family would be upset if they knew the person was receiving help for a mental or emotional problem (16 percent of those who had depression and 18 percent of those who did not). Even smaller proportions said that someone in their family would object if the person wanted to go for treatment of a mental or emotional problem (11 and 7 percent, respectively) or that they would avoid treatment of a mental or emotional problem because friends might find out (5 and 1 percent, respectively). Nearly one-third of both groups said they believed that "you should always handle mental and emotional problems by yourself." Nearly one-quarter (24 percent) of those who had depression and 17 percent of those who did not have depression said that mental and emotional problems will get better by themselves.

The findings from this study are reflected to varying degrees in findings from surveys conducted in national, population-based samples. The National Comorbidity Survey Replication (NCS-R) (see Box 2-2) found that more than 80 percent of community-living older adults had positive

BOX 2-6
Suicide Prevention Programs in the VA

Suicide prevention is a major national priority of the VA, and the agency has implemented a comprehensive array of systemwide suicide prevention programs. These programs include suicide monitoring and risk assessment, a national suicide crisis line, full-time suicide prevention coordinators in every VA medical center, and electronic medical record flags to notify clinicians of suicide risk.

Suicide monitoring and risk assessment. The VA conducts ongoing comprehensive, systemwide suicide monitoring and risk assessment for veterans who use VA health care services. Findings from suicide monitoring activities show that in fiscal years 2000 and 2001, age- and sex-adjusted suicide rates among VA users were elevated in comparison with rates in the general U.S. population, with a standardized suicide ratio of 1.66 for male veterans and 1.87 for female veterans (McCarthy et al., 2009). Trends in suicide rates among VA users show a slight reduction between fiscal years 2000 and 2007, with male veterans age 30 to 64 being at the highest risk of suicide (Blow et al., 2012). Risk assessment activities have identified various factors associated with elevated suicide risk, including recent psychiatric hospitalizations, the start of antidepressant medication, and dosage changes (Valenstein et al., 2009). Mental disorders have been found to be strongly associated with elevated risk of suicide. For example, suicide risk for male veterans with bipolar disorder was found to be three times higher than for other male veterans (Ilgen et al., 2010). Suicide risk has also been found to be elevated for veterans living in rural areas, even after adjusting for clinical factors and distance to nearest VA mental health providers (McCarthy et al., 2012). These and other findings from the VA's ongoing suicide monitoring and risk assessment activities are routinely shared with VA admin-

help-seeking attitudes: 86 percent of the survey respondents age 65-74 and 82 percent of those age 75 and older said they would seek professional help if they had serious emotional problems (Mackenzie et al., 2008). Likewise, 82 percent of those age 65-74 and 76 percent of those age 75 and older said they would be comfortable talking about personal problems with a professional. Most of the respondents age 65 and older also had positive treatment beliefs: more than 70 percent said they believed that half or more of people who see a professional for serious emotional istrators at all levels, and medical and mental health clinicians and other frontline service providers.

National suicide crisis line. In 2007, the VA established a national 24/7 crisis hotline that has received more than 600,000 calls and made more than 21,000 life-saving rescues. Initially named the National Veterans Suicide Prevention Hotline, the call line was renamed as the Veterans Crisis Line to reduce perceived stigma and facilitate use by veterans and their families and friends. In 2009, VA added an anonymous online chat service that has been used by more than 50,000 people.

Suicide prevention coordinators. The VA has placed suicide prevention coordinators at all medical centers. The coordinators have a full-time commitment to suicide prevention activities. They collaborate with VA mental health clinicians to support suicide prevention efforts for individuals at high risk and to ensure that these individuals receive increased monitoring and enhanced care. Specific activities include tracking and reporting on veterans found to be at high risk for suicide and those who have attempted suicide; training staff who have contact with veterans so that they know how to get immediate assistance if veterans express any suicide plan or intent; collaborating with community organizations and partners and providing training to their staff who have contact with veterans; and providing consultations to providers regarding resources for suicidal individuals.

Clinical flags for high-risk veterans. The VA uses electronic medical record flags to identify veterans at high risk for suicide. High risk is defined by various factors, including a history of suicide attempts and recent discharge from an inpatient mental health unit. For veterans identified as having high risk for suicide, VA clinicians can contact the suicide prevention coordinator about services and need for closer monitoring. Clinicians are also trained to recognize that absence of a positive flag does not imply the veteran is not at risk for suicide.

problems are helped. Nevertheless, 31 percent of those age 65-74 and 26 percent of those age 75 and older said they would be embarrassed if their friends knew they were getting professional help for an emotional problem.

The 2001 NSDUH found that among community-living older adults with mental health conditions, only 10 percent reported receiving any mental health services (Karlin et al., 2008). The two primary reasons older adults gave for not using mental health services were (1) not knowing where to go for services (28 percent), and (2) lack of affordability (19 percent). Less than 1 percent said they needed but did not receive mental health services in the previous year. On the other hand, older adults who used mental health services were at least as likely as younger adults who used the services to say the services benefited them.

Several studies have found that substantial proportions of older adults with mental health conditions do not perceive a need for mental health services and are not interested in using such services. One study of more than 9,500 adults with probable mental disorders found that only 28 percent of those age 65 and older perceived a need for mental health services, compared with higher proportions of those under age 65 (49 percent of those age 18-29 and 43 percent of those age 30-64) (Klap et al., 2003). Another study of 268 community-living people age 57-97 found that more than half of those with depressive symptoms were not receiving any mental health services, and only 34 percent of them expressed interest in receiving such services (Cohen-Mansfield and Frank, 2008).

Older people differ in their beliefs about the causes of mental health conditions. One study of 90 older people with depression found that 28 percent attributed the condition to "old age" rather than to an illness. Those who attributed their depressive symptoms to old age were four times less likely than those who attributed the symptoms to an illness to say that it is important to discuss such symptoms with a doctor (Sarkisian et al., 2003). A recent analysis of the beliefs of white, black, Hispanic/Latino, and Asian American older adults about the causes of mental health conditions found significant variation among groups that is likely to affect help-seeking behaviors (Jimenez et al., 2012).

Interviews and focus groups conducted in San Diego with 165 mental health service providers, family caregivers, consumers age 55 and older, and other older adults identified many factors associated with unmet needs for mental health services for older adults (Palinkas et al., 2007). Of the 66 consumers age 55 and older and other older adults, more than 60 percent were from racial and ethnic minority groups. Factors identified by the consumers and other older adults included the following:

- stigma (63 percent);
- lack of information about available services (50 percent);
- lack of age-appropriate and culturally and linguistically appropriate services, including translators in mental health settings (44 percent);
- lack of transportation to services (38 percent); and
- lack of money or insurance to pay for services (25 percent).

As noted earlier, the available research shows that many older adults perceive stigma associated with MH/SU conditions and MH/SU services. Beliefs and attitudes, such as that mental and emotional problems will get better by themselves and that it is better to handle these problems by oneself, could be thought of as separate from, caused by, or resulting in perceived stigma. Likewise, lack of awareness of one's mental health condition and lack of interest in receiving services for a mental health condition could be thought of as separate from, contributing to, or caused by perceived stigma. Other factors, such as lack of information about available services, lack of age- and culturally and linguistically appropriate services, lack of transportation, and lack of money or insurance to pay for services, undoubtedly reflect current reality. In the context of older adults' positive beliefs about the importance of obtaining mental health services and the likely effectiveness of such services, however, these other factors interact with perceived stigma and related attitudes and beliefs to reduce older adults' willingness to use MH/SU services. Professional and other service providers who interact with older adults in specialty MH/SU, general medical, residential, and home- and community-based care settings should be aware of the array of attitudes, beliefs, and other factors that influence older adults' decisions about MH/SU service use and able to identify and implement approaches to reduce such barriers to needed services.

Older Adults' Use of MH/SU Services

Comprehensive information is not available about the proportion or number of older adults with MH/SU conditions that use any of the kinds of MH/SU, and much less information is available about detection than about diagnosis, treatment, ongoing management and monitoring. In general, by the time an older adult uses services provided by specialty MH/SU organizations and settings, the person's MH/SU condition has already been detected by someone and may have been diagnosed. The MH/SU services needed by the person at that point are diagnosis, if not already completed, treatment, ongoing management, and monitoring. In contrast, MH/SU conditions in older adults may not have been detected in general medical, residential, and home- and community-based care settings. From a workforce perspective, it is important to consider this fundamental difference in needed MH/SU services by type of setting and its implications for training and workforce competencies.

Studies of detection of MH/SU conditions in older adults in general medical, residential, and home- and community-based care settings indicate that the conditions are frequently not detected (see, e.g., Brown et al., 2003; Rosenblatt et al., 2004). Such studies are difficult to conduct because they require both a process to determine which older adults have an MH/SU condition and a process to determine whether the condition has been detected. Moreover, study findings differ, depending on the type of setting, particular provider, and how "detection" is measured, for example, by a notation in a person's medical record, a diagnostic code on a billing or claim form, the report of the person or a family member that a physician has said the person has the condition, or the report of a service provider who has worked with the person. Nevertheless, frequent calls to implement screening for various MH/SU conditions in general medical, residential, and home- and community-based care settings reflect many service providers' experience that the conditions are often missed.

A convincing body of evidence shows that older adults are less likely than younger adults to receive treatment for their MH/SU conditions (Dixon et al., 2001; German et al., 1985; Karlin et al., 2008; Klap et al., 2003; Shapiro et al., 1984; Wang et al., 2000, 2005) and that they are less likely than younger adults to receive MH/SU treatment in a specialty setting and more likely to receive treatment in general medical, residential, and home- and community-based service care settings (German et al., 1985; Shapiro et al., 1984; Wang et al., 2005). Large-scale, population-based surveys conducted over the past 30 years in the United States have found that only small proportions of older adults with MH/SU conditions receive any services for these conditions. Most of the surveys do not include institutionalized people; thus, they do not include people living in nursing homes. The surveys differ somewhat in the MH/SU conditions and kinds of services they include. They all use structured diagnostic interviews to identify people with MH/SU conditions but generally do not ask whether the people have received a diagnostic evaluation or a formal diagnosis of the condition.

From 1980 to 1984, the National Institute of Mental Health Epidemiologic Catchment Area (ECA) Program conducted interviews with more than 18,500 adults age 18 and older, including 5,700 adults age 65 and older, in five sites across the country. The survey found that about one-third of adults age 18 and older who had a MH/SU condition received any treatment for the condition in a 1-year period (Narrow et al., 2000; Regier et al., 1993), and those age 65 and older were less likely than those under age 65 to receive treatment (Shapiro et al., 1984). In the Baltimore site, where older adults were oversampled, only 1 percent of adults age 65-74 with MH/SU conditions and no one age 75 and older with these conditions had received treatment in a specialty setting, compared with 17 percent of adults age 18-64 with the conditions (German et al., 1985). About the same proportions of adults age 18-64 and 65-74 with MH/SU conditions (17 percent and 18 percent, respectively) said they had discussed emotional problems with a primary care provider during a general medical care visit, but only 10 percent of those age 75 and older said they had such discussions.

Two studies conducted in the late 1990s found that older adults with mental health conditions were less likely than younger people to receive treatment for the conditions:

- The 1996 Midlife Development in the United States (MIDUS) study used a telephone interview and mail questionnaire to assess use of mental health treatment in a nationally representative sample of 3,000 adults age 25-74; the study found that adults age 65-74 with mental health conditions were 40 percent to 140 percent less likely than those under age 65 with the conditions to receive any treatment for the conditions (Wang et al., 2000).
- The 1997-1998 Health Care for Communities (HCC) household study used a telephone interview and mailed questionnaire to assess use of mental health treatment in a stratified random sample of 9,585 adults age 18 and older. The study found that adults age 65 and older with mental health conditions were less likely than those age 30-64 with the conditions to receive mental health treatment (53 versus 60 percent, respectively), but they were more likely to receive mental health treatment than adults age 18-29 (53 percent versus 49 percent, respectively) (Klap et al., 2003). Among adults who received any mental health treatment, only 7 percent of older adults, compared with 18 percent of adults age 18-29 and 26 percent of those age 30-64 received treatment in a specialty mental health setting. Fewer older adults reported being asked by a primary care provider if they felt tense or anxious (15 percent compared with 23 percent for younger people); fewer older adults reported that a primary care provider had spent 5 minutes or more on mental health counseling (4 percent compared with 7 percent to 8 percent for younger people); and only 1 percent of older adults reported that a primary care provider had referred them to a mental health specialist in the past year for evaluation or treatment, compared with 3 percent of younger people.

Large-scale surveys conducted in the early 2000s continued to find relatively low use of MH/SU treatment by older adults. As noted earlier, the 2001 NSDUH found that only 10 percent of adults age 65 and older with mental health conditions received MH/SU treatment, compared with 25 percent of younger adults with the conditions (Karlin et al., 2008). Among those with SMI, the difference was greater (9 percent for adults age 65 and older compared with 32 percent for people under age 65).

One analysis of data from the NCS-R, which was conducted in 2001-

2002, found a lower overall rate of treatment for older adults with any of the MH/SU conditions included in the study and a lower likelihood of receiving treatment in a specialty setting for older adults (Wang et al., 2005). Another analysis of data from the three surveys that are part of the CPES conducted from 2001 to 2003, found that 66 percent of older adults with major depressive disorder and 72 percent of older adults with anxiety disorders had not received any treatment for these conditions in the previous year (Garrido et al., 2011). Importantly, only 50 percent of older adults with major depressive disorder and only 43 percent of those with anxiety disorders perceived a need for treatment; of those who perceived a need for treatment, 17 percent did not seek treatment at all, and 21 percent delayed seeking treatment for at least 4 weeks.

As noted earlier, it is sometimes said that the greater tendency of older adults to use MH/SU services provided in general medical, residential, and home- and community-based settings versus specialty MH/SU settings is due to perceived stigma. Other interrelated factors probably also contribute to this longstanding pattern of service use. Coexisting physical health conditions in older people with MH/SU conditions mean that they are often receiving care in general medical settings and are, therefore, familiar with and perhaps comfortable in these settings. Similarly, coexisting physical health conditions and cognitive and functional impairments mean that some older adults with MH/SU conditions are receiving care in general residential and home- and community-based settings. They are familiar with these settings, and many of them have physical and other difficulties getting to specialty MH/SU settings. Lack of knowledge about specialty mental health organizations and settings among older adults, their families, and even the medical, residential, and home- and community-based care providers who interact with them are probably also factors. People in the baby boom generation have had higher average rates of mental health service use throughout their lives, including use of specialty mental health services, and their willingness to use such services is expected to continue as they age. As a result, older adults' use of specialty mental health services may increase in the future. At present, however, there is no clear consensus among geriatric MH/SU experts about which older people with MH/SU conditions would be better served in specialty versus general medical, residential, and home and community-based care settings. Moreover, concerns about whether the available MH/SU services are age-appropriate and culturally and linguistically appropriate pertain to both specialty and general care settings.

Box 2-7 describes older adults' use of public mental health services provided by the public mental health system in San Diego County, California. The findings show low use of mental health services overall but high use of emergency psychiatric services provided by a mobile team of law enforcement and mental health personnel.

BOX 2-7
Older Adults' Use of Mental Health Services Provided by the San Diego County Public Mental Health System

The San Diego County public mental health system provides various specialty mental health services, including psychiatric hospitalization, emergency psychiatric unit, outpatient clinic, day treatment, and case management (Jin et al., 2003). A study of use of these services by adults with schizophrenia in 1999 and 2000 found that those age 65 and older were less likely than those under age 65 to use any of the services except case management. The researchers hypothesized that the older adults may have needed case management more than younger adults because of their coexisting medical conditions and functional impairments, and that as a service, case management may be more acceptable than the other services to older adults with schizophrenia.

Another study conducted in the San Diego county public mental health system from 2002 to 2006 found that adults age 60 and older were more likely than those under age 60 to enter the system through the Psychiatric Emergency Response Team (PERT), which responds to psychiatric-related 911 calls (Gilmer et al., 2009). Older adults were less likely than younger adults to use follow-up outpatient or inpatient mental health services in the next 90 days but more likely to have another encounter with the PERT. The researchers emphasize the need for better linkages between the PERT and outpatient mental health service providers to facilitate sustained follow-up care.

Trends in Older Adults' Use of MH/SU Services

In recent years, the proportion and number of older adults receiving treatment for depression has increased substantially. Between 1992 and 1998, the proportion of community-living older adults with a diagnosis of depression that was receiving any treatment for the condition remained about the same, but the proportion that received only antidepressant medications increased, while the proportion that received only psychotherapy decreased (Crystal et al., 2003). This trend has continued, and in the period from 2002 to 2005, 67 percent of older adults with a diagnosis of depression received antidepressant medications, while only 15 percent received psychotherapy (Akincigil et al., 2011). In the period from 2005 to 2008, 15 percent of all community-living adults age 60 and over were taking antidepressants, including 9 percent of men and 19 percent of women in that age group (Pratt et al., 2011).

The trends for increased use of antidepressants and decreased use of psychotherapy in older adults mirror changes that have taken place in treatment of depression in people of all ages (Marcus and Olfson, 2010; Olfson and Marcus, 2010) and have led some commentators to lament the reduction in potentially valuable treatment options (Akincigil et al., 2011; Druss, 2010). The high use of antidepressants in older people has likewise led to concerns about overuse, inappropriate use, and side effects (Hanlon et al., 2011; Mark et al., 2011). These concerns are increased by national data showing that among medical visits for people of all ages in which antidepressants were prescribed, the proportion in which there was no diagnosis of depression increased from 60 percent in 1996 to 73 percent in 2007 (Mojtabai and Olfson, 2011). Moreover, visits in which antidepressants were prescribed without a diagnosis of depression were significantly more frequent for people age 65 and older than for those under age 65.

Older African Americans with depression are less likely than older whites, Hispanic/Latinos, and Asian Americans to use antidepressants, thus raising concerns about possible underuse in this group. One study of more than 7,000 Medicaid beneficiaries age 65-84 with a diagnosis of depression found that in 1998, African Americans were significantly less likely than other groups to use antidepressants (Strothers et al., 2005). Another study that compared use of antidepressants by older people in five North Carolina counties in 1986 and 1996 found that use was lower for African Americans than whites in 1986 (2.3 percent versus 4.6 percent, respectively), and the difference between the groups increased over the next decade. In 1996, 5 percent of African Americans and 14 percent of whites were using antidepressants (Blazer et al., 2000a).

Aside from depression, it is not clear that treatment for other MH/SU conditions has increased in general for older adults. On the other hand, national data show that the use of antianxiety medications by community-living older adults increased from 8 percent in the period from 1999 to 2002 to 10 percent in the period from 2005 to 2008 (NCHS, 2011c). Use of antipsychotic medications for older people with dementia decreased from 1999 to 2007 (Kales et al., 2011), but concerns remain about overuse, inappropriate use and negative effects of all these medications, especially in older people who are taking multiple medications for other physical health conditions (McLendon and Shelton, 2012).

FACTORS THAT COULD AFFECT THE FUTURE MH/SU SERVICE NEEDS OF OLDER ADULTS

U.S. Census Bureau projections show that the population age 65 and older will increase from 40.3 million in 2010 to 54.8 million in 2020 and 72.1 million in 2030 (Census Bureau, 2011b). As discussed earlier in this chapter, the committee estimates that at least 5.6 million to 8 million adults age 65 and older, or 14 percent to 20 percent of the older population, had one or more MH/SU conditions in 2010 (see Table 2-5). Even without future changes in the proportion of older adults with MH/SU conditions, projected growth in the older population will result in large increases in the number of older adults with these conditions. Applying the 14 percent to 20 percent figures to the projected population for 2020, 54.8 million older adults, indicates there will be at least 7.7 million to 11 million older adults with one or more MH/SU conditions in 2020. Applying the same figures to the projected population for 2030, 72.1 million older adults, indicates there will be at least 10.1 million to 14.4 million older adults with one or more MH/SU conditions in 2030.

These figures for 2020 and 2030 are conservative because the 2010 figures on which they are based include only 13 of the 27 MH/SU conditions identified by the committee. Data presented earlier in this chapter show that several million older adults may have one or more of three other conditions—depressive symptoms, anxiety symptoms, and at-risk drinking. These people are not included in the committee's 2010 estimates, mainly because information is not available to account for comorbidity. The numbers for the other 11 conditions are smaller or not available, but adding people with any of the conditions that were not included in the committee's estimates would increase the totals for 2010 and, in turn, the estimated proportions and numbers of older adults that will have MH/SU conditions in 2020 and 2030.

Large increases in future numbers of older adults with MH/SU conditions due to growth in the size of the older population will clearly create a need for more MH/SU services and a substantially larger workforce capable of providing the services. If, in addition to growth in the size of the older population, there are also increases in the proportion of older adults that has particular conditions, those increases would further expand the total number of older adults with the conditions and related service needs and workforce requirements.

In the past, population-based surveys of MH/SU conditions have found much higher rates for most MH/SU conditions in younger people than in older people. Table 2-13 illustrates this pattern. The table shows 12-month prevalence rates for 10 DSM-IV-TR mental disorders

TABLE 2-13
12-Month Prevalence of Selected MH/SU Conditions in Community-Living People in the United States by Age Group

	Age Group				
	35-44 (%)	45-54 (%)	55-64 (%)	65-74 (%)	75+ (%)
Mental health conditions					
Depressive disorders	10.0	8.8	6.4	3.7	2.1
Major depressive episode	9.8	8.4	6.4	3.7	2.0
Dysthymic disorder	2.9	3.5	2.1	0.9	0.7
Panic disorder	3.3	3.2	2.1	0.5	1.8
Agoraphobia without panic	1.0	1.3	0.8	0.4	0.2
Social phobia	8.2	7.0	5.2	3.6	1.1
Generalized anxiety disorder	4.7	4.8	4.2	1.8	1.3
Posttraumatic stress disorder	3.4	4.6	3.7	0.8	0.4
Substance use conditions					
Alcohol dependence or abuse	3.0	1.9	0.7	[a]	[a]
Other drug dependence or abuse	1.1	0.5	[a]	[a]	[a]
Summary figures					
One or more of the disorders	20.4	19.8	14.1	8.2	4.8
Two or more of the disorders	9.4	8.4	5.8	2.5	1.8
Three or more of the disorders	4.7	4.3	3.3	0.8	0.5

[a] The prevalence rate from the CPES is less than 0.2 percent.
SOURCE: Center for Multicultural Mental Health Research, 2011.

for community-living people in five age groups. The data come from the CPES conducted from 2001 to 2003 (see Box 2-2).

As shown in the table, rates for each disorder are higher in the groups under age 65 than in the groups age 65-74 and 75 and older. For each of the summary variables, the rates drop steadily from a high in people age 35-44 to a low in people age 75 and older.

Findings from other population-based surveys of MH/SU conditions that have included older adults, such as the ECA survey conducted in the early 1980s, and the NESARC 1, conducted from 2001 to 2002, show the same pattern of higher rates in younger people and a drop-off after age 65. One might expect that the higher rates in younger age groups, for example, the groups age 45-54 and 55-64, would be maintained as people in those age groups become age 65 and older. In fact, rates for some MH/SU conditions in adults age 65 and older have increased since the 1980s, but the increases have been smaller than would be expected if the higher rates in younger age groups had been maintained as they grew older.

The extent to which the pattern of higher rates in younger people and a drop-off after age 65 will be maintained in the future is unclear. A major factor in this context is the aging of the baby boomer cohort. This large cohort of individuals born between 1946 and 1964 was age 46 to 64 in 2010, and its oldest members turned 65 in 2011. Many researchers, clinicians, and others believe that prevalence rates for some MH/SU conditions, particularly alcohol-related and drug-related conditions, will rise substantially in the older population as the baby boomers age. The committee agrees that the prevalence of these conditions will increase in coming decades, but concludes that it is not possible at present to predict the rates or number of older adults who will have the conditions in 2020 or 2030.

Table 2-14 shows 12-month prevalence rates for self-reported alcohol-related and drug-related conditions in community-living adults age 65 and older at 2-year intervals from 2000 and 2010. The data come from the NSDUH.

As shown in the table, rates of alcohol-related conditions in older adults increased by small amounts from 2000 through 2010, with slight variations in the intervening years. Rates for three of the drug-related conditions also increased by small amounts over that period, and rates for drug dependence or abuse were the same in 2000 and 2010. Rates for nonmedical use of prescription pain relievers were not reported for 2000, but were the same in 2002 and 2010, with slight variations in the intervening years.

Tracking changes in age cohorts as they grow older is complicated. It is interesting to note, however, that in 2000, the self-reported rates for binge drinking were 15.8 percent in the group age 55-59 and 11.3 percent

TABLE 2-14
12-Month Prevalence Rates for Alcohol- and Drug-Related Conditions in Adults Age 65 and Older in 2000, 2002, 2004, 2006, 2008, and 2010

	Year					
	2000 N = 2,946 (%)	2002 N = 2,239 (%)	2004 N = 2,393 (%)	2006 N = 2,665 (%)	2008 N = 2,527 (%)	2010 N = 2,500 (%)
Alcohol-related conditions						
Binge alcohol use in the past month[a]	6.1	7.5	6.9	7.6	8.2	7.6
Heavy alcohol use in the past month[b]	1.5	1.4	1.8	1.6	2.2	1.6
Alcohol dependence/abuse in the past year[c]	1.4	1.2	1.4	1.3	1.0	2.0
Drug-related conditions						
Illicit drug use in the past year[d]	0.7	1.3	0.9	1.1	1.4	1.7
Marijuana use in the past month	[e]	0.5	0.3	0.5	0.4	1.0
Nonmedical use of prescription drugs in the past year	0.6	0.7	0.6	0.6	0.9	0.9
Nonmedical use of prescription pain relievers in the past year	[f]	0.4	0.4	0.5	0.8	0.4
Drug dependence/abuse in the past year[c]	0.1	[e]	[e]	0.1	0.2	0.1

[a] Binge alcohol use is defined as drinking five or more drinks on the same occasion (i.e., at the same time or within a couple of hours of each other) on at least 1 day in the past 30 days.

[b] Heavy alcohol use is defined as drinking five or more drinks on the same occasion on each of 5 or more days in the past 30 days; all heavy alcohol users are also binge alcohol users.

[c] See Box 2-1 for definitions.

[d] Illicit drugs are marijuana, cocaine, heroin, hallucinogens, inhalants, and prescription-type psychotherapeutic drugs, including pain relievers, that are used for nonmedical purposes.

[e] Numbers were not reported because of low precision.

[f] Nonmedical use of prescription pain relievers is not reported for the 2000 NSDUH.

SOURCES: CBHSQ, 2012f; Center for Behavioral Health Statistics and Quality, unpublished data from the 2010 National Survey on Drug Use and Health provided to the IOM committee, 2011.

in the group age 60-64. In 2010, when people in these groups were age 65-69 and 70-74, the self-reported rates for binge drinking were 11.0 percent in the group age 65-69 and 8.6 percent in the group age 70-74, compared with only 4 percent in the group age 75 and older. For nonmedical use of prescription drugs, the self-reported rates in 2000 were 2.5 percent in the group age 55-59 and 0.9 percent in the group age 60-64. In 2010, when people in these groups were age 65-69 and 70-74, the self-reported rates for nonmedical use of prescription drugs were 1.3 percent in the group age 65-69, 0.7 percent in the group age 70-74, and 0.7 percent in the group age 75 and older.

One research team has estimated the growth in the number of people with nonmedical use of prescription drugs from 1999 to 2020 for various age groups (Colliver et al., 2006). The researchers predict that the number of people with this condition in the group age 60-69 will increase more than fivefold, from 170,000 people in 1999 to 991,000 people in 2020. The comparable figures are 131,000 to 321,000 people in the group age 70-79 and 31,000 to 70,000 people in the group age 80-89.

Several recent reports on various aspects of illicit drug use also suggest future increases in the older population:

- A 2009 report shows that use of illicit drugs almost doubled, from 5.1 to 9.4 percent, for adults age 50-59 in the period from 2002 and 2007 (Han et al., 2009). The researchers point out that nearly 90 percent of adults age 50-59 who were using illicit drugs in 2007 began using such drugs before age 30, suggesting that illicit drug use is a lifelong habit that is likely to continue as this age group gets older.
- A 2011 report, based on data from the Drug Abuse Warning Network surveillance system, shows that 61 percent of the 1.1 million emergency department (ED) visits for adverse drug reactions in 2008 involved a person age 65 or older and nearly one-quarter of these ED visits were for adverse reactions to central nervous system drugs, including narcotic and nonnarcotic pain relievers (CBHSQ, 2011a).
- A 2011 report on substance use treatment for adults age 55 and older found that the proportion of adults in that age group with first admissions for substance use treatment increased from 2.9 percent in 1998 to 4.4 percent in 2008 (Arndt et al., 2011). Admissions for alcohol treatment were more common than admissions for other drug treatment throughout the 10-year period, but admissions for treatment of marijuana, cocaine, and heroin abuse increased from 1998 to 2008.
- A 2010 report on urine screens for drug use that were conducted in an academic suburban hospital shows that in the period from

2004 to 2009, 2.3 percent of screens for adults age 65 and older were positive for cocaine (Chait et al., 2010).

Another condition for which recent reports suggest possible increases in future prevalence rates in the older population is suicide. As discussed earlier in this section, reported suicide rates have been higher for white men age 85 and older than for any other group for at least the past 60 years, and suicide rates for white men age 75-84 have been second highest in that period (NCHS, 2011a). From 1999 to 2005, average annual suicide rates for whites of all ages increased by 1.1 percent, while average annual suicide rates for blacks decreased by 1.1 percent (Hu et al., 2008). Among whites, average annual suicide rates increased by 3 percent in those age 40-64 and decreased by 1.2 percent for those age 65 and older, and among whites age 40-64, the average annual increase in suicide rates was higher for women than men (3.9 percent versus 2.7 percent, respectively). For women in that age group, suicides by poisoning, including drug-related suicides, increased by an average annual rate of 19.3 percent.

Recent data also show a 49 percent increase in emergency department visits for drug-related suicide attempts in women age 50 and older between 2005 and 2009 (CBHSQ, 2011b). For women in this age group, statistically significant increases were found for ED visits for suicide attempts involving drugs used to treat anxiety and insomnia and some narcotic pain relievers.

In addition to increases in the number of older adults with MH/SU conditions that result from growth in the size of the older population and increases in prevalence rates for particular MH/SU conditions, another factor that will affect the future number of older adults with these conditions is changes in the age composition of the older population. As noted earlier in this chapter, 54 percent of the 40.3 million adults age 65 and older in 2010 were age 65-74, 32 percent were age 75-84, and 14 percent were age 85 and older (Census Bureau, 2011b). As the baby boomer cohort ages, the proportion of the older population that is age 65-74 is projected to increase to 59 percent in 2020 and return to 54 percent in 2030 (Census Bureau, 2011b). The proportion that is age 75-84 is projected to decrease to 29 percent in 2020 and then increase to 34 percent in 2030. The proportion that is age 85 and older is projected to decrease from 14 to 12 percent in 2020 and remain at that level until after 2031, when the oldest baby boomers begin to reach age 85.

Because the prevalence of dementia increases with age (Plassman et al., 2007), growth in the proportion of adults age 75-84 by 2030 is likely to result in larger numbers of older adults with dementia-related behavioral and psychiatric symptoms. It is unclear what, if any, other MH/SU conditions are more prevalent in adults age 75-84 than in those age 65-74 and would therefore increase disproportionately as the oldest baby boomers begin to reach age 75 in 2021.

Likewise, it is unclear what conditions other than suicide and dementia are more prevalent in adults age 85 and older than in those ages 65-74 and 75-84. As the total number of people in the oldest old age group grows from 5.5 million in 2010 to a projected 6.6 million in 2020 and 8.7 million in 2030 (Census Bureau, 2011b), the number with MH/SU conditions is likely to grow proportionately. For particular conditions with high prevalence in this age group, the numbers will likely grow even faster after 2031. More information is needed about the prevalence of particular MH/SU conditions in adults age 75-84 and 85 and older to plan for the services and workforce required to meet their service needs now and in the future.

Changes in the racial and ethnic composition of the older population will probably also affect the number of older adults with MH/SU conditions. From 2010 to 2030, the number of whites age 65 and older will increase by about 60 percent, but the proportion of whites in the older population will decrease from about 80 percent to about 71 percent. In the same period, the number of people in all other racial and ethnic groups will increase by larger proportions: the number of blacks will increase by about 115 percent, and the number of Hispanic/Latinos will increase by more than 200 percent. Blacks, Hispanic/Latinos, and other racial/ethnic groups will also increase as a proportion of the older population. In 2030, blacks will constitute about 10 percent of the older population, up from about 8.5 percent in 2010, and Hispanic/Latinos will constitute about 12 percent of the older population, up from 8 percent in 2010 (Census Bureau, 2008).

Analyses conducted for the committee by the Center for Multicultural Mental Health Research show that the prevalence of DSM-IV-TR mental disorders varies in different racial and ethnic groups. As shown previously (see Table 2-7), prevalence rates for some disorders and for one or more, two or more, and three or more disorders seems to be higher for older Hispanic/Latinos than for older adults in other groups, but these differences have not been tested for statistical significance. If it is true that prevalence rates are higher in the Hispanic/Latino group, the expected growth in the number of older Hispanic/Latinos from 2010 to 2030 will result in further increases in the total number and proportion of older adults with MH/SU conditions. As discussed earlier, various factors have been found to be related to the prevalence of MH/SU conditions in older adults in different racial and ethnic groups, for example, whether the person was born in the United States or elsewhere; how long the person has been in the United States; and the person's gender, education, income, perceived financial strain, and life events. Epidemiologic research is needed to clarify these relationships and their likely impact on future proportions and numbers of older adults with MH/SU conditions in racial and ethnic groups.

Lastly, for veterans who are enrolled in the VA health care system and use VA services, available data on the prevalence of some MH/SU conditions in younger age groups suggest large future increases in the number of veterans with these conditions. Table 2-15 shows the 12-month prevalence of selected MH/SU diagnoses in veterans who used VA health care services in FY 2011 for five age groups.

As shown in the table, the prevalence of each condition and one or more, two or more, and three or more conditions is higher in the groups under age 65 than in the groups ages 65-74 and 75 and older. The prevalence of diagnosed PTSD is very high in the groups ages 35-44 and 55-64. Prevalence rates for some other conditions, notably diagnosed alcohol-related and drug-related conditions, are higher in the group age 45-54. These data indicate that expanded VA services will be required in the future to the meet the needs of larger numbers of older veterans with MH/SU conditions in general, and workforce competencies to address particular conditions will have to be increased.

As noted earlier, people in the baby boom generation have had higher average rates of mental health service use throughout their lives, and their willingness to use such services is expected to continue as they age. No data are available to test this expectation now, but accurate and timely information about service use will be needed in the future for service and workforce planning.

TABLE 2-15
12-Month Prevalence of Selected MH/SU Diagnoses in Veterans Who Used VA Health Care Services in FY 2011 by Age Group

MH/SU Diagnoses	Age Group				
	35-44	45-54	55-64	65-74	75+
Mental health diagnoses					
Major depressive disorder	8.2	8.5	7.0	3.3	1.4
Dysthymic disorder	2.5	2.9	2.8	1.7	1.1

TABLE 2-15 Continued

MH/SU Diagnoses	Age Group				
	35-44	45-54	55-64	65-74	75+
Other mood spectrum disorders	18.0	18.8	16.7	9.7	6.9
Schizophrenia	1.7	3.1	2.4	1.0	0.5
Bipolar disorder	4.3	4.7	2.5	1.2	0.4
Other psychoses	1.0	1.4	1.1	0.6	0.9
Panic disorder	2.0	1.6	1.1	0.5	0.2
Agoraphobia without panic	[a]	[a]	[a]	[a]	[a]
Social phobia	0.2	0.2	0.1	[a]	[a]
Generalized anxiety disorder	2.3	2.1	1.8	1.1	0.8
Posttraumatic stress disorder	15.0	9.6	16.4	6.7	2.5
Substance use diagnoses					
Alcohol dependence or abuse	8.2	12.2	9.7	4.3	1.2
Other drug dependence or abuse	6.0	10.0	5.4	1.1	0.2
Summary figures					
One or more of the diagnoses	35.5	37.8	37.5	20.6	12.2
Two or more of the diagnoses	19.3	20.5	18.2	7.4	2.9
Three or more of the diagnoses	8.9	10.1	7.5	2.4	0.7

[a] Proportion is less than 0.1 percent.

SOURCE: VA, 2012.

SUMMARY OF FINDINGS AND IMPLICATIONS FOR THE GERIATRIC MENTAL HEALTH WORKFORCE

Many older adults have MH/SU conditions. Analyses conducted for this IOM report indicate that in 2010, at least 5.6 million to 8 million adults age 65 and older had one or more of the 27 conditions identified by the committee as likely to have a substantial negative effect on the person's emotional well-being, functional and self-care abilities, and quality of life. These figures represent 14 to 20 percent of the 40.3 million older adults in 2010. The figures constitute a conservative estimate of the number and proportion of older adults with MH/SU conditions for two reasons. First, they are based primarily on data from surveys conducted in nationally representative, population-based samples, and these surveys do not assess all the conditions identified by the committee. In addition, the figures include only older adults with conditions for which adequate information was available to avoid double counting people with more than one condition. As a result, the figures do not include large numbers of older adults with conditions for which information about comorbidity could not be found.

Accurate, up-to-date information about the number and proportion of older adults with MH/SU conditions is essential for analyzing their service needs and planning for a workforce capable of meeting those needs. Assembling the available information about the frequency of these conditions for this report was difficult. Some of the needed information existed but was not readily accessible, and much of the needed information was not available at all. More comprehensive information is essential to support planning for MH/SU services for older adults and related workforce requirements. Much of this planning occurs at the state and local levels, so the needed information includes not only national-level data, but also state- and local-level data.

The 27 MH/SU conditions identified by the committee include 15 conditions that are defined as mental disorders in the DSM-IV-TR. The other 12 conditions are symptoms or clusters of symptoms that are not defined as mental disorders in the DSM-IV-TR. In general, more information is available about the proportion and number of older adults with DSM-IV-TR-defined mental disorders, but the committee did not find data to support estimates of the number or proportion of older adults with two of the DSM-IV-TR mental disorders, and the accuracy of the available data on three other DSM-IV-TR conditions is unclear.

For the 5.6 million to 8 million adults age 65 and older with one or more MH/SU conditions, the most prevalent conditions were DSM-IV-TR depressive disorders and behavioral and psychiatric symptoms associated with dementia. The available data indicate that 1.8 million to 2.4 million older adults had depressive disorders in 2010, and 2.2 million to 2.9 million older adults had behavioral and psychiatric symptoms associated with dementia. The numbers are smaller but still substantial for other conditions included in the totals, for example, social phobia and generalized anxiety disorder, each of which affects up to 800,000 or more older adults. The range of figures for these conditions is wide, however. The ranges for PTSD and alcohol dependence or abuse are even wider (200,000 to 1 million older adults for PTSD and less than 50,000 to 700,000 for alcohol dependence or abuse).

Several DSM-IV-TR mental disorders, including bipolar disorder and schizophrenia, constitute the core of a category of conditions, SMI, that create a high need for treatment, usually involving specialty mental health providers and services. The committee defined SMI to include those two conditions plus nonaffective psychoses and major depressive disorder that is not responsive to treatment. Based on this definition and information assembled for this report, the committee estimates that 1.4 million to 1.9 million older adults had SMI in 2010. These figures represent 3 to 4.8 percent of the older population.

Large proportions of older adults who have MH/SU conditions also have coexisting acute and chronic physical health conditions, and some have cognitive and functional impairments. These coexisting conditions are a defining feature of the geriatric mental health and substance use fields. They often complicate the detection, diagnosis, treatment, and ongoing management of MH/SU conditions; they also result in difficult caregiving situations for families, physicians, and other health care professionals, and residential care and home- and community-based service providers; and they may affect the types of MH/SU treatments and other services that are likely to work best and the care settings where these treatments and services should be delivered. Certainly they create important requirements for workforce competencies, including ability to detect possible MH/SU conditions in older adults with coexisting physical health conditions and cognitive and functional impairments; ability to diagnosis the conditions or knowledge about how to refer the person for a diagnostic evaluation; and ability to adapt treatments and ongoing management to accommodate the coexisting conditions.

A substantial proportion of older adults with MH/SU conditions live in nursing homes and other congregate-living settings, such as assisted living, senior housing, and public housing facilities. Practical and effective approaches for delivering MH/SU services differ for older adults in congregate-living settings versus older adults in single-family housing in the community, but the needed skills and competencies for staff working with older adults with MH/SU conditions in various kinds of congregate-living settings are similar. The development of a workforce with these skills and competencies is a high priority for improving care for older adults with MH/SU conditions.

Race and ethnicity are associated not only with likely differences in the prevalence of MH/SU conditions, but also with the kinds of treatment and services that are needed and will be used. As the racial and ethnic diversity of the older population increases, the need for diversity training and language competencies will also increase. MH/SU assessment procedures and service models will have to be adapted to meet the needs of the wide array of racial and ethnic subgroups.

Finally, it is clear that older veterans, at least those who are enrolled in the VA health care system and use VA health care services, are more likely than other older adults to have MH/SU conditions and to have particular conditions that influence their service needs. Workforce competencies within the VA health care system and awareness among non-VA health care professionals and service providers of referral procedures for veterans who will benefit from VA MH/SU services are essential to meet the needs of these veterans.

REFERENCES

Abrams, R. C., M. Lachs, G. McAvay, D. J. Keohane, and M. L. Bruce. 2002. Predictors of self-neglect in community-dwelling elders. *American Journal of Psychiatry* 159(10):1724-1730.

Acierno, R., K. Brady, M. Gray, D. Kilpatrick, D. Resnick, and C. Best. 2002. Psychopathology following interpersonal violence: A comparison of risk factors in older and younger adults. *Journal of Clinical Geropsychology* 8:13-23.

AHCA (American Health Care Association). 2010. *OSCAR data report: Nursing facility patient characteristics report.* June update. http://www.ahcancal.org/research_data/oscar_data/NursingFacilityPatientCharacteristics/HISTORICAL_HSNF_OSCAR%20Data%20Report_2010Q2.pdf (accessed June 6, 2012).

AHRQ (Agency for Healthcare Research and Quality). 2009a. Online data tables, Table 1: Number of people with care for selected conditions by type of service, United States, 2009, age 65-90. Medical Expenditure Panel Survey. http://meps.ahrq.gov/mepsweb/data_stats/tables_compendia_hh_interactive.jsp?File=HCFY2009&Table=HCFY2009_CNDXP_A&TCOPT1=&TCOPT2=&ModPopCheck=Yes&ModPop=Yes&_Debug=&DDAGELOW=65&DDAGEHIGH=90&Action.x=196&Action.y=19 (accessed February 22, 2012).

———. 2009b. Online data tables, Table 3: Total expenses and percent distribution for selected conditions by type of service, United States, 2009, age 65-90. Medical Expenditure Panel Survey. http://meps.ahrq.gov/mepsweb/data_stats/tables_compendia_hh_interactive.jsp?File=HCFY2009&Table=HCFY2009_CNDXP_C&TCOPT1=&TCOPT2=&ModPopCheck=Yes&ModPop=Yes&_Debug=&DDAGELOW=65&DDAGEHIGH=90&Action.x=191&Action.y=12 (accessed February 22, 2012).

———. 2009c. Online data tables, Table 4: Total expenses and percent distribution for selected conditions by source of payment, United States, 2009, age 65-90. Medical Expenditure Panel Survey. http://meps.ahrq.gov/mepsweb/data_stats/tables_compendia_hh_interactive.jsp?File=HCFY2009&Table=HCFY2009_CNDXP_D&TCOPT1=&TCOPT2=&ModPopCheck=Yes&ModPop=Yes&_Debug=&DDAGELOW=65&DDAGEHIGH=90&Action.x=123&Action.y=12 (accessed February 22, 2012).

Akincigil, A., M. Olfson, J. T. Walkup, M. J. Siegel, E. Kalay, S. Amin, K. A. Zurlo, and S. Crystal. 2011. Diagnosis and treatment of depression in older community-dwelling adults: 1992-2005. *Journal of the American Geriatrics Society* 59(6):1042-1051.

Alegria, M., N. Mulvaney-Day, M. Torres, A. Polo, Z. Cao, and G. Canino. 2007. Prevalence of psychiatric disorders across Latino subgroups in the United States. *American Journal of Public Health* 97(1):68-75.

Alexopoulos, G. S. 2005. Depression in the elderly. *Lancet* 365(9475):1961-1970.

APA (American Psychological Association). 2000. *Diagnostic and statistical manual of mental disorders: DSM-IV-TR, 4th ed.* Washington, DC: APA.

———. 2010. *DSM-5 development: F 02 hoarding disorder.* http://www.dsm5.org/ProposedRevision/Pages/proposedrevision.aspx?rid=398 (accessed February 22, 2012).

Aranda, M. P., D. H. Chae, K. D. Lincoln, R. J. Taylor, A. T. Woodward, and L. M. Chatters. 2011. Demographic correlates of DSM-IV major depressive disorder among older African Americans, black Caribbeans, and non-Hispanic whites: Results from the National Survey of American Life. *International Journal of Geriatric Psychiatry.* Epub. Oct. 28, doi:10:1002/gps.2805.

Arndt, S., C. L. Turvey, and M. Flaum. 2002. Older offenders, substance abuse, and treatment. *American Journal of Geriatric Psychiatry* 10(6):733-739.

Arndt, S., R. Clayton, and S. K. Schultz. 2011. Trends in substance abuse treatment 1998-2008: Increasing older adult first-time admissions for illicit drugs. *American Journal of Geriatric Psychiatry* 19(8):704-711.

Aschbrenner, K., D. C. Grabowski, S. Cai, S. J. Bartels, and V. Mor. 2011. Nursing home admissions and long-stay conversions among persons with and without serious mental illness. *Journal of Aging and Social Policy* 23(3):286-304.

Ayers, C. R., S. Saxena, S. Golshan, and J. L. Wetherell. 2010. Age at onset and clinical features of late life compulsive hoarding. *International Journal of Geriatric Psychiatry* 25(2):142-149.

Banta, J. E., R. M. Andersen, A. S. Young, G. Kominski, and W. E. Cunningham. 2010. Psychiatric comorbidity and mortality among veterans hospitalized for congestive heart failure. *Military Medicine* 175(10):732-741.

Bartels, S. J. 2004. Caring for the whole person: Integrated health care for older adults with severe mental illness and medical comorbidity. *Journal of the American Geriatrics Society* 52(Suppl.12):S249-S257.

———. 2011. Commentary: The forgotten older adult with serious mental illness: The final challenge in achieving the promise of Olmstead? *Journal of Aging and Social Policy* 23(3):244-257.

Bartels, S. J., E. Coakley, T. E. Oxman, G. Constantino, D. Oslin, H. Chen, C. Zubritsky, K. Cheal, U. N. B. Durai, J. J. Gallo, M. Llorente, and H. Sanchez. 2002. Suicidal and death ideation in older primary care patients with depression, anxiety, and at-risk alcohol use. *American Journal of Geriatric Psychiatry* 10(4):417-427.

Beck, A. T., M. Kovacs, and A. Weissman. 1979. Assessment of suicidal intention: The Scale for Suicide Ideation. *Journal of Consulting and Clinical Psychology* 47(2):343-352.

Becker, M., L. Schonfeld, and P. G. Stiles. 2002. Assisted living: The new frontier for mental health care. *Generations* 26(1):72-77.

Berks, J., and R. McCormick. 2008. Screening for alcohol misuse in elderly primary care patients: A systematic literature review. *International Psychogeriatrics* 20(6):1090-1103.

Black, S. A., K. S. Markides, and T. Q. Miller. 1998. Correlates of depressive symptomatology among older community-dwelling Mexican Americans: The Hispanic EPESE. *Journals of Gerontology, Series B: Psychological Sciences and Social Sciences* 53(4):S198-S208.

Blazer, D. G. 2000. Psychiatry and the oldest old. *American Journal of Psychiatry* 157(12):1915-1924.

———. 2003. Depression in late life: Review and commentary. *Journals of Gerontology, Series A: Biological Sciences and Medical Sciences* 58(3):M249-M265.

Blazer, D. G., and L. T. Wu. 2009a. The epidemiology of at-risk and binge drinking among middle-aged and elderly community adults: National Survey on Drug Use and Health. *American Journal of Psychiatry* 166(10):1162-1169.

———. 2009b. The epidemiology of substance use and disorders among middle aged and elderly community adults: National Survey on Drug Use and Health. *American Journal of Geriatric Psychiatry* 17(3):237-245.

———. 2009c. Nonprescription use of pain relievers by middle-aged and elderly community-living adults: National Survey on Drug Use and Health. *Journal of the American Geriatrics Society* 57(7):1252-1257.

———. 2011. The epidemiology of alcohol use disorders and subthreshold dependence in a middle-aged and elderly community sample. *American Journal of Geriatric Psychiatry* 19(8):685-694.

Blazer, D., D. C. Hughes, and L. K. George. 1987. The epidemiology of depression in an elderly community population. *Gerontologist* 27(3):281-287.

Blazer, D., C. Hybels, E. Simonsick, and J. T. Hanlon. 2000a. Marked differences in antidepressant use by race in an elderly community sample: 1986-1996. *American Journal of Psychiatry* 157(7):1089-1094.

———. 2000b. Sedative, hypnotic, and antianxiety medication use in an aging cohort over ten years: A racial comparison. *Journal of the American Geriatrics Society* 48(9):1073-1079.

Blazer, D., C. Hybels, and J. Hays. 2004. Demography and epidemiology of psychiatric disorders in late life. In *Textbook of geriatric psychiatry*, edited by D. G. Blazer and E. W. Busse. Arlington, VA: American Psychiatric Publishing, Inc.

Blow, F. C. 1998. *Substance abuse among older adults: Treatment improvement protocol (TIP) series 26.* Pub. No. (SMA) 98-3179. Rockville, MD: Substance Abuse and Mental Health Services Administration.

Blow, F. C., and K. L. Barry. 2002. Use and misuse of alcohol among older women. *Alcohol Research and Health* 26(4):308-315.

Blow, F. C., A. S. B. Bohnert, M. A. Ilgen, R. V. Ignacio, J. F. McCarthy, M. Valenstein, and K. Knox. 2012. Suicide mortality among patients treated by the Veterans Health Administration from 2000 to 2008. *American Journal of Public Health* 102(Suppl. 1):S98-S104.

Booth, B. M., F. C. Blow, and C. A. Cook. 1998. Functional impairment and co-occurring psychiatric disorders in medically hospitalized men. *Archives of Internal Medicine* 158(14): 1551-1559.

Booth, B. M., F. C. Blow, and C. A. Loveland Cook. 2001. Persistence of impaired functioning and psychological distress after medical hospitalization for men with co-occurring psychiatric and substance use disorders. *Journal of General Internal Medicine* 16(1):57-65.

Borson, S. 2010. Posttraumatic stress disorder and dementia: A lifelong cost of war. *Journal of the American Geriatrics Society* 58(9):1798-1799.

Borson, S., S. J. Bartels, C. C. Colenda, G. L. Gottlieb, and B. Meyers. 2001. Geriatric mental health services research: Strategic plan for an aging population: Report of the Health Services Work Group of the American Association for Geriatric Psychiatry. *American Journal of Geriatric Psychiatry* 9(3):191-204.

Boustani, M., S. Zimmerman, C. S. Williams, A. L. Gruber-Baldini, L. Watson, P. S. Reed, and P. D. Sloane. 2005. Characteristics associated with behavioral symptoms related to dementia in long-term care residents. *Gerontologist* 45(Spec. 1):56-61.

Brady, K. T. 1997. Posttraumatic stress disorder and comorbidity: Recognizing the many faces of PTSD. *Journal of Clinical Psychiatry* 58(Suppl. 9):12-15.

Breslau, J., and D. F. Chang. 2006. Psychiatric disorders among foreign-born and U.S.-born Asian-Americans in a U.S. national survey. *Social Psychiatry and Psychiatric Epidemiology* 41(12):943-950.

Brookmeyer, R., S. Gray, and C. Kawas. 1998. Projections of Alzheimer's disease in the United States and the public health impact of delaying disease onset. *American Journal of Public Health* 88(9):1337-1342.

Brown, E. L., G. J. McAvay, P. J. Raue, S. Moses, and M. L. Bruce. 2003. Recognition of depression among elderly recipients of home care services. *Psychiatric Services* 54(2):208-213.

Bruce, M. L., and P. J. Leaf. 1989. Psychiatric disorders and 15-month mortality in a community sample of older adults. *American Journal of Public Health* 79(6):727-730.

Bruce, M. L., T. E. Seeman, S. S. Merrill, and D. G. Blazer. 1994. The impact of depressive symptomatology on physical disability: Macarthur Studies of Successful Aging. *American Journal of Public Health* 84(11):1796-1799.

Bruce, M. L., G. J. McAvay, P. J. Raue, E. L. Brown, B. S. Meyers, D. J. Keohane, D. R. Jagoda, and C. Weber. 2002. Major depression in elderly home health care patients. *American Journal of Psychiatry* 159(8):1367-1374.

Bryant, C., H. Jackson, and D. Ames. 2008. The prevalence of anxiety in older adults: Methodological issues and a review of the literature. *Journal of Affective Disorders* 109(3):233-250.

———. 2009. Depression and anxiety in medically unwell older adults: Prevalence and short-term course. *International Psychogeriatrics* 21(4):754-763.

Caffrey, C., M. Sengupta, E. Park-Lee, A. J. Moss, E. Rosenoff, and L. D. Harris-Kojetin. 2012. Residents living in residential care facilities: United States, 2010. NCHS Data Brief No. 91, National Center for Health Statistics, Centers for Disease Control and Prevention, Hyattsville, MD, April.

Casey, P., and S. Bailey. 2011. Adjustment disorders: The state of the art. *World Psychiatry* 10(1):11-18.

CBHSQ (Center for Behavioral Health Statistics and Quality). 2011a. National Survey on Drug Use and Health. 2011a. *The DAWN Report. Emergency department visits involving adverse reactions to medications among older adults.* Substance Abuse and Mental Health Services Administration. Rockville, MD: SAMHSA.

———. 2011b. National Survey on Drug Use and Health. *The DAWN Report. Trends in emergency department visits for drug-related suicide attempts among females: 2005 and 2009.* Rockville, MD: SAMHSA.

———. 2011c. National Survey on Drug Use and Health. *Table 1.11A—illicit drug use in lifetime, past year, and past month, by detailed age category: Numbers in thousands, 2009 and 2010.* http://oas.samhsa.gov/NSDUH/2k10NSDUH/tabs/Sect1peTabs1to46.htm#Tab1.11A (accessed February 22, 2012).

———. 2011d. National Survey on Drug Use and Health. *Table 1.11B—illict drug use in lifetime, past year, and past month, by detailed age category: Percentages, 2009 and 2010.* http://oas.samhsa.gov/NSDUH/2k10NSDUH/tabs/Sect1peTabs1to46.htm#Tab1.11B (accessed February 22, 2012).

———. 2011e. National Survey on Drug Use and Health. *Table 1.12A—marijuana use in lifetime, past year, and past month, by detailed age category: Numbers in thousands, 2009 and 2010.* http://oas.samhsa.gov/NSDUH/2k10NSDUH/tabs/Sect1peTabs1to46.htm#Tab1.12A (accessed February 22, 2012).

———. 2011f. National Survey on Drug Use and Health. *Table 1.12B—marijuana use in lifetime, past year, and past month, by detailed age category: Percentages, 2009 and 2010.* http://oas.samhsa.gov/NSDUH/2k10NSDUH/tabs/Sect1peTabs1to46.htm#Tab1.12B (accessed February 22, 2012).

———. 2011g. National Survey on Drug Use and Health. *Table 1.17A—nonmedical use of prescription-type psychotherapeutics in lifetime, past year, and past month, by detailed age category: Numbers in thousands, 2009 and 2010.* http://oas.samhsa.gov/NSDUH/2k10NSDUH/tabs/Sect1peTabs1to46.htm#Tab1.17A (accessed February 22, 2012).

———. 2011h. National Survey on Drug Use and Health. *Table 1.17B—nonmedical use of prescription-type psychotherapeutics in lifetime, past year, and past month, by detailed age category: Percentages, 2009 and 2010.* http://oas.samhsa.gov/NSDUH/2k10NSDUH/tabs/Sect1peTabs1to46.htm#Tab1.17B (accessed February 22, 2012).

———. 2011i. National Survey on Drug Use and Health. *Table 1.18A—nonmedical use of pain relievers in lifetime, past year, and past month, by detailed age category: Numbers in thousands, 2009 and 2010.* http://oas.samhsa.gov/NSDUH/2k10NSDUH/tabs/Sect1peTabs1to46.htm#Tab1.18A (accessed February 22, 2012).

———. 2011j. National Survey on Drug Use and Health. *Table 1.18B—nonmedical use of pain relievers in lifetime, past year, and past month, by detailed age category: Percentages, 2009 and 2010.* http://oas.samhsa.gov/NSDUH/2k10NSDUH/tabs/Sect1peTabs1to46.htm#Tab1.18B (accessed February 22, 2012).

———. 2011k. National Survey on Drug Use and Health. *Table 2.16A—alcohol use, binge alcohol use, and heavy alcohol use in the past month, by detailed age category: Numbers in thousands, 2009 and 2010.* http://oas.samhsa.gov/NSDUH/2k10NSDUH/tabs/Sect2peTabs1to42.htm#Tab2.16A (accessed February 22, 2012).

———. 2011l. National Survey on Drug Use and Health. *Table 2.16B—alcohol use, binge alcohol use, and heavy alcohol use in the past month, by detailed age category: Percentages, 2009 and 2010.* http://oas.samhsa.gov/NSDUH/2k10NSDUH/tabs/Sect2peTabs1to42.htm#Tab2.16B (accessed February 22, 2012).

———. 2011m. National Survey on Drug Use and Health. *Table 5.3A—substance dependence or abuse in the past year, by detailed age category: in thousands, 2009 and 2010.* http://oas.samhsa.gov/NSDUH/2k10NSDUH/tabs/Sect5peTabs1to13.pdf (accessed February 22, 2012).

———. 2011n. National Survey on Drug Use and Health. *Table 8.IN—survey sample size for respondents aged 12 or older, by general and detailed age category: 2009 and 2010.* http://oas.samhsa.gov/NSDUH/2k10NSDUH/tabs/Sect8peTabs1to13.htm (accessed February 22, 2012).

———. 2012a. *Mental health, United States, 2010.* HHS Pub No.(SMA) 12-4681, Rockville, MD: Substance Abuse and Mental Health Services Administration.

———. 2012b. National Survey on Drug Use and Health. Appendix B.4.3: Estimation of serious and other levels of mental illness. In *Results from the 2010 National Survey on Drug Use and Health: Mental health findings.* http://www.samhsa.gov/data/nsduh/2k10MH_Findings/2k10MHResults.htm (accessed February 22, 2012)

———. 2012c. National Survey on Drug Use and Health. *Table 1.46B—had serious thoughts of suicide in the past year among persons aged 18 or older, by gender and detailed age category: Percentages, 2009 and 2010.* http://www.samhsa.gov/data/NSDUH/2k10MH_Findings/2k10MH_DTables/Sect1peMHtabs.htm#Tab1.46B (accessed February 22, 2012).

———. 2012d. National Survey on Drug Use and Health. *Table 1.6B—serious mental illness in the past year among persons aged 18 or older, by gender and detailed age category: Percentages, 2009 and 2010.* http://www.samhsa.gov/data/NSDUH/2k10MH_Findings/2k10MH_Dtables/Sect1peMHtabs.htm#Tab1.6B (accessed February 22, 2012).

———. 2012e. National Survey on Drug Use and Health. *Table 1.61A—serious psychological distress in the past month among persons aged 18 or older, by gender and detailed age category: Numbers in thousands, 2009 and 2010.* http://www.samhsa.gov/data/NSDUH/2k10MH_Findings/2k10MH_DTables/Sect1peMHtabs.htm#Tab1.61A (accessed February 22, 2012).

———. 2012f. National Survey on Drug Use and Health. *Detailed tables from the National Surveys on Drug Use and Health.* http://www.oas.samhsa.gov/WebOnly.htm#NSDUHtabs (accessed February 22, 2012).

CDC (Centers for Disease Control and Prevention) and National Association of Chronic Disease Directors. 2008. *The state of mental health and aging in America. Issue Brief 1: What do the data tell us?* http://www.cdc.gov/aging/pdf/mental_health.pdf (accessed February 23, 2012).

Census Bureau. 2008. *U.S. population projections, released 2008 (based on Census 2000), calculated from summary tables 14, 15, 16, 17, 18, 19, and 20.* http://www.census.gov/population/www/projections/summarytables.html (accessed June 8, 2012).

———. 2010a. *Decennial management division glossary.* http://www.census.gov/dmd/www/glossary.html (accessed February 22, 2012).

———. 2010b. *Table qt-p13, group quarters population by sex, age, and type of group quarters: 2010.* Economic and Statistics Administration. http://factfinder2.census.gov/faces/tableservices/jsf/pages/productview.xhtml?pid=DEC_10_SF1_QTP13&prodType=table (accessed February 22, 2012).

———. 2010c. *Table s2101: Veteran status: 2010 American community survey 1-year estimates.* http://factfinder2.census.gov/faces/tableservices/jsf/pages/productview.xhtml?pid=ACS_10_1YR_S2101&prodType=table (accessed March 7, 2012).

———. 2010d. *Table s2601b: Characteristics of the group quarters population by group quarters type.* http://factfinder2.census.gov/faces/tableservices/jsf/pages/productview.xhtml?pid=ACS_10_1YR_S2601B&prodType=table (accessed February 22, 2012).

———. 2011a. *Age and sex composition: 2010.* 2010 Census Briefs. Washington, DC: Economics and Statistics Administration, May.

———. 2011b. *Statistical abstract of the United States: 2011. Table 8. Resident population projections by sex and age: 2010 to 2050.* http://www.census.gov/prod/2011pubs/11statab/pop.pdf (accessed February 22, 2012).

———. 2011c. *Statistical abstract of the United States: 2011. Table 11. Resident population projections by race, Hispanic-origin status, and age: 2010 and 2015.* http://www.census.gov/prod/2011pubs/11statab/pop.pdf (accessed February 22, 2012).

Center for Multicultural Mental Health Research. 2011. Data provided to the IOM committee, Cambridge Health Alliance and Harvard Medical School, Somerville, MA, November.

Chachamovich, E., M. Fleck, K. Laidlaw, and M. Power. 2008. Impact of major depression and subsyndromal symptoms on quality of life and attitudes toward aging in an international sample of older adults. *Gerontologist* 48(5):593-602.

Chait, R., S. Fahmy, and J. Caceres. 2010. Cocaine abuse in older adults: An underscreened cohort. *Journal of the American Geriatrics Society* 58(2):390-391.

Chan, D. C., J. D. Kasper, B. S. Black, and P. V. Rabins. 2003. Prevalence and correlates of behavioral and psychiatric symptoms in community-dwelling elders with dementia or mild cognitive impairment: The Memory and Medical Care Study. *International Journal of Geriatric Psychiatry* 18(2):174-182.

Chiriboga, D. A., S. A. Black, M. Aranda, and K. Markides. 2002. Stress and depressive symptoms among Mexican American elders. *Journals of Gerontology, Series B: Psychological Sciences and Social Sciences* 57(6):P559-P568.

Chung, M. C., J. Werrett, Y. Easthope, and S. Farmer. 2004. Coping with post-traumatic stress: Young, middle-aged and elderly comparisons. *International Journal of Geriatric Psychiatry* 19(4):333-343.

Chung, M. C., K. J. McKee, C. Austin, H. Barkby, H. Brown, S. Cash, J. Ellingford, L. Hanger, and T. Pais. 2009. Posttraumatic stress disorder in older people after a fall. *International Journal of Geriatric Psychiatry* 24(9):955-964.

Clark, R. E., Y. Leung, W.-C. Lin, F. C. Little, and E. O'Connell. 2009. *Twelve-month diagnosed prevalence of mental illness, substance use disorders, and medical comorbidity in Massachusetts Medicare and Medicaid members aged 55 and over.* Shrewsbury, MA: UMass Medical School, Center for Health Policy and Research.

Clemans-Cope, L., and T. Waidmann. 2011. Improving care for dual eligibles through innovations in financing. *New England Journal of Medicine* 365(11):e21.

CMS (Centers for Medicare & Medicaid Services). 2010. *Medicare & Medicaid statistical supplement, table 2.1. Medicare enrollment: Hospital insurance and/or supplemental medical insurance programs for total, fee-for-service, and managed care enrollees as of July 1, 2009: Selected calendar years 1966-2009.* https://www.cms.gov/MedicareMedicaidStatSupp/09_2010.asp (accessed June 6, 2012).

———. 2011. *Chronic conditions among Medicare beneficiaries, chart book, chronic conditions data tables, section_1_Data_Tables, data table for figures 1.1a-1.1d. Percentage of Medicare beneficiaries with the 15 selected chronic conditions, 2008.* http://www.cms.gov/TheChartSeries/02_5_ChronicConditionsChartBook.asp (accessed June 6, 2012).

Cohen, B. J., G. Nestadt, J. F. Samuels, A. J. Romanoski, P. R. McHugh, and P. V. Rabins. 1994. Personality disorder in later life: A community study. *British Journal of Psychiatry* 165(4):493-499.

Cohen, C. I., G. D. Cohen, K. Blank, C. Gaitz, I. R. Katz, A. Leuchter, G. Maletta, B. Meyers, K. Sakauye, and C. Shamoian. 2000. Schizophrenia and older adults. An overview: Directions for research and policy. *American Journal of Geriatric Psychiatry* 8(1):19-28.

Cohen, G. D. 1996. The special case of mental health in later life—the obvious has been overlooked. *American Journal of Geriatric Psychiatry* 4(1):17-23.

Cohen-Mansfield, J., and J. Frank. 2008. Relationship between perceived needs and assessed needs for services in community-dwelling older persons. *Gerontologist* 48(4):505-516.

Cohen-Mansfield, J., M. S. Marx, and A. S. Rosenthal. 1989. A description of agitation in a nursing home. *Journals of Gerontology* 44(3):M77-M84.

Colliver, J. D., W. M. Compton, J. C. Gfroerer, and T. Condon. 2006. Projecting drug use among aging baby boomers in 2020. *Annals of Epidemiology* 16(4):257-265.

Colton, C. W., and R. W. Manderscheid. 2006. Congruencies in increased mortality rates, years of potential life lost, and causes of death among public mental health clients in eight states. *Preventing Chronic Disease* 3(2):A42.

Cook, J. M., J. I. Ruzek, and E. Cassidy. 2003. Possible association of posttraumatic stress disorder with cognitive impairment among older adults. *Psychiatric Services* 54(9):1223-1225.

Cook, J. M., J. D. Elhai, E. L. Cassidy, J. I. Ruzek, G. D. Ram, and J. I. Sheikh. 2005. Assessment of trauma exposure and post-traumatic stress in long-term care veterans: Preliminary data on psychometrics and post-traumatic stress disorder prevalence. *Military Medicine* 170(10):862-866.

Cooley, S. G., and S. Asthana. 2010. Dementia care for veterans: Enhancing comprehensive, coordinated services. *Generations* 34(2):57-63.

Coryell, W., J. Fiedorowicz, D. Solomon, and J. Endicott. 2009. Age transitions in the course of bipolar I disorder. *Psychological Medicine* 39(8):1247-1252.

Coughlin, T., T. Waidmann, and M. O. Watts. 2009. *Where does the burden lie? Medicaid and Medicare spending for dual eligible beneficiaries.* Kaiser Family Foundation, April.

Crosby, A. E., L. Ortega, and M. R. Stevens. 2011. Suicides—United States, 1999-2007. *MMWR Surveillance Summary* 60(Suppl.):56-59.

Crystal, S., U. Sambamoorthi, J. T. Walkup, and A. Akincigil. 2003. Diagnosis and treatment of depression in the elderly Medicare population: Predictors, disparities, and trends. *Journal of the American Geriatrics Society* 51(12):1718-1728.

Cummings, J. L., M. Mega, K. Gray, S. Rosenberg-Thompson, D. A. Carusi, and J. Gornbein. 1994. The neuropsychiatric inventory: Comprehensive assessment of psychopathology in dementia. *Neurology* 44(12):2308-2314.

Dallam, D. L., T. A. Mellman, A. Bhatnagar, S. Nguyen, and M. Kurukumbi. 2011. Trauma reenactments in aging veterans with dementia. *Journal of the American Geriatrics Society* 59(4):766-768.

Degenhardt, L., W. T. Chiu, N. Sampson, R. C. Kessler, and J. C. Anthony. 2007. Epidemiological patterns of extra-medical drug use in the United States: Evidence from the National Comorbidity Survey Replication, 2001-2003. *Drug and Alcohol Dependence* 90(2-3):210-223.

Delbaere, K., J. C. T. Close, H. Brodaty, P. Sachdev, and S. R. Lord. 2010. Determinants of disparities between perceived and physiological risk of falling among elderly people: Cohort study. *British Medical Journal* 341:c4165.

Depp, C. A., and D. V. Jeste. 2004. Bipolar disorder in older adults: A critical review. *Bipolar Disorders* 6(5):343-367.

Devanand, D. P., N. Turret, B. J. Moody, L. Fitzsimons, S. Peyser, K. Mickle, M. S. Nobler, and S. P. Roose. 2000. Personality disorders in elderly patients with dysthymic disorder. *American Journal of Geriatric Psychiatry* 8(3):188-195.

Dirkzwager, A. J., I. Bramsen, and H. M. van der Ploeg. 2001. The longitudinal course of posttraumatic stress disorder symptoms among aging military veterans. *Journal of Nervous and Mental Disease* 189(12):846-853.

Dixon, L., A. Lyles, C. Smith, J. S. Hoch, M. Fahey, L. Postrado, A. Lucksted, and A. Lehman. 2001. Use and costs of ambulatory care services among Medicare enrollees with schizophrenia. *Psychiatric Services* 52(6):786-792.

Dong, X. Q., M. Simon, and D. Evans. 2010. Cross-sectional study of the characteristics of reported elder self-neglect in a community-dwelling population: Findings from a population-based cohort. *Gerontology* 56(3):325-334.

Dowling, G. J., S. R. Weiss, and T. P. Condon. 2008. Drugs of abuse and the aging brain. *Neuropsychopharmacology* 33(2):209-218.

Druss, B. G. 2010. The changing face of U.S. mental health care. *American Journal of Psychiatry* 167(12):1419-1421.

Druss, B. G., and S. A. von Esenwein. 2006. Improving general medical care for persons with mental and addictive disorders: Systematic review. *General Hospital Psychiatry* 28(2):145-153.

Druss, B. G., and E. R. Walker. 2011. *Mental disorders and medical comorbidity.* Synthesis Project, Research Synthesis Report No. 21, Princeton, NJ: Robert Wood Johnson Foundation.

Druss, B. G., L. Zhao, S. Von Esenwein, E. H. Morrato, and S. C. Marcus. 2011. Understanding excess mortality in persons with mental illness: 17-year follow up of a nationally representative U.S. survey. *Medical Care* 49(6):599-604.

Epstein, E. E., K. Fischer-Elber, and Z. Al-Otaiba. 2007. Women, aging, and alcohol use disorders. *Journal of Women & Aging* 19(1/2):31-48.

Flint, A. J. 2002. The complexity and challenge of non-major depression in late life. *American Journal of Geriatric Psychiatry* 10(3):229-232.

Ford, B. C., K. M. Bullard, R. J. Taylor, A. K. Toler, H. W. Neighbors, and J. S. Jackson. 2007. Lifetime and 12-month prevalence of Diagnostic and Statistical Manual of Mental Disorders, 4th edition disorders among older African Americans: Findings from the national survey of American life. *American Journal of Geriatric Psychiatry* 15(8):652-659.

Forstmeier, S., and A. Maercker. 2007. Comparison of two diagnostic systems for complicated grief. *Journal of Affective Disorders* 99:203-211.

Frost, R. O., G. Steketee, and L. Williams. 2000. Hoarding: A community health problem. *Health and Social Care in the Community* 8(4):229-234.

Fullerton, C. A., T. G. McGuire, Z. Feng, V. Mor, and D. C. Grabowski. 2009. Trends in mental health admissions to nursing homes, 1999-2005. *Psychiatric Services* 60(7):965-971.

Gaboda, D., J. Lucas, M. Siegel, E. Kalay, and S. Crystal. 2011. No longer undertreated? Depression diagnosis and antidepressant therapy in elderly long-stay nursing home residents, 1999 to 2007. *Journal of the American Geriatrics Society* 59(4):673-680.

Gallo, J. J., J. C. Anthony, and B. O. Muthen. 1994. Age differences in the symptoms of depression: A latent trait analysis. *Journals of Gerontology* 49(6):P251-P264.

Gallo, J. J., P. V. Rabins, and J. C. Anthony. 1999. Sadness in older persons: 13-year follow-up of a community sample in Baltimore, Maryland. *Psychological Medicine* 29(2):341-350.

Garfield, R. L. 2011. *Mental health financing in the United States: A primer.* Kaiser Commission on Medicaid and the Uninsured, Washington, DC, April.

Garrido, M. M., R. L. Kane, M. Kaas, and R. A. Kane. 2011. Use of mental health care by community-dwelling older adults. *Journal of the American Geriatrics Society* 59(1):50-56.

Gauthier, S., J. Cummings, C. Ballard, H. Brodaty, G. Grossberg, P. Robert, and C. Lyketsos. 2010. Management of behavioral problems in Alzheimer's disease. *International Psychogeriatrics* 22(3):346-372.

German, P. S., S. Shapiro, and E. A. Skinner. 1985. Mental health of the elderly: Use of health and mental health services. *Journal of the American Geriatrics Society* 33(4):246-252.

Gilmer, T. P., V. D. Ojeda, D. Fuentes, V. Criado, and P. Garcia. 2009. Access to public mental health services among older adults with severe mental illness. *International Journal of Geriatric Psychiatry* 24(3):313-318.

Gleason, P. P., R. Schulz, N. L. Smith, J. T. Newsom, P. D. Kroboth, F. J. Kroboth, and B. M. Psaty. 1998. Correlates and prevalence of benzodiazepine use in community-dwelling elderly. *Journal of General Internal Medicine* 13(4):243-250.

Goldman, H. H., and G. N. Grob. 2006. Defining "mental illness" in mental health policy. *Health Affairs (Millwood)* 25(3):737-749.

Gonzalez, H. M., W. Tarraf, K. E. Whitfield, and W. A. Vega. 2010. The epidemiology of major depression and ethnicity in the United States. *Journal of Psychiatric Research* 44(15):1043-1051.

Grabowski, D. C., K. A. Aschbrenner, Z. Feng, and V. Mor. 2009. Mental illness in nursing homes: Variations across states. *Health Affairs (Millwood)* 28(3):689-700.

Grant, B. F., and D. A. Dawson. 2006. Introduction to the national epidemiologic survey on alcohol and related conditions. *Alcohol Research & Health* 29(2):74-78.

Grant, B. F., D. A. Dawson, and D. S. Hasin. 2001. *The alcohol use disorder and associated disabilities interview schedule—DSM-IV version.* Bethesda, MD: National Institute on Alcohol Abuse and Alcoholism.

Grant, B. F., D. S. Hasin, F. S. Stinson, D. A. Dawson, S. P. Chou, W. J. Ruan, and R. P. Pickering. 2004. Prevalence, correlates, and disability of personality disorders in the United States: Results from the national epidemiologic survey on alcohol and related conditions. *Journal of Clinical Psychiatry* 65(7):948-958.

Gray, S. L., A. E. Eggen, D. Blough, D. Buchner, and A. Z. LaCroix. 2003. Benzodiazepine use in older adults enrolled in a health maintenance organization. *American Journal of Geriatric Psychiatry* 11(5):568-576.

Grenier, S., M. Preville, R. Boyer, K. O'Connor, S.-G. Beland, O. Potvin, C. Hudon, and J. Brassard. 2011. The impact of DSM-IV symptom and clinical significance criteria on the prevalence estimates of subthreshold and threshold anxiety in the older adult population. *American Journal of Geriatric Psychiatry* 19(4):316-326.

Gruber-Baldini, A. L., M. Boustani, P. D. Sloane, and S. Zimmerman. 2004. Behavioral symptoms in residential care/assisted living facilities: Prevalence, risk factors, and medication management. *Journal of the American Geriatrics Society* 52(10):1610-1617.

Gum, A. M., B. King-Kallimanis, and R. Kohn. 2009. Prevalence of mood, anxiety, and substance-abuse disorders for older Americans in the National Comorbidity Survey-Replication. *American Journal of Geriatric Psychiatry* 17(9):769-781.

Han, B., J. Gfroerer, and J. Colliver. 2009. *An examination of trends in illicit drug use among adults aged 50 to 59 in the United States. OAS data review.* http://www.samhsa.gov/data/2k11/DataReview/OAS_data_review_OlderAdults.pdf (accessed February 23, 2012).

Hanlon, J. T., X. Wang, N. G. Castle, R. A. Stone, S. M. Handler, T. P. Semla, M. J. Pugh, D. R. Berlowitz, and M. W. Dysken. 2011. Potential underuse, overuse, and inappropriate use of antidepressants in older veteran nursing home residents. *Journal of the American Geriatrics Society* 59(8):1412-1420.

Harris, Y., and J. K. Cooper. 2006. Depressive symptoms in older people predict nursing home admission. *Journal of the American Geriatrics Society* 54(4):593-597.

Hebert, L. E., P. A. Scherr, J. L. Bienias, D. A. Bennett, and D. A. Evans. 2003. Alzheimer disease in the U.S. population: Prevalence estimates using the 2000 Census. *Archives of Neurology* 60(8):1119-1122.

Heeringa, S. G., J. Wagner, M. Torres, N. Duan, T. Adams, and P. Berglund. 2004. Sample designs and sampling methods for the Collaborative Psychiatric Epidemiology Studies (CPES). *International Journal of Methods in Psychiatric Research* 13(4):221-240.

Hegel, M. T., J. Unützer, L. Tang, P. A. Arean, W. Katon, P. H. Noel, J. W. Williams, Jr., and E. H. Lin. 2005. Impact of comorbid panic and posttraumatic stress disorder on outcomes of collaborative care for late-life depression in primary care. *American Journal of Geriatric Psychiatry* 13(1):48-58.

Hirschfeld, R. M. A., and L. A. Vornik. 2004. Recognition and diagnosis of bipolar disorder. *Journal of Clinical Psychiatry* 65(Suppl. 15):5-9.

Horowitz, M. J., B. Siegel, A. Holen, G. A. Bonanno, C. Milbrath, and C. H. Stinson. 1997. Diagnostic criteria for complicated grief disorder. *American Journal of Psychiatry* 154(7):904-910.

Howard, R., P. V. Rabins, M. V. Seeman, and D. V. Jeste. 2000. Late-onset schizophrenia and very-late-onset schizophrenia-like psychosis: An international consensus. The international late-onset schizophrenia group. *American Journal of Psychiatry* 157(2):172-178.

Hu, G., H. C. Wilcox, L. Wissow, and S. P. Baker. 2008. Mid-life suicide: An increasing problem in U.S. whites, 1999-2005. *American Journal of Preventive Medicine* 35(6):589-593.

HUD (U.S. Department of Housing and Urban Development). 2011. *The 2010 annual homeless assessment report to Congress.* Washington, DC, June.

———. 2012. *Resident characteristics report as of February 29, 2012.* https://pic.hud.gov/pic/RCRPublic/rcrmain.asp (accessed April 2, 2012).

Human Rights Watch. 2012. *Old behind bars: The aging prison population in the United States.* http://www.hrw.org/sites/default/files/reports/usprisons0112webwcover_0.pdf (accessed February 22, 2012).

Hybels, C. F., C. F. Pieper, and D. G. Blazer. 2009. The complex relationship between depressive symptoms and functional limitations in community-dwelling older adults: The impact of subthreshold depression. *Psychological Medicine* 39(10):1677-1688.

Ilgen, M. A., A. S. B, Bohnert, R. Ignacio, J. F. McCarthy, M. Valenstein, H. M. Kim, and F. C. Blow. 2010. Psychiatric diagnoses and risk of suicide in veterans. *Archives of General Psychiatry* 67(11):1152-1158.

Jacobsen, L. K., S. M. Southwick, and T. R. Kosten. 2001. Substance use disorders in patients with posttraumatic stress disorder: A review of the literature. *American Journal of Psychiatry* 158(8):1184-1190.

James, D. J., and L. E. Glaze. 2006. *Mental health problems of prison and jail inmates.* Bureau of Justice Statistics Special Report. http://bjs.ojp.usdoj.gov/content/pub/pdf/mhppji.pdf (accessed February 21, 2012).

Jeste, D. V., and S. I. Finkel. 2000. Psychosis of Alzheimer's disease and related dementias. Diagnostic criteria for a distinct syndrome. *American Journal of Geriatric Psychiatry* 8(1):29-34.

Jeste, D. V., G. S. Alexopoulos, S. J. Bartels, J. L. Cummings, J. J. Gallo, G. L. Gottlieb, M. C. Halpain, B. W. Palmer, T. L. Patterson, C. F. Reynolds, and B. D. Lebowitz. 1999. Consensus statement on the upcoming crisis in geriatric mental health: Research agenda for the next 2 decades. *Archives of General Psychiatry* 56(9):848-853.

Jeste, D. V., D. G. Blazer, and M. First. 2005. Aging-related diagnostic variations: Need for diagnostic criteria appropriate for elderly psychiatric patients. *Biological Psychiatry* 58(4):265-271.

Jimenez, D. E., S. J. Bartels, V. Cardenas, S. S. Dhaliwal, and M. Alegria. 2012. Cultural beliefs and mental health treatment preferences of ethnically diverse older adult consumers in primary care. *American Journal of Geriatric Psychiatry* 20(6):533-542.

Jin, H., D. P. Folsom, l. Lindamer, A. Bailey, W. Hawthrone, P. Garcia, and D. V. Jeste. 2003. Patterns of public mental health service use by age in patients with schizophrenia. *American Journal of Geriatric Psychiatry* 11(5):525-533.

Johnston, D. 2000. A series of cases of dementia presenting with PTSD symptoms in World War II combat veterans. *Journal of the American Geriatrics Society* 48(1):70-72.

Jorstad, E. C., K. Hauer, C. Becker, and S. E. Lamb. 2005. Measuring the psychological outcomes of falling: A systematic review. *Journal of the American Geriatrics Society* 53(3):501-510.

Judd, L. L., M. P. Paulus, K. B. Wells, and M. H. Rapaport. 1996. Socioeconomic burden of subsyndromal depressive symptoms and major depression in a sample of the general population. *American Journal of Psychiatry* 153(11):1411-1417.

Kales, H. C., K. Zivin, H. M. Kim, M. Valensein, C. Chiang, R.V. Ignacio, D. Ganoczy, F. Cunningham, L. S. Schneider, and F. C. Blow. 2011. Trends in antipsychotic use in dementia 1999-2007. *Archives of General Psychiatry* 68(2):190-197.

Kanny, D., Y. Liu, R. D. Brewer, W. S. Garvin, and L. Balluz. 2012. Vital signs: Binge drinking prevalence, frequency, and intensity among adults—United States, 2010. *MMWR* 61(1):14-19.

Karlin, B. E., and M. P. Norris. 2006. Public mental health care utilization by older adults. *Administration and Policy in Mental Health and Mental Health Services Research* 33(6):730-736.

Karlin, B. E., M. Duffy, and D. H. Gleaves. 2008. Patterns and predictors of mental health service use and mental illness among older and younger adults in the United States. *Psychological Services* 5(3):275-294.

Kasper, J., M. O. Watts, and B. Lyons. 2010. *Chronic disease and co-morbidity among dual eligibles: Implications for patterns of Medicaid and Medicare service use and spending.* Washington, DC: Kaiser Commission on Medicaid and the Uninsured, Henry J. Kaiser Family Foundation.

Katz, I. R. 1996. On the inseparability of mental and physical health in aged persons—lessons from depression and medical comorbidity. *American Journal of Geriatric Psychiatry* 4(1):1-16.

Kelly, P. A., C. B. Dyer, V. Pavlik, R. Doody, and G. Jogerst. 2008. Exploring self-neglect in older adults: Preliminary findings of the self-neglect severity scale and next steps. *Journal of the American Geriatrics Society* 56(Suppl. 2):S253-S260.

Kersting, A., E. Brahler, H. Glaesmer, and B. Wagner. 2011. Prevalence of complicated grief in a representative population-based sample. *Journal of Affective Disorders* 131(1-3):339-343.

Kessler, R. C., and T. B. Ustun. 2004. The World Mental Health (WMH) Survey Initiative version of the World Health Organization (WHO) Composite International Diagnostic Interview (CIDI). *International Journal of Methods in Psychiatric Research* 13(2):93-121.

Kessler, R. C., H. Birnbaum, O. Demler, I. R. H. Falloon, E. Gagnon, M. Guyer, M. J. Howes, K. S. Kendler, L. Shi, E. Walters, and E. Q. Wu. 2005. The prevalence and correlates of nonaffective psychosis in the National Comorbidity Survey-Replication (NCS-R). *Biological Psychiatry* 58(8):668-676.

Kilbourne, A. M., J. R. Cornelius, X. Han, G. L. Haas, I. Salloum, J. Conigliaro, and H. A. Pincus. 2005. General-medical conditions in older patients with serious mental illness. *American Journal of Geriatric Psychiatry* 13(3):250-254.

Kim, H. J., G. Steketee, and R. O. Frost. 2001. Hoarding by elderly people. *Health and Social Work* 26(3):176-184.

Klap, R., K. T. Unroe, and J. Unützer. 2003. Caring for mental illness in the United States: A focus on older adults. *American Journal of Geriatric Psychiatry* 11(5):517-524.

Knight, B. G. 2004. *Psychotherapy with older adults, 3rd ed.* Thousand Oaks, CA: Sage.

Koenig, H. G., and L. K. George. 1998. Depression and physical disability outcomes in depressed medically ill hospitalized older adults. *American Journal of Geriatric Psychiatry* 6(3):230-247.

Kohn, R., I. Levav, I. D. Garcia, M. E. Machuca, and R. Tamashiro. 2005. Prevalence, risk factors and aging vulnerability for psychopathology following a natural disaster in a developing country. *International Journal of Geriatric Psychiatry* 20(9):835-841.

Kronick, R. G., M. Bella, and T. P. Gilmer. 2009. *The faces of Medicaid III: Refining the portrait of people with multiple chronic conditions.* Hamilton, NJ: Center for Health Care Strategies, Inc.

Lach, H. W. 2005. Incidence and risk factors for developing fear of falling in older adults. *Public Health Nursing* 22(1):45-52.

Lantz, M. 2008. Adjustment disorders in the older adult. *Clinical Geriatrics* 16(5):17-19.

Lapp, L. K., C. Agbokou, and F. Ferreri. 2011. PTSD in the elderly: The interaction between trauma and aging. *International Psychogeriatrics* Mar. 22, Epub ahead of print: 1-11.

Lavretsky, H., and A. Kumar. 2002. Clinically significant non-major depression: Old concepts, new insights. *American Journal of Geriatric Psychiatry* 10(3):239-255.

Lemke, S. P., and J. A. Schaefer. 2010. Recent changes in the prevalence of psychiatric disorders among VA nursing home residents. *Psychiatric Services* 61(4):356-363.

Lenze, E. J., and J. L. Wetherell. 2011. Anxiety disorders: New developments in old age. *American Journal of Geriatric Psychiatry* 19(4):301-304.

Lenze, E. J., B. H. Mulsant, M. K. Shear, H. C. Schulberg, M. A. Dew, A. E. Begley, B. G. Pollock, and C. F. Reynolds. 2000. Comorbid anxiety disorders in depressed elderly patients. *American Journal of Psychiatry* 157(5):722-728.

Li, L. W., and Y. Conwell. 2007. Mental health status of home care elders in Michigan. *Gerontologist* 47(4):528-534.

Lin, W.-C., J. Zhang, G. Y. Leung, and R. E. Clark. 2011. Chronic physical conditions in older adults with mental illness and/or substance use disorders. *Journal of the American Geriatrics Society* 59(10):1913-1921.

Lyketsos, C. G., M. Steinberg, J. T. Tschanz, M. C. Norton, D. C. Steffens, and J. C. Breitner. 2000. Mental and behavioral disturbances in dementia: Findings from the Cache County Study on Memory in Aging. *American Journal of Psychiatry* 157(5):708-714.

Lyketsos, C. G., O. Lopez, B. Jones, A. L. Fitzpatrick, J. Breitner, and S. DeKosky. 2002. Prevalence of neuropsychiatric symptoms in dementia and mild cognitive impairment: Results from the cardiovascular health study. *JAMA* 288(12):1475-1483.

Lyketsos, C. G., M. C. Carrillo, J. M. Ryan, A. S. Khachaturian, P. Trzepacz, J. Amatniek, J. Cedarbaum, R. Brashear, and D. S. Miller. 2011. Neuropsychiatric symptoms in Alzheimer's disease. *Alzheimer's & Dementia* 7(5):532-539.

Lyness, J. M., A. Niculescu, X. Tu, C. F. Reynolds, III, and E. D. Caine. 2006. The relationship of medical comorbidity and depression in older, primary care patients. *Psychosomatics* 47(5):435-439.

Lyness, J. M., B. P. Chapman, J. McGriff, R. Drayer, and P. R. Duberstein. 2009. One-year outcomes of minor and subsyndromal depression in older primary care patients. *International Psychogeriatrics* 21(1):60-68.

Mackenzie, C. S., T. Scott, A. Mather, and J. Sareen. 2008. Older adults' help-seeking attitudes and treatment beliefs concerning mental health problems. *American Journal of Geriatric Psychiatry* 16(12):1010-1019.

Maercker, A., S. Forstmeier, A. Enzler, G. Krusi, E. Horler, C. Maier, and U. Ehlert. 2008. Adjustment disorders, posttraumatic stress disorder, and depressive disorders in old age: Findings from a community survey. *Comprehensive Psychiatry* 49(2):113-120.

Marcus. S. C., and M. Olfson. 2010. National trends in the treatment for depression from 1998-2007. *Archives of General Psychiatry* 67(12):1265-1273.

Mark, T. L., V. N. Joish, J. W. Hay, D. V. Sheehan, S. S. Johnson, and Z. Cao. Antidepressant use in geriatric populations: The burden of side effects and interactions and their impact on adherence and costs. *American Journal of Geriatric Psychiatry* 19(3):211-221.

McCarthy, J. F., F. C. Blow, and H. C. Kales. 2004. Disruptive behaviors in Veterans Affairs nursing home residents: How different are residents with serious mental illness? *Journal of the American Geriatrics Society* 52(12):2031-2038.

McCarthy, J. F., M. Valenstein, H. M. Kim, M. Ilgen, K. Zivin, and F. C. Blow. 2009. Suicide mortality among patients receiving care in the Veterans Health Administration health system. *American Journal of Epidemiology* 169(8):1033-1038.

McCarthy, J. F., F. C. Blow, R. V. Ignacio, M. A. Ilgen, K. L. Austin, and M. Valenstein. 2012. Suicide among patients in the Veterans Affairs health system: Rural-urban differences in rates, risks and methods. *American Journal of Public Health* 102:S111-S117.

McKeith, I., and J. Cummings. 2005. Behavioural changes and psychological symptoms in dementia disorders. *Lancet Neurology* 4(11):735-742.

McLendon, A. N., and P. S. Shelton. 2012 New symptoms in older adults: Disease or drug? *Generations* 35(4):25-30.

McNeese, T. D., A. L. Snow, L. P. Rehm, P. J. Massman, J. A. Davila, A. Walder, R. O. Morgan, and M. E. Kunik. 2009. Type, frequency, and disruptiveness of aggressive behavior in persons with dementia. *Alzheimer's Care Today* 10(4):204-211.

MedPAC (Medicare Payment Advisory Commission). 2010. *Coordinating the care of dual-eligible beneficiaries, In Report to Congress: Aligning incentives in Medicare.* Washington, DC, June 2010.

Mehta, K. M., E. M. Simonsick, B. W. Penninx, R. Schulz, S. M. Rubin, S. Satterfield, and K. Yaffe. 2003. Prevalence and correlates of anxiety symptoms in well-functioning older adults: Findings from the Health Aging and Body Composition Study. *Journal of the American Geriatrics Society* 51(4):499-504.

Merrick, E. L., C. M. Horgan, D. Hodgkin, D. W. Garnick, S. F. Houghton, L. Panas, R. Saitz, and F. C. Blow. 2008. Unhealthy drinking patterns in older adults: Prevalence and associated characteristics. *Journal of the American Geriatrics Society* 56(2):214-223.

Mittal, D., R. Torres, A. Abashidze, and N. Jimerson. 2001. Worsening of post-traumatic stress disorder symptoms with cognitive decline: Case series. *Journal of Geriatric Psychiatry and Neurology* 14(1):17-20.

Mojtabai, R., and M. Olfson. 2011. Proportion of antidepressants prescribed without a psychiatric diagnosis is growing. *Health Affairs (Milwood)* 30(8):1434-1444.

Morrow-Howell, N., E. Proctor, S. Choi, L. Lawrence, A. Brooks, L. Hasche, P. Dore, and W. Blinne. 2008. Depression in public community long-term care: Implications for intervention development. *Journal of Behavioral Health Services & Research* 35(1):37-51.

Murphy, S. L., J. A. Dubin, and T. M. Gill. 2003. The development of fear of falling among community-living older women: Predisposing factors and subsequent fall events. *Journals of Gerontology, Series A: Biological Sciences and Medical Sciences* 58(10):M943-M947.

Narrow, W. E., D. A. Regier, G. Norquist, D. S. Rae, C. Kennedy, and B. Arons. 2000. Mental health service use by Americans with severe mental illnesses. *Social Psychiatry and Psychiatric Epidemiology* 35(4):147-155.

NCEA (National Center on Elder Abuse). 2011. *Types of elder abuse: Self neglect.* http://www.ncea.aoa.gov/ncearoot/Main_Site/FAQ/Basics/Types_Of_Abuse.aspx (accessed May 25, 2012).

NCHS (National Center for Health Statistics). 2011a. *Health, United States, 2010: With special feature on death and dying. Table 39—death rates for suicide, by sex, race, Hispanic origin, and age: United States, selected years 1950-2007.* Hyattsville, MD: NCHS.

———. 2011b. *Health, United States, 2010: With special feature on death and dying. Table 65—heavier drinking and drinking five or more drinks in a day among adults 18 years of age and older by selected characteristics: United States, selected years, 1997-2009*. Hyattsville, MD: NCHS.

———. 2011c. *Health, United States 2010: With special feature on death and dying. Table 95—selected prescription drug classes, used in the past month by sex and age: United States, selected years 1988-1994 through 2005-2008*. Hyattsville, MD: NCHS.

———. 2011d. *Health, United States 2011: With special feature on socioeconomic status and health. Table 59: Serious psychological distress in the past 30 days among adults age 18 years and over, by selected characteristics: United States, average annual, selected years 1997-1998 through 2009-2010*. http://www.cdc.gov/nchs/data/hus/2011/059.pdf (accessed June 6, 2012).

Nelson, E., and J. Rice. 1997. Stability of diagnosis of obsessive-compulsive disorder in the Epidemiologic Catchment Area study. *American Journal of Psychiatry* 154(6):826-831.

Ng, T., C. Harrington, and M. Kitchener. 2010. Medicare and Medicaid in long-term care. *Health Affairs (Millwood)* 29(1):22-28.

NIAAA (National Institute on Alcohol Abuse and Alcoholism). 2010. Alcohol use and alcohol use disorders in the United States, a 3-year follow-up: Main findings from the 2004-2005 Wave 2 National Epidemiologic Survey on Alcohol and Related Conditions (NESARC). In *U.S. alcohol epidemiologic data reference manual*, Vol. 8. Bethesda, MD: NIAAA.

Noel, P. H., J. W. Williams, J. Unützer, J. Worchel, S. Lee, J. Cornell, W. Katon, L. H. Harpole, and E. Hunkeler. 2004. Depression and comorbid illness in elderly primary care patients: Impact on multiple domains of health status and well-being. *Annals of Family Medicine* 2(6):555-562.

NRI (National Association of State Mental Health Program Directors Research Institute, Inc.). 2009. *Mental health services provided across state government agencies*. HHS Pub. No. SMA09-44.64, Rockville, MD: Substance Abuse and Mental Health Services Administration.

Oh-Park, M., X. Xue, R. Holtzer, and J. Verghese. 2011. Transient versus persistent fear of falling in community-dwelling older adults: Incidence and risk factors. *Journal of the American Geriatrics Society* 59(7):1225-1231.

Okura, T., B. L. Plassman, D. C. Steffens, D. J. Llewellyn, G. G. Potter, and K. M. Langa. 2010. Prevalence of neuropsychiatric symptoms and their association with functional limitations in older adults in the United States: The Aging, Demographics, and Memory Study. *Journal of the American Geriatrics Society* 58(2):330-337.

Olfson, M., and S. C. Marcus. 2010. National trends in outpatient psychotherapy. *American Journal of Psychiatry* 167(12):1456-1463.

Ostling, S., and I. Skoog. 2002. Psychotic symptoms and paranoid ideation in a nondemented population-based sample of the very old. *Archives of General Psychiatry* 59(1):53-59.

Ostling, S., A. Borjesson-Hanson, and I. Skoog. 2007. Psychotic symptoms and paranoid ideation in a population-based sample of 95-year-olds. *American Journal of Geriatric Psychiatry* 15(12):999-1004.

Owens, G. P., D. G. Baker, J. Kasckow, J. A. Ciesla, and S. Mohamed. 2005. Review of assessment and treatment of PTSD among elderly American Armed Forces veterans. *International Journal of Geriatric Psychiatry* 20(12):1118-1130.

Ozer, E. J., S. R. Best, T. L. Lipsey, and D. S. Weiss. 2003. Predictors of posttraumatic stress disorder and symptoms in adults: A meta-analysis. *Psychological Bulletin* 129(1):52-73.

Palinkas, L. S., V. Criado, D. Fuentes, S. Shepherd, H. Milian, D. Folsom, and D. V. Jeste. 2007. Unmet needs for services for older adults with mental illness: Comparison of views of different stakeholder groups. *American Journal of Geriatric Psychiatry* 15(6):530-540.

Palmer, B. W., D. V. Jeste, and J. I. Sheikh. 1997. Anxiety disorders in the elderly: DSM-IV and other barriers to diagnosis and treatment. *Journal of Affective Disorders* 46(3):183-190.

Palmer, B. W., S. C. Heaton, and D. V. Jeste. 1999. Older patients with schizophrenia: Challenges in the coming decades. *Psychiatric Services* 50(9):1178-1183.

Park-Lee, E., C. Caffrey, M. Sengupta, A. J. Moss, E. Rosenoff, and L. D. Harris-Kojetin. 2011. *Residential care facilities: A key sector in the spectrum of long-term care providers in the United States.* NCHS Data Brief No. 78, National Center for Health Services Research, Centers for Disease Control and Prevention, Hyattsville, MD, December.

Parks, J., D. Svendsen, P. Singer, and M. E. Foti. 2006. *Morbidity and mortality in people with serious mental illness.* Alexandria, VA: National Association of State Mental Health Program Directors, October.

Pavlik, V. N., D. J. Hyman, N. A. Festa, and C. Bitondo Dyer. 2001. Quantifying the problem of abuse and neglect in adults—analysis of a statewide database. *Journal of the American Geriatrics Society* 49(1):45-48.

Paykel, E. S., J. K. Myers, J. J. Lindenthal, and J. Tanner. 1974. Suicidal feelings in the general population: A prevalence study. *British Journal of Psychiatry* 124:460-469.

Pertusa, A., M. A. Fullana, S. Singh, P. Alonso, J. M. Menchon, and D. Mataix-Cols. 2008. Compulsive hoarding: OCD symptom, distinct clinical syndrome, or both? *American Journal of Psychiatry* 165(10):1289-1298.

Pietrzak, R. H., R. B. Goldstein, S. M. Southwick, and B. F. Grant. 2012. Physical health conditions associated with posttraumatic stress disorder in U.S. older adults: Results from Wave 2 of the National Epidemiologic Survey on Alcohol and Related Conditions. *Journal of the American Geriatrics Society* 60(2):296-303.

Pittman, R. K. 2010. Posttraumatic stress disorder and dementia: What is the origin of the association? *JAMA* 303(22):2287-2288.

Plassman, B. L., K. M. Langa, G. G. Fisher, S. G. Heeringa, D. R. Weir, M. B. Ofstedal, J. R. Burke, M. D. Hurd, G. G. Potter, W. L. Rodgers, D. C. Steffens, R. J. Willis, and R. B. Wallace. 2007. Prevalence of dementia in the United States: The Aging, Demographics, and Memory Study. *Neuroepidemiology* 29(1-2):125-132.

Polzer, K. 2011. *Assisted living state regulatory review 2011.* Washington, DC: National Center for Assisted Living, March.

Porensky, E. K., M. A. Dew, J. F. Karp, E. Skidmore, B. L. Rollman, M. K. Shear, and E. J. Lenze. 2009. The burden of late-life generalized anxiety disorder: Effects on disability, health-related quality of life, and health care utilization. *American Journal of Geriatric Psychiatry* 17(6):473-482.

Port, C. L., B. Engdahl, and P. Frazier. 2001. A longitudinal and retrospective study of PTSD among older prisoners of war. *American Journal of Psychiatry* 158(9):1474-1479.

Pratt, L., D. Brody, and Q. Gu. 2011. *Antidepressant use in persons aged 12 and over: United States, 2005–2008.* NCHS Data Brief No. 76, National Center for Health Statistics, Hyattsville, MD.

Proctor, E. K., N. L. Morrow-Howell, P. Dore, J. Wentz, E. H. Rubin, S. Thompson, and H. Li. 2003. Comorbid medical conditions among depressed elderly patients discharged home after acute psychiatric care. *American Journal of Geriatric Psychiatry* 11(3):329-338.

Qureshi, S. U., T. Kimbrell, J. M. Pyne, K. M. Magruder, T. J. Hudson, N. J. Petersen, H. J. Yu, P. E. Schulz, and M. E. Kunik. 2010. Greater prevalence and incidence of dementia in older veterans with posttraumatic stress disorder. *Journal of the American Geriatrics Society* 58(9):1627-1633.

Rabins, P. V., B. Black, P. German, R. Roca, M. McGuire, L. Brant, and J. Cook. 1996. The prevalence of psychiatric disorders in elderly residents of public housing. *Journals of Gerontology, Series A: Biological Sciences and Medical Sciences* 51A(6):M319-M324.

Raue, P. J., B. S. Meyers, J. L. Rowe, M. Heo, and M. L. Bruce. 2007. Suicidal ideation among elderly homecare patients. *International Journal of Geriatric Psychiatry* 22(1):32-37.

Regier, D. A., W. E. Narrow, D. S. Rae, R. W. Manderscheid, B. Z. Locke, and F. K. Goodwin. 1993. The de facto U.S. mental and addictive disorders service system. Epidemiologic Catchment Area prospective 1-year prevalence rates of disorders and services. *Archives of General Psychiatry* 50(2):85-94.

Reinhard, S. C., E. Kassner, A. Houser, and R. Mollica. 2011. *Rising expectations: A state scorecard on long-term services and supports for older adults, people with physical disabilities, and family caregivers.* Washington, DC: AARP, September.

Reynolds, C. F., G. S. Alexopoulos, and I. R. Katz. 2002. Geriatric depression: Diagnosis and treatment. *Generations* 26(1):28-31.

Richardson, T. M., A. Simning, H. He, and Y. Conwell. 2011. Anxiety and its correlates among older adults accessing aging services. *International Journal of Geriatric Psychiatry* 26(1):31-38.

Rodriguez, C. A., L. Schonfeld, B. King-Kallimanis, and A. M. Gum. 2010. Depressive symptoms and alcohol abuse/misuse in older adults: Results from the Florida BRITE project. *Best Practice in Mental Health* 6(1):90-102.

Rosenblatt, A., Q. M. Samus, C. D. Steele, A. S. Baker, M. G. Harper, J. Brandt, P. V. Rabins, and C. G. Lyketsos. 2004. The Maryland Assisted Living Study: Prevalence, recognition, and treatment of dementia and other psychiatric disorders in the assisted living population of central Maryland. *Journal of the American Geriatrics Society* 52(10):1618-1625.

Sajatovic, M., F. C. Blow, and R. V. Ignacio. 2006. Psychiatric comorbidity in older adults with bipolar disorder. *International Journal of Geriatric Psychiatry* 21(6):582-587.

SAMHSA (Substance Abuse and Mental Health Services Administration). 1993. Final notice [final definitions for: (1) children with a serious emotional disturbance, and (2) adults with a serious mental illness]. *Federal Register* 58(96):29422-29425.

———. 2009. *Funding and characteristics of state mental health agencies, 2009.* HHS Pub. No. (SMA) 11-4655 Rockville, MD: SAMHSA.

Samus, Q. M., A. Rosenblatt, C. Steele, A. Baker, M. Harper, J. Brandt, L. Mayer, P. V. Rabins, and C. G. Lyketsos. 2005. The association of neuropsychiatric symptoms and environment with quality of life in assisted living residents with dementia. *Gerontologist* 45(Spec. 1):19-26.

Sansone, R. A., and L. A. Sansone. 2011. Personality disorders: A nation-based perspective on prevalence. *Innovations in Clinical Neuroscience* 8(4):13-18.

Sarkisian, C. A., M. H. Lee-Henderson, and C. M. Mangione. 2003 Do depressed older adults who attribute depression to "old age" believe it is important to seek care? *Journal of General Internal Medicine* 18:1001-1005.

Schnurr, P. P., A. Spiro, and A. H. Paris. 2000. Physician-diagnosed medical disorders in relation to PTSD symptoms in older male military veterans. *Health Psychology* 19(1):91-97.

Schnurr, P., A. Spiro, M. Vielhauer, M. Findler, and J. Hamblen. 2002. Trauma in the lives of older men: Findings from the Normative Aging Study. *Journal of Clinical Geropsychology* 8(3):175-187.

Schultz, S. K. 2011. The hazardous territory of late-life depression: A challenge to geropsychiatry. *American Journal of Geriatric Psychiatry* 19(3):197-200.

Seitz, D., N. Purandare, and D. Conn. 2010. Prevalence of psychiatric disorders among older adults in long-term care homes: A systematic review. *International Psychogeriatrics* 22(7):1025-1039.

Shapiro, S., E. A. Skinner, L. G. Kessler, M. Von Korff, P. S. German, G. L. Tischler, P. J. Leaf, L. Benham, L. Cottler, and D. A. Regier. 1984. Utilization of health and mental health services. Three epidemiologic catchment area sites. *Archives of General Psychiatry* 41(10):971-978.

Shear, K., E. Frank, P. R. Houck, and C. F. Reynolds. 2005. Treatment of complicated grief: A randomized controlled trial. *JAMA* 293(21):2601-2608.

Simoni-Wastila, L. 2000. The use of abusable prescription drugs: The role of gender. *Journal of Women's Health and Gender-Based Medicine* 9(3):289-297.

Simoni-Wastila, L., and H. K. Yang. 2006. Psychoactive drug abuse in older adults. *American Journal of Geriatric Pharmacotherapy* 4(4):380-394.

Sloane, P. D., S. Zimmerman, A. L. Gruber-Baldini, J. R. Hebel, J. Magaziner, and T. R. Konrad. 2005. Health and functional outcomes and health care utilization of persons with dementia in residential care and assisted living facilities: Comparison with nursing homes. *Gerontologist* 45(Spec. 1):124-132.

Smith, M., and K. Buckwalter. 2005. Behaviors associated with dementia: Whether resisting care or exhibiting apathy, an older adult with dementia is attempting communication. Nurses and other caregivers must learn to "hear" this language. *American Journal of Nursing* 105(7):40-52.

Snowdon, J., and G. Halliday. 2011. A study of severe domestic squalor: 173 cases referred to an old age psychiatry service. *International Psychogeriatrics* 23(2):308-314.

Snowdon, J., A. Shah, and G. Halliday. 2007. Severe domestic squalor: A review. *International Psychogeriatrics* 19(1):37-51.

Spiro, A., P. P. Schnurr, and C. M. Aldwin. 1994. Combat-related posttraumatic stress disorder symptoms in older men. *Psychology and Aging* 9(1):17-26.

Spitzer, C., S. Barnow, H. Volzke, U. John, H. J. Freyberger, and H. J. Grabe. 2008. Trauma and posttraumatic stress disorder in the elderly: Findings from a German community study. *Journal of Clinical Psychiatry* 69(5):693-700.

Spitzer, R. L., K. Kroenke, M. Linzer, S. R. Hahn, J. B. Williams, F. V. deGruy III, D. Brody, and M. Davies. 1995. Health-related quality of life in primary care patients with mental disorders. Results from the Prime-MD 1000 Study. *JAMA* 274(19):1511-1517.

Steffens, D. C., I. Skoog, M. C. Norton, A. D. Hart, J. T. Tschanz, B. L. Plassman, B. W. Wyse, K. A. Welsh-Bohmer, and J. C. S. Breitner. 2000. Prevalence of depression and its treatment in an elderly population—the Cache County Study. *Archives of General Psychiatry* 57(6):601-607.

Strothers, H. S., G. Rust, P. Minor, E. Fresh, B. Druss, and D. Satcher. 2005. Disparities in antidepressant treatment in Medicaid elderly diagnosed with depression. *Journal of the American Geriatrics Society* 53(3):456-461.

Suicide Prevention Resource Center and SPAN USA. 2010. *Charting the future of suicide prevention: A 2010 progress review of the national strategy and recommendations for the decade ahead,* edited by D. Litts. Newton, MA: Education Development Center, Inc.

Teri, L., P. Truax, R. Logsdon, J. Uomoto, S. Zarit, and P. P. Vitaliano. 1992. Assessment of behavioral problems in dementia: The Revised Memory and Behavior Problems Checklist. *Psychology and Aging* 7(4):622-631.

Thomson Reuters. 2011. *Analysis of Medicare claims data for 2009,* conducted for the Substance Abuse and Mental Health Services Administration (SAMHSA). Washington, DC.

Trappler, B., C. I. Cohen, and R. Tulloo. 2007. Impact of early lifetime trauma in later life: Depression among Holocaust survivors 60 years after the liberation of Auschwitz. *American Journal of Geriatric Psychiatry* 15(1):79-83.

Trull, T. J., S. Jahng, R. L. Tomko, P. K. Wood, and K. J. Sher. 2010. Revised NESARC personality disorder diagnoses: Gender, prevalence, and comorbidity with substance dependence disorders. *Journal of Personality Disorders* 24(4):412-426.

Valenstein, M., H. M. Kim, D. Ganoczy, J. F. McCarthy, K. Zivin, K. Austin, K. Hoggatt, D. Eisenberg, J. Piette, F. C. Blow, and M. Olfson. 2009. Higher-risk periods for suicide among VA patients receiving depression treatment: Prioritizing suicide prevention efforts. *Journal of Affective Disorders* 112(1-3):50-58.

van Achterberg, M. E., R. M. Rohrbaugh, and S. M. Southwick. 2001. Emergence of PTSD in trauma survivors with dementia. *Journal of Clinical Psychiatry* 62(3):206-207.

van Zelst, W. H., E. de Beurs, A. T. Beekman, D. J. Deeg, I. Bramsen, and R. van Dyck. 2003a. Criterion validity of the Self-Rating Inventory for Posttraumatic Stress Disorder (SRIP) in the community of older adults. *Journal of Affective Disorders* 76(1-3):229-235.

van Zelst, W. H., E. de Beurs, A. T. Beekman, D. J. Deeg, and R. van Dyck. 2003b. Prevalence and risk factors of posttraumatic stress disorder in older adults. *Psychotherapy and Psychosomatics* 72(6):333-342.

Wang, P. S., P. Berglund, and R. C. Kessler. 2000. Recent care of common mental disorders in the United States: Prevalence and conformance with evidence-based recommendations. *Journal of General Internal Medicine* 15(5):284-292.

Wang, P. S., M. Lane, M. Olfson, H. A. Pincus, K. B. Wells, and R. C. Kessler. 2005. Twelve-month use of mental health services in the United States: Results from the National Comorbidity Survey Replication. *Archives of General Psychiatry* 62(6):629-640.

Watson, L. C., J. M. Garrett, P. D. Sloane, A. L. Gruber-Baldini, and S. Zimmerman. 2003. Depression in assisted living: Results from a four-state study. *American Journal of Geriatric Psychiatry* 11(5):534-542.

Weissman, M. M., P. J. Leaf, G. L. Tischler, D. G. Blazer, M. Karno, M. L. Bruce, and L. P. Florio. 1988. Affective disorders in five United States communities. *Psychological Medicine* 18(1):141-153.

Wolitzky-Taylor, K. B., N. Castriotta, E. J. Lenze, M. A. Stanley, and M. G. Craske. 2010. Anxiety disorders in older adults: A comprehensive review. *Depression and Anxiety* 27(2):190-211.

Woo, B. K. P., J. W. Daly, E. C. Allen, D. V. Jeste, and D. D. Sewell. 2003. Unrecognized medical disorders in older psychiatric inpatients in a senior behavioral health unit in a university hospital. *Journal of Geriatric Psychiatry and Neurology* 16(2):121-125.

Wu, E. Q., L. Shi, H. Birnbaum, T. Hudson, and R. Kessler. 2006. Annual prevalence of diagnosed schizophrenia in the USA: A claims data analysis approach. *Psychological Medicine* 36(11):1535-1540.

Wu, L.-T., and D. G. Blazer. 2011. Illicit and nonmedical drug use among older adults: A review. *Journal of Aging and Health* 23(3):481-504.

Xu, J., K. D. Kochanek, S. L. Murphy, and B. Tejada-Vera. 2010. *Deaths: Final data for 2007. National Vital Statistics Reports* 58(19). National Center for Health Statistics, Hyattsville, MD, May 20.

Yaffe, K., E. Vittinghoff, K. Lindquist, D. Barnes, K. E. Covinsky, T. Neylan, M. Kluse, and C. Marmar. 2010. Posttraumatic stress disorder and risk of dementia among U.S. veterans. *Archives of General Psychiatry* 67(6):608-613.

Yardley, L., and H. Smith. 2002. A prospective study of the relationship between feared consequences of falling and avoidance of activity in community-living older people. *Gerontologist* 42(1):17-23.

Yehuda, R., J. Schmeidler, E. Labinsky, A. Bell, A. Morris, S. Zemelman, and R. A. Grossman. 2009. Ten-year follow-up study of PTSD diagnosis, symptom severity and psychosocial indices in aging Holocaust survivors. *Acta Psychiatrica Scandinavica* 119(1):25-34.

Zimmerman, S., K. Love, P. D. Sloane, L. W. Cohen, D. Reed, and P. C. Carder. 2011. Medication administration errors in assisted living: Scope, characteristics, and the importance of staff training. *Journal of the American Geriatrics Society* 59(6):1060-1068.

Zisook, S., and S. R. Shuchter. 1991. Depression through the first year after the death of a spouse. *American Journal of Psychiatry* 148(10):1346-1352.

Zubenko, G. S., L. J. Marino, Jr., R. A. Sweet, A. H. Rifai, B. H. Mulsant, and R. E. Pasternak. 1997. Medical comorbidity in elderly psychiatric inpatients. *Biological Psychiatry* 41(6): 724-736.

3

The Geriatric Mental Health and Substance Use Workforce

Abstract: *The geriatric mental health and substance use (MH/SU) workforce is a loosely defined set of providers who assess, diagnose, treat, manage, and care for older adults who have or are at risk for MH/SU conditions. Members of this workforce have shifting and overlapping roles, as older adults may see many types of health providers to deal with their complex array of physical and mental health concerns. Current education and training for most health care providers do not cover the skills and competencies necessary to provide adequate care for older adults who need MH/SU care. Geriatric MH/SU specialists, who are the most highly trained to handle complex MH/SU cases, are in very short supply. Direct care workers, peer support providers, and consumers and their families are playing increasingly vital roles in the MH/SU workforce. Training for these groups is less systematic and thus more difficult to analyze. Though the challenges facing the geriatric MH/SU workforce are numerous and complex, many stakeholders have initiated efforts to build and strengthen the workforce, with various degrees of success.*

This chapter addresses the Institute of Medicine (IOM) committee's most fundamental challenge: to assess the capacity and competence of the mental health and substance use (MH/SU) workforce to meet the needs of the rapidly growing older population. Yet, this workforce is not easy to define, document, or examine. The term "workforce" often connotes a cohesive, definable group of professionals, paraprofessionals, and others who are employed with a common purpose. However, the geriatric MH/SU workforce is more aptly described as a de facto group (Robiner, 2006) of diverse professionals and others who care for older adults in a wide variety of settings under many different working conditions. Some members of the MH/SU workforce are highly trained individuals with advanced graduate training while others have associate's or bachelor's degrees, high school diplomas, or less formal education (Hoge et al., 2007). Each profession has its own history, unique educational requirements and curriculum, career path, certification and licensure requirements, earning potential, and employment options, though these may vary significantly within some professions. In addition, the MH/SU workforce is blurred by the ambiguous boundaries among the numerous professions. Mental health providers, such as psychiatrists and psychologists, advanced practice nurses and physician assistants, and counselors and social workers, often have overlapping roles and scopes of practice, which may differ by state.

Many researchers have described the difficulties in trying to ascertain the nature, location, qualifications, and size of the MH/SU workforce for patients of any age (Hoge et al., 2007; IOM, 2006; Robiner, 2006). Focusing on the workforce with specific skills who are providing geriatric MH/SU services is even more of a challenge. The committee discussed these challenges at its first meeting and addressed two questions: first, how to define the geriatric MH/SU workforce and, second, how to estimate workforce demands and supply. These decisions are explained below. The chapter then presents a review of the key sectors of the workforce. The following sections will describe some of the primary challenges in improving the geriatric MH/SU workforce and include relevant efforts that have been implemented to strengthen the workforce.

DEFINING THE GERIATRIC MH/SU WORKFORCE[1]

Older adults are diagnosed and treated for MH/SU conditions by an array of providers in a wide variety of settings, including primary care offices, hospitals, individuals' homes, long-term care facilities, and specialty settings (both outpatient and residential), which makes defining the "geriatric MH/SU workforce" difficult. The committee focused on those who provide services specifically in the diagnosis, treatment, care,

[1]This report uses the term "geriatric MH/SU workforce" to refer to the full range of personnel providing services to older adults with mental health and substance use conditions.

BOX 3-1
Geriatric Mental Health and Substance Abuse Workforce Professions

- Physicians
  - Primary care physicians
  - Psychiatrists
- Nurses
  - Licensed practical nurses
  - Registered nurses (RNs)
  - Advanced practice RNs
- Physician assistants
- Psychologists
- Social workers
- Marriage and family therapists
- Counselors
- Pharmacists
- Occupational therapists
- Peer support specialists
- Community health workers
- Direct care workers
- Family and other unpaid caregivers

and management of MH/SU conditions in the geriatric population. This includes primary care providers, MH/SU professionals, and professionals providing other types of therapies for MH/SU conditions, direct care workers (DCWs), community providers, and family caregivers, as listed in Box 3-1. Many other groups also work closely with older adults and are integral to the overall health and well-being of this population. Their role in identifying MH/SU symptoms and referring older adults to appropriate services is vitally important, but will not be discussed in this review.

ESTIMATING WORKFORCE SUPPLY AND DEMAND

Questions about demand/need and their relationship to supply emerge naturally in any discussion of workforce issues. At first blush, it might seem straightforward to translate data on illness prevalence into estimates of service need and then, in turn, to estimates of required workforce supply. Throughout the history of health care, however, such efforts have been fraught with methodological challenges and serious questions about the validity of estimates that have been generated.

A previous IOM committee, which focused on the provision of psychosocial services to cancer patients, grappled with this issue and drew the following conclusions:

> Ideally, one might want to estimate carefully the level of need for these services and then attempt to predict accurately the necessary workforce supply to meet that need. However, experts in health care workforce issues note decades of failure of efforts to estimate the size, composition, and distribution of the nation's health care workforce. . . . Even in countries with centrally managed, universal health care systems, progress in medical technology and changes in the organization of care can create large forecasting errors. Predicting workforce supply in the United States is further complicated by the fact that demand for services is not tightly controlled, and the distribution of the workforce is neither controlled nor actively shaped through reimbursement mechanisms. . . . To complicate the matter, data on health professions are not collected in a routine, standardized fashion across the multiple disciplines . . . and the dramatic growth in selected disciplines, such as clinical psychology and counseling, has reshaped the composition of the health care workforce. Another limitation on a forecasting effort is that the same function (e.g., care coordination, case management, or patient navigation) may be carried out by different types of professionals, paraprofessionals, or volunteers in different organizations or systems. Thus, workforce needs are heavily influenced at the local level by the assignment of functions to providers. For these and other reasons . . . the development of estimates of the overall workforce capacity required to meet psychosocial health needs through modeling or other methods was not a feasible activity for this study. (IOM, 2008a, pp. 287-288)

Data on the geriatric MH/SU workforce is even more elusive because the majority of workers who provide services to the geriatric population do not have recognized credentials in this specialty, and are thus more difficult to count, track, and analyze. The committee used information from professional organizations, government agencies such as the Bureau of Labor Statistics (BLS) and the Health Resources and Services Administration (HRSA), and other sources to obtain estimates of the existing workforce. However, the committee chose not to make predictions of workforce capacity or demands because the data to inform these estimates are severely lacking.

REVIEW OF THE GERIATRIC MH/SU WORKFORCE

This portion of the chapter will provide an overview of the main professions that comprise the geriatric MH/SU workforce. Each section will describe the general scope of the profession, the nature of the profession's work with older adults and patients or clients with MH/SU conditions, and workforce characteristics. Required training and competency in geriatric MH/SU will be discussed briefly for each group. Detailed requirements for each profession in the areas of older adult care, mental health, substance use, co-occurring MH/SU conditions, and geriatric MH/SU are listed in Appendix C.

Overview on Accreditation, Licensure, Examination, and Certification

A wide variety of organizations and entities, at both the national and state levels, play a role in setting standards and requirements for the education and training of health care providers. Accreditation, licensure, examination, and certification are the primary processes used to ensure quality training and minimum competencies for a provider. The process, structure, and requirements for each vary among professions. However, there are some commonalities, and they will be described generally here. The entities responsible for accreditation, licensure, examination, and certification for each profession are listed in Table 3-1.

Accreditation is the primary process by which higher education institutions and programs ensure quality to the public. Accreditation is carried out by private, nonprofit organizations. Institutions, specific programs, or freestanding schools (e.g., schools of medicine) may be accredited. While accreditation is voluntary, it is often used as an indicator of academic quality, and may be a condition of federal and state funding or professional licensure. Accreditation bodies are held accountable by receiving recognition from the Council for Higher Education Accreditation (nongovernmental) or the U.S. Department of Education (Eaton, 2011).

Licensure is state regulated and required for individual practitioners. Where a profession is licensed, it is illegal for an individual to practice without a license (Hartigan, 2011). State licensing boards establish scopes of practice, minimum standards for education and training, examination requirements, and standards for professional behavior and ethics (NCSBN, 2011b).

Examination is a process that is typically required for licensure. Because state licensing boards are the primary user of exam scores, many licensing exams are created by nonprofit associations of state licensing boards, such as the Association of Social Work Boards and the National Coalition of State Boards of Nursing. Most professions use the same exam nationwide to ensure consistency and to improve the portability of credentials across state lines. However, individual state boards may have different criteria for passing.

TABLE 3-1
Accreditation, Licensure, Examination, and Certification Bodies for the Mental Health and Substance Use Workforce

Workforce Sector	Accreditation	Licensure	Licensure Examination	Certification (Voluntary Credentialing)
Physicians: Allopathic (MD)	Liaison Committee on Medical Education (undergraduate); Accreditation Council for Graduate Medical Education (graduate)	State medical boards	Federation of State Medical Boards and National Board of Medical Examiners (U.S. Medical Licensing Exam)	American Board of Medical Specialties
Physicians: Osteopathic (DO)	American Osteopathic Association	State medical boards	National Board of Osteopathic Medical Examiners (Comprehensive Osteopathic Licensure Examination)	American Osteopathic Association Specialty Certifying Boards
Nursing: Licensed practical nurses	State boards of nursing; National League of Nursing Accrediting Commission (voluntary)	State boards of nursing	National Council of State Boards of Nursing (National Council Licensure Examination for Practical Nurses)	None

Nursing: Registered nurses (RNs)	State boards of nursing; Commission on Collegiate Nursing Education (voluntary); National League of Nursing Accrediting Commission (voluntary)	State boards of nursing	National Council of State Boards of Nursing (National Council Licensure Examination for Registered Nurses)	American Nurses Credentialing Center
Nursing: Advanced practice RNs	State boards of nursing; Commission on Collegiate Nursing Education (voluntary); National League of Nursing Accrediting Commission (voluntary)	State boards of nursing	None	American Nurses Credentialing Center; American Academy of Nurse Practitioners; American Association of Critical-Care Nurses Certification Corporation
Physician assistants (PAs)	Accreditation Review Commission on Education for the Physician Assistant	State PA or medical boards	National Commission on Certification of Physician Assistants (PA National Certifying Exam)	National Commission on Certification of Physician Assistants
Psychology	American Psychological Association Commission on Accreditation	State boards of psychology	Association of State and Provincial Psychology Boards (Examination for Professional Practice in Psychology)	Association Board of Professional Psychology

continued

TABLE 3-1 Continued

Workforce Sector	Accreditation	Licensure	Licensure Examination	Certification (Voluntary Credentialing)
Social work	Council on Social Work Education	State boards of social work, behavioral health professionals	Association of Social Work Boards (bachelor's, master's, advanced generalist, and clinical social work licensure examinations)	National Association of Social Workers
Marriage and family therapists (MFTs)	Commission on Accreditation for Marriage and Family Therapy Education	State boards of MFT, counseling, or behavioral health professionals	Association of Marriage and Family Therapy Regulatory Boards (AMFTRB Examination in Marriage and Family Therapy)	None
Counselors	Council for the Accreditation of Counseling and Related Educational Programs; Council on Rehabilitation Education	State boards of counseling, or behavioral health professionals	National Board for Certified Counselors (National Counselor Examination, National Clinical Mental Health Counseling Examination, Examination for Master's Addiction Counseling); Commission on	National Board for Certified Counselors; Commission on Rehabilitation Counselor Certification

			Rehabilitation Counselor Certification (Certified Rehabilitation Counselor Examination)	
Pharmacists	Accreditation Council for Pharmacy Education; American Society of Health System Pharmacists (residency programs)	State boards of pharmacy	National Association of Boards of Pharmacy (North American Pharmacist Licensure Examination, Multistate Pharmacy Jurisprudence Examination); state boards of pharmacy (may have separate state jurisprudence examination)	Board of Pharmacy Specialties; Commission for Certification in Geriatric Pharmacy
Occupational therapists	Accreditation Council for Occupational Therapy Education	State boards of occupational therapy	National Board for Certification in Occupational Therapy (NBCOT Certification Examination)	National Board for Certification in Occupational Therapy, American Occupational Therapy Association

continued

TABLE 3-1 Continued

Workforce Sector	Accreditation	Licensure	Licensure Examination	Certification (Voluntary Credentialing)
Direct care workers, certified nurse assistants	State boards of nursing or departments of public health; Medicare- or Medicaid-qualified nursing homes must follow federal requirements for minimum training	State boards of nursing or departments of public health	Evaluation developed by state regulatory body; some states use National Council of State Boards of Nursing program (National Nurse Aide Assessment Program) Medicare- or Medicaid-qualified nursing homes must follow federal requirements for evaluation	None
Home health aides	State boards of nursing, departments of public health; Medicare- or Medicaid-qualified home health agencies must follow federal requirements for minimum training	Some states do not credential home health aides; where credentialing exists, it is regulated by state boards of nursing or departments of public health	Evaluation requirements established by state regulatory body Medicare- or Medicaid-qualified home health agencies must follow federal requirements for evaluation	None

Personal and home care aides	Most states do not regulate personal and home care aide training programs	Most states do not credential personal or home care aides; federal legislation requires states to establish personnel qualifications for Medicaid-funded personal care services, but does not establish specific standards	Most states do not require evaluation or examination of personal or home care aides	National Association for Home Care and Hospice (Home Care Aide Certification); Direct Care Alliance (Personal Care and Support Credential); CertifiedCare (Basic Caregiving, Advanced Health and Safety, and Alzheimer's-Dementia Specialist Certification)

SOURCES: 42 C.F.R. Parts 483 and 484, State Medicaid Manual (Chapter 4, Section 4480, paragraph E).

Unlike licensure, certification is a voluntary, nongovernmental process that allows practitioners to publicly attest that they have met the professional competence standards of specific credentialing organizations (ACA, 2012). Certification is often used to document competency in a specialty or subspecialty, such as psychiatry or geriatric psychiatry. Certification may require examination as well. While certification is a voluntary credential in most professions, in some contexts, certification is required in order to practice. For example, certified nursing assistants and certified substance abuse counselors must obtain certification to practice in these roles, and the certification is regulated by a government entity (CSAT, 2005; Maryland Board of Nursing, 2010).

Physicians

This section will focus on primary care physicians, psychiatrists, and geriatric specialists, although it is recognized that physicians of numerous specialties play an important role in the care of older adults with MH/SU disorders. The nature of our health care system often renders physicians as the principals in patient care within ambulatory, inpatient, and long-term care settings. Thus, for many episodes of patient care, a specialist physician (e.g., cardiologist, oncologist, emergency medicine physician) without specific training in MH/SU disorders may be the first-contact provider of care for older adults with MH/SU disorders. These specialist providers, who clearly play a role in the care of older adults with MH/SU, are not included in the discussion below. Furthermore, when referring to physicians, the term is meant to encompass both medical doctors (MDs) and doctors of osteopathic medicine (DOs), including foreign medical graduates.

Undergraduate Medical Education

Every state licensing board requires physicians to graduate from an accredited 4-year medical school program and to pass either the U.S. Medical Licensing Exam or the Comprehensive Osteopathic Licensure Examination in order to practice. Allopathic programs are required to include clinical experience in psychiatry (Liaison Committee on Medical Education, 2011); on average, psychiatry clerkships last 7 weeks (Barzansky and Etzel, 2001). However, the extent of medical students' specific exposure to geriatric mental health is not well documented. Medical licensing examinations assess general knowledge of early identification, diagnosis, and treatment of mental disorders and substance-related disorders, and the normal physical and mental changes associated with aging (Federation of

State Medical Boards of the United States and National Board of Medical Examiners, 2011; NBOME, 2011).

Primary Care Physicians

Primary care physicians[2] are trained to provide comprehensive and continuous care for patients without limitation to diagnosis, organ system, or problem origins. They often serve as the first point of entry into the health system, and assist individuals in navigating other health services as needed (AAFP, 2011). In 2008, there were an estimated 208,000 general internal medicine or family medicine physicians—the principal primary care medical specialties—in the United States (AAMC, 2008).

Few details are available on the geriatric MH/SU content of postgraduate primary care education. In a 2008 survey, about 50 percent of family medicine and 29 percent of internal medicine residency program directors reported that their programs required fewer than 12 days of clinical geriatrics during the entire 3-year residency training period (GWPSC, 2009a,b,c). Family medicine residency directors indicated that their programs also required some training in geriatric psychiatry.

Geriatricians There were about 7,500 certified geriatricians in 2011 (ABFM, 2011; ABIM, 2011; AOA, 2010). Geriatricians are physicians who complete 1 to 3 years of geriatric fellowship after a 3-year residency in internal medicine or family practice. Geriatric fellowships typically require didactic and clinical experience in geriatric psychiatry, including knowledge of depressive, psychotic, anxiety, personality, and substance disorders and treatment options as well as the assessment of physical and mental status in older adults (ACGME, 2006, 2007; AOA, 2011b).

Opportunities to train in geriatrics appear to far exceed demand for training slots. In the 2011-2012 academic year, 362 fellows held 149 accredited geriatric fellowships (ACGME, 2012). Since 2000, 25 to 46 percent of geriatric fellowship positions have not been filled (GWPSC, 2010a). In 2009-2010, the American Osteopathic Association had 12 accredited geriatric fellowship programs with 46 positions available; only 2 were filled (GWPSC, 2010b).

Psychiatrists

Psychiatrists are physicians who specialize in the prevention, diagnosis, and treatment of mental, addictive, and emotional disorders upon

[2]The term "primary care physician" is used throughout this report to refer to general internal medicine or family medicine physicians.

completion of a 4-year residency program (ACGME, 2009). Psychiatric residencies include some contact with older adults with mental health or substance use conditions. Allopathic residencies specifically require 1 month in both geriatric psychiatry and substance use, including patients with dual diagnoses (ACGME, 2009). The osteopathic psychiatric residency also includes geriatric experience in psychiatric disorders and substance abuse problems for an unspecified time period (Ross and Goldner, 2009).

Geriatric psychiatrists Geriatric psychiatrists specialize in the treatment and diagnosis of mental health conditions in older adults. They work with older adults, families and caregivers, and other health professionals to address co-occurring medical conditions, medication management, family concerns, and social or environmental issues specific to older adults (Geriatric Mental Health Foundation, 2012). Subspecialization in geriatric psychiatry requires a 1-year fellowship after residency (ACGME, 2003b). Although the fellowships in geriatric psychiatry have been available since 1991, few psychiatrists have pursued additional training, and interest in the subspecialty appears to be waning. In the most recent academic year (2011-2012), there were 58 geriatric psychiatry fellows nationwide (ACGME, 2012). Since 2006, less than half of the available geriatric psychiatry fellowships have been filled (GWPSC, 2010b).

Psychiatrists who subspecialize in geriatric psychiatry have the option to become board certified in geriatric psychiatry. Since 1991, when the credential was introduced, 3,067 psychiatrists have been certified in geriatric psychiatry (ABPN, 2010a). Certification must be renewed after 10 years (ABPN, 2007). As of 2010, 1,382 geriatric certificates were still active (ABPN, 2010b).

Addiction psychiatrists Psychiatrists also have the option to subspecialize in addiction psychiatry. The 1-year fellowships include training in geriatrics and may offer some experience with the diagnosis and care of older adults with substance use conditions (ACGME, 2003a; AOA, 2011a). The American Board of Psychiatry and Neurology has awarded 2,102 certificates in addiction psychiatry since 1993 (ABPN, 2010a). Only 40 percent of them have been maintained (ABPN, 2010b).

Nurses

Nursing is a multilevel profession focused primarily on caring for and dealing with individual responses to health problems (ANA, 2011). This section will focus on licensed practical nurses (LPNs), registered nurses (RNs), and advanced practice registered nurses (APRNs). Certified nursing assistants (CNAs) will be discussed in the direct care worker section below.

A new role—the clinical nurse leader (CNL)—has recently been added to nursing master's-level education. Nurses in this role are viewed as "advanced generalists." The first CNL certification exams were offered in December 2008 (AACN Commission on Nurse Certification, 2011; CNC, 2011).

Licensed Practical Nurses[3]

LPNs are nurses who care for people under the direction of RNs and physicians. The role of the LPN varies by state and by job setting; most often LPNs provide basic patient care such as recording vital signs, dressing wounds, assisting with bathing and dressing, and collecting health histories. Experienced LPNs may supervise nursing assistants and aides and help physicians and RNs perform tests and procedures. In some states, LPNs are permitted to administer prescribed medicines (Lafer and Moss, 2007). Nursing homes employ the largest number of LPNs, followed by hospitals, physician offices, home health services, and community care facilities for the elderly (BLS, 2011).

There were more than 730,000 LPNs in the United States in 2010 (BLS, 2010). LPN training is obtained through 12- to 18-month programs in vocational/technical schools or community colleges. The programs are accredited by state boards of nursing with varying levels of coordination with national accrediting bodies (NCSBN, 2004). There is a national licensing exam that tests knowledge in geriatric and psychiatric care, including identifying symptoms of mental health and substance abuse problems, supporting patients in seeking and receiving treatment, and providing care for the special needs of older adults (NCSBN, 2011a). Whether the exam includes competencies in geriatric MH/SU is unclear.

Registered Nurses

The vast majority of nurses—more than 3 million in 2008—are registered nurses (HRSA, 2010). RNs are trained to treat, educate, and support patients in a variety of health care settings. RNs work more independently than LPNs and have the added responsibilities of developing and adjusting plans of care and supervising other nursing staff. Most RNs (62 percent) work in hospital settings; nearly 12 percent (190,000) of hospital-based RNs report spending the majority of their time with older adults. About 5 percent of hospital-based nurses work primarily

[3]In some states, LPNs are referred to as licensed vocational nurses, or LVNs.

in psychiatry and mental health (HRSA, 2010). RNs are also commonly employed by nursing facilities, home health agencies, physician offices, schools, and public health clinics. One in four RNs in nonhospital settings (240,000) report that their time is predominantly devoted to geriatric patients (HRSA, 2010).

To achieve the RN title, an individual must complete a nursing program—either a 4-year bachelor's degree program (BSN), a 2-year associate degree program (ADN), or a 3-year diploma program. All three routes lead to the same license (Center to Champion Nursing in America, 2010). An estimated 45 percent of RNs have 2-year degrees (HRSA, 2010). However, interest in bachelor's-level training is growing. Between 1980 to 2008, the percentage of RNs with bachelor's degrees doubled from 17 to 34 percent (HRSA, 2010). Baccalaureate students receive more training in population health, leadership, and the translation of research into practice. RN programs are accredited by state boards of nursing. Two national groups offer voluntary accreditation (NCSBN, 2004). One requires baccalaureate programs to provide clinical experience with the frail elderly, including depression and other mental disorders (AACN, 2008), while the other does not specify standards for geriatric MH/SU curricula.

RNs must pass a national licensure examination. The exam includes geriatric and psychiatric topics and tests candidates' abilities in handling clients' reactions to MH/SU diagnoses, support and monitoring of adherence to treatment plans, recognizing changes in mood and behavior, evaluating abnormal responses to aging, and tailoring care and patient education to older adults' special needs (NCSBN, 2010a).

Nursing specialty certification RNs may specialize in gerontological nursing, adult psychiatric and mental health nursing, and family psychiatric and mental health nursing. Specialty certification requires an active RN license; 2 years of experience; 2,000 hours of clinical nursing experience in the specialty area; and 30 hours of continuing education in the specialty area. The gerontological exam assesses knowledge of tools and techniques for psychological assessment of older adults, and identification of risk factors for self-harm and variations from normal behavior (ANCC, 2010a). The psychiatric and mental health exam includes normal and abnormal mental changes across the life span and the use of age-appropriate assessment tools and techniques (ANCC, 2010b). An estimated 9,000 RNs are certified in gerontology; 19,000 are certified in psychiatric/mental health (HRSA, 2010). Certifications are valid for 5 years (ANCC, 2012).

Advanced Practice Registered Nurses

APRNs have master's degrees or PhDs in nursing and work with a high level of independence. In most states, they have authority to diagnose, to order tests, and to refer patients in collaboration with or under physician supervision. In some states, APRNs can work and prescribe medications without physician oversight (Christian et al., 2007).

There were approximately 250,000 APRNs in the United States in 2008 (HRSA, 2010). Training and certification of APRNs are evolving. By 2015, all APRNs will be required to have a graduate degree, national certification, and licensure from a state board (NCSBN, 2010c). APRNs will be licensed and certified in specific areas of practice (nurse practitioner [NP], clinical nurse specialist, midwife, or anesthetist) and patient populations (family/individual, adult-gerontology, neonatal, pediatrics, women's health/gender, or psychiatric-mental health). Adult-gerontology nurse practitioners may further focus on acute or primary care (NCSBN, 2011c). The required degree for APRNs will be a doctorate in nursing practice. There are currently 150 doctoral nursing programs, with 100 in development (AACN, 2004).

Advanced specialty nursing Few APRNs have specialty certification in gerontological or psychiatric/mental health nursing. Two percent are certified in gerontology (HRSA, 2010); of these, only half work full-time as a gerontological nurse practitioner (Kennedy Malone et al., 2008). Core competencies for primary care gerontology include diagnosing and treating mental disorders, assessing patients with comorbid physical and mental conditions, and discussing substance use with patients (AACN, 2010a,b). Four percent of APRNs are certified in psychiatric/mental health (HRSA, 2010). In 2004, more than a quarter of advanced practice psychiatric nurses reported working in the field for at least 30 years (Hanrahan and Hartley, 2008).

Physician Assistants

Physician assistants (PAs) are credentialed or licensed health care professionals who practice medicine under physician supervision. Most states allow PAs to work autonomously if communication with a physician is available (Hooker, 2006). PAs usually perform patient assessments, order and interpret diagnostic tests, develop diagnoses, establish and manage treatment plans, and prescribe and manage medications. They have prescription privileges nationwide (AAPA, 2010a).

PAs are typically employed in hospitals and physician offices (AAPA, 2010b), where they often care for older patients. However, fewer than 1 percent of PAs work in specialty geriatrics. Fewer than 5 percent of PAs report working in nursing homes or other long-term care facilities; even fewer work in specialty psychiatry (1 percent) or addiction medicine (0.4 percent) (AAPA, 2010b).

The PA workforce has quadrupled in the past two decades, growing from just over 20,000 PAs in practice in 1991 to nearly 83,500 in 2010 (AAPA, 2010b; Morgan and Hooker, 2010). During the same period, the number of accredited PA training programs increased from 54 to 154 (ARCEPA, 2010b).

Through the 1990s most PA programs offered bachelor's degrees as their highest credential. By 2009, nearly 90 percent offered master's degrees (Physician Assistant Education Association, 2009). Accreditation curriculum standards include instruction on detection and treatment of substance abuse; palliative and end-of-life care; basic counseling and patient education; issues of death, dying, and loss; and psychiatric/behavioral conditions. Supervised clinical practice in care for the elderly and for behavioral and mental health conditions is also required (ARCEPA, 2010a). An earlier requirement for clinical experience in long-term care settings was dropped in 2010 (ARCEPA, 2010a).

PA programs are typically 27 months long. Graduates may opt for additional 12- to 24-month clinical postgraduate training, although most do not (Brugna et al., 2007). More than half of PA postgraduate programs focus on surgery, surgical specialties, critical care, or emergency medicine. In 2010, there were only two PA programs in psychiatry, and none in geriatrics or addiction medicine (Association of Postgraduate PA Programs, 2010).

Psychiatry Certification

As of 2011, PAs can obtain certificates of added qualifications in five areas. The psychiatry certificate requires an unrestricted PA license; general PA certification; 150 specialty-focused continuing medical education hours; at least 2,000 hours of PA practice in the specialty; attestation of skill and knowledge from a physician in the specialty; and a passing score on the psychiatry qualifying exam (NCCPA, 2009b). The psychiatry exam blueprint indicates that knowledge and skills in "age issues" may be tested (NCCPA, 2009a).

Pharmacists

Pharmacists are trained in the safe, effective, and appropriate use of medications (Council on Credentialing in Pharmacy, 2009). In community-based settings, pharmacists provide direct patient care by evaluating the appropriateness of prescriptions and providing counseling and education to the patient on proper usage, side effects, and potential interactions. In institutional settings, pharmacists may play a role in medication selection and monitor medication distribution within the institution (Council on Credentialing in Pharmacy, 2009). In 2009, 54 percent of practicing pharmacists reported working in community settings (e.g., independent pharmacies, chains, or supermarkets); 27 percent in hospitals; 3 percent in nursing facilities or other long-term care settings; and 16 percent in other settings including industry and nonpatient care (Midwest Pharmacy Workforce Research Consortium, 2010).

Pharmacists must earn a doctor of pharmacy (PharmD) degree from an accredited program and pass exams as determined by their state (ACPE, 2011). Graduate pharmacy education typically takes 4 years to complete (AACP, 2010). Accreditation for pharmacy schools does not require training in mental health, substance use, or geriatrics. However, advanced practice experience in the last year of education must include primary, acute, chronic, and preventive care among patients of all ages in community pharmacy, hospital or health-system pharmacy, ambulatory care, and inpatient/acute care general medicine. In a 2007 survey of all accredited pharmacy schools, 100 percent of the 49 out of 91 schools that responded reported teaching about depression, schizophrenia, bipolar disorder, and generalized anxiety disorder. Eighty-one percent said they covered substance use disorders (Cates et al., 2007).

Graduates may do 1 or 2 years of residency to prepare them for clinical work or specialty fields (Council on Credentialing in Pharmacy, 2009). As of 2011, there were 12 geriatric and 23 psychiatric residency programs (ASHSP, 2011). In the 2011 residency match process, 9 out of 14 geriatric positions were filled; 26 of 31 psychiatric positions were filled (National Matching Services, 2011). Psychiatry residents are required to understand the clinical presentation, pharmacotherapeutic treatments, and monitoring parameters for therapeutic effects, adverse reactions, and toxicity of psychiatric disorders in the elderly (ASHSP, 2007).

Psychiatric Pharmacy

Pharmacists may obtain specialty certification in psychiatric pharmacy. The certification exam likewise covers psychiatric disorders and medications seen in the elderly and in long-term care settings (BPS, 2005). As of 2010 there were 627 board-certified psychiatric pharmacists in the United States (BPS, 2011). Psychiatric pharmacists work with other health professionals to develop optimal drug therapy plans for patients with psychiatric or neurologic disorders. They may conduct mental status examinations, interview patients, and analyze health history data to design or recommend treatment and monitoring strategies (BPS, 2005).

Geriatric Pharmacy

Geriatric pharmacists are often called consultant pharmacists. Certification as a geriatric pharmacist requires knowledge of psychiatric disorders, including depression and other mood disorders; schizophrenia and other psychotic disorders; sleep disturbances; anxiety disorders; behavioral disorders; and alcohol and drug abuse (CCGP, 2011). There are currently nearly 1,700 certified geriatric pharmacists; an estimated 36 percent are actively working in long-term care, 21 percent in hospital pharmacies.[4]

Psychologists

Professional psychologists provide an array of prevention, assessment, intervention, and consultation services designed to promote the behavioral health of individuals and populations. There are an estimated 93,000 clinically trained psychologists in the United States (APA, 2011a). Clinical psychology is the largest general provider specialty in this profession. Clinical psychologists assess, diagnose, prevent, and treat a wide variety of mental disorders and abnormal behaviors across the life span. Counseling psychology is another general provider specialty. Counseling psychologists focus more on development and personal functioning, and generally work on healthy aspects and strengths of the client (APA, 2011b,c). In the 2008 American Psychological Association (APA) Survey of Psychology Health Service Providers, 67 percent of psychologists reported graduating in clinical psychology, and 19 percent in counseling psychology. Practicing psychologists have reported that 9 percent of their practice time is dedicated to adult clients over the age of 65 (Michalski et al., 2010). While only 4.2 percent of licensed members of the APA identified geropsychology as a focus, 39 percent of all psychologists surveyed reported delivering services to adults over 65 during a sample week.

Psychologists are licensed by the professional board for psychology in the state in which they practice. To independently practice as a clinical or counseling psychologist, most states require a doctoral degree in psychology, postdoctoral experience, and passing of a licensing exam. Some states allow individuals with master's degrees to practice as psychologist associates, psychologist assistants, or school psychologists (ASPPB, 2011b). Accreditation standards for doctoral, internship, and postdoctoral residency programs in clinical, counseling, and school psychology are not highly prescriptive about curriculum (APA Commission on Accreditation, 2009).

---

[4]T. Clark, Executive Director, Commission for Certification in Geriatric Pharmacy, personal communication, August 18, 2011.

Twelve percent of the psychology licensing exam is devoted to life span development, which includes psychosocial factors, individual and family development, and diseases/disorders that affect people across the life span. It is unclear how much is specifically related to older adults. The exam also covers comorbidity of mental illness with substance abuse and medical disorders, including rates of occurrence and age ranges affected (ASPPB, 2011a).

Geropsychology

Geropsychology applies the knowledge and methods of psychology to understanding and helping older persons and their families address behavioral health problems and achieve maximum potential during later life. The APA formally recognized geropsychology as a specialty area in 2010; it was previously designated as an area of professional proficiency (APA, 2011d; Hinrichsen, 2010). The American Board of Professional Psychology does not offer specialty certification in geropsychology (ABPP, 2012). Psychologists who identified as geropsychologists in the 2008 APA survey reported a broad range of work settings, including private practice (35.1 percent), nursing homes (16.3 percent), group private practices (11.7 percent), and Department of Veterans Affairs (VA) medical centers (7.9 percent) (Michalski et al., 2010). Few geropsychologists reported working in primary care offices or community health centers.

Specialized training in geropsychology may occur through graduate, internship, fellowship, and/or postlicensure continuing education (Hinrichsen et al., 2010; Karel et al., 2010b; Qualls et al., 2005a). Such training usually includes a didactic curriculum on normal versus illness-related aging experiences; orientation to the ethical and legal issues in geropsychology; supervised clinical experience with older adults in varied care settings; membership on an interprofessional team; and experiences designed to promote self-awareness regarding personal responses to aging and the diverse life histories of older adults.

Relatively few opportunities are available for formal geropsychology training at the graduate level, with only 10-15 programs offering a special geropsychology track (Perry and Boccaccini, 2009; Qualls et al., 2005a). Many psychologists-in-training have their first opportunity to specialize in the care of older adults during the internship year, through intensive geropsychology rotations in settings that include VA medical centers, outpatient clinics, psychiatric hospitals, and rehabilitation hospitals. The 2011 Association of Psychology Postdoctoral and Internship Centers directory listed 86 accredited U.S. programs as providing a major rotation in geropsychology, and 223 programs as offering a minor rotation. Formal postdoctoral fellowship programs provide the most intensive, specialized training in the field, typically through a year of full-time training after completion of the doctoral degree. In 2010, there were approximately 22 full-time fellowships in geropsychology. Continuing professional education opportunities in geropsychology are growing, but still limited (Karel et al., 2010b).

Social Workers

Social workers "assist individuals, groups, or communities to restore or enhance their capacity for social functioning, while creating societal conditions favorable to their goals" (NASW, 2011d, p. 1). They provide a wide array of services across the life span, helping people cope with and overcome challenges such as poverty, addiction, disability, and mental illness. Social workers play a large role in the care of older adults in nursing homes. Federal law requires that skilled nursing facilities provide medically related social services.[5] Nursing homes with more than 120 beds are required to employ a full-time social worker with at least a bachelor's degree in social work or "similar professional qualifications." Facilities with 120 beds or fewer must still provide social services, but do not need to have a full-time social worker on staff (Social Work Policy Institute, 2010).

The United States has an estimated 642,000 social workers (BLS, 2009b). The Association of Social Work Boards (ASWB) offers licensing exams in five general categories of social work practice: associate's, bachelor's, master's, advanced generalist, and clinical. Individual state licensing boards may offer licensing at some or all of these levels. Associate-level licensing is only offered in four states, for the titles of social work associate, assistant, or technician. The ASWB offers the same exam for associate's- and bachelor's-level candidates, though the passing score is lower for the former (ASWB, 2011).

Bachelor's-level positions typically include outreach, case management, and resource linkage duties. At this level most states require a bachelor's of social work (BSW) degree from an accredited program, and a passing score on the ASWB bachelor's licensing exam. Some states will license individuals with non-BSW bachelor's degrees if they have compensating work experience. Some states do not license bachelor's-level social workers at all (ASWB, 2008). The licensing exam includes questions on mental health, substance use disorders, co-occurring conditions, and older adult behavior. It also covers the intersection of aging and MH/SU,

[5] 42 C.F.R. § 483.15.

including the symptoms of mental illness across the life span and the effects of aging on specific interventions (ASWB, 2011).

A master's in social work (MSW) is required for more advanced social work practice and management. Though the MSW is considered the terminal degree for social workers, about 2 percent of social workers have doctoral degrees (Whitaker et al., 2006). The ABSW master's licensing exam covers aging processes and more advanced mental health topics, such as the DSM[6] framework and intervention planning, though the content outline does not explicitly include MH/SU in the elderly. In states that license advanced generalists and clinical social workers, an MSW or doctorate is required, plus 2 years of postgraduate work experience. Advanced generalists are expected to have more developed training in supervision and leadership, research use, and administration. Clinical social workers apply the principles and goals of social work to the diagnosis, treatment, and prevention of mental and behavioral disorders. They are trained to provide psychotherapy to clients (NASW, 2005).

Mental Health and Substance Abuse Social Work

The 2006 National Association of Social Workers (NASW) workforce study estimates that 37 percent of social workers work in mental health, making it by far the largest practice area (Whitaker et al., 2006). Social workers also constitute the largest proportion of mental health providers in the United States. Social workers who practice in the fields of mental health and/or substance abuse typically assess and treat individuals in recovery from mental illness and/or substance abuse, and provide a bridge to needed services and resources in the community. These services may include outreach and engagement; assessment and service planning; case management; treatment with individuals, families, and groups; discharge planning; and program planning and implementation across home, community-based, and institutional settings.

The NASW offers voluntary credentials for specialty social work practice. Clinical social workers can apply for the Certified Clinical Alcohol, Tobacco, and Other Drug (ATOD) Social Worker credential. Social workers in this specialty area have advanced knowledge and skills in ATOD epidemiology, physiology, pharmacology, treatment, and policy issues. An MSW, 2 years of postgraduate experience, 180 hours of continuing education, a state license, and adherence to NASW standards are required

[6]DSM, or DSM-IV-TR, refers to the *Diagnostic and Statistical Manual of Mental Disorders*. During the course of this study, the Fourth Edition-Text Revision (DSM-IV-TR) was in use. A fifth edition is expected in 2013 (American Psychiatric Association, 2012).

(NASW, 2011b). All NASW specialty credentials must be renewed every 2 years.

Gerontological Social Work

Seventy-eight percent of social workers report working with older adults, and 9 percent report aging as their primary area of practice (Whitaker et al., 2006). Social workers who work with older adults may assist with advance care planning, loss and grief, independent living, and lifestyle adjustments, among many other issues that older adults may face. They also provide support for family caregivers of older adults.

Gerontology is one of two specialty credentials that the NASW offers at the BSW level. The credential requires a bachelor's degree, 3 years of work experience with older adults, 20 hours of continuing education, a state license (passing licensing exam score or extra work experience and education may substitute), and adherence to NASW standards of practice (NASW, 2011e). NASW also offers credentials in gerontology for advanced social workers and clinical social workers, which require an MSW, 2 years of postgraduate experience, 20 (advanced) or 30 (clinical) hours of continuing education, a state license, and adherence to NASW standards (NASW, 2011a,c).

Marriage and Family Therapists

Marriage and family therapists (MFTs) diagnose and treat mental health and behavioral disorders within the context of marriage and family relationships. They provide psychotherapy to individuals, couples, or families, with emphasis on how relationships impact an individual's behavior. Marriage and family therapy is meant to be brief, lasting 9 to 13 weeks, and oriented toward specific therapeutic goals (AAMFT, 2011b). BLS estimates that there were 33,050 MFTs in 2010 (BLS, 2012c).

All 50 states and the District of Columbia recognize and license MFTs (AAMFT, 2011a). Most states require a master's or doctoral degree from an accredited MFT program, at least 2 years of postgraduate clinical experience, and successful completion of a licensing exam. Educational accreditation guidelines and the licensing exam content include elements on age diversity, life stages, and human development, but do not explicitly mention MH/SU care for older adults (Commission for Accreditation of Marriage and Family Therapy Education, 2005; Professional Examination Service, 2011).

Medicare does not cover mental health services provided by MFTs, thus limiting opportunities for MFTs to work with older adults. This exclusion from Medicare is inconsistent with other federal policy, since marriage and family therapy is recognized as one of five core mental health professions (psychiatry, psychology, mental health nursing, clinical social work, and MFT) by HRSA's Bureau of Health Professions in determining mental health provider shortage areas (AAMFT, 2006; HRSA, 2012).

Counselors

Counselors are trained to helped people accomplish mental health, wellness, education, and career goals. There are several types of counselors. The specialties most relevant to geriatric MH/SU are mental health, substance abuse, rehabilitation, gerontological, and pastoral counseling.

State licensure requirements for counselors vary greatly, and may differ by the type of counseling. Typically, one must obtain a master's degree or higher to be a licensed professional counselor (LPC).[7] BLS estimates there were more than 100,000 mental health counselors and nearly 78,000 substance use counselors in 2011. Estimates for the other counseling specialties were not identified.

Mental Health Counseling

Mental health counselors are trained to work with individuals, families, and groups to prevent, assess, and treat mental health, substance use, behavioral, and emotional disorders (BLS, 2009a). For mental health and addiction counseling programs, core curricula must include theories, strategies, and interventions for addiction, as well as individual and family development over the life span. Counselors should also have knowledge of screening and assessment for addictive disorders, and an understanding of the presentation and treatment of co-occurring mental health and substance use conditions (CACREP, 2010).

Addiction and Substance Abuse Counseling

Counselors specializing in addiction and substance abuse counseling are typically licensed by a state agency or board different from mental health counselors. State regulation of this profession is more widely varied than for other types of counselors or mental health providers. For example, North Dakota has only one licensed addiction counseling position, while California has at least nine credentials that can be obtained

[7]In some states, LPCs are referred to as licensed clinical professional counselors or licensed mental health counselors. Rehabilitation and pastoral counselors may have different licenses in some states.

in alcohol and drug counseling (CAADAC, 2011; North Dakota Board of Addiction Counseling Examiners, 2000). In many states, individuals can become certified or licensed as an addiction or substance abuse counselor with an associate's degree or less (ATTC, 2011).

Gerontological Counseling

Accreditation for gerontological counseling programs was dropped in 2009 (CACREP, 2011). Certification in gerontological counseling has also been discontinued due to low levels of interest (Bobby and Urofsky, 2008).

Rehabilitation Counseling

Rehabilitation counselors are trained to work with people with physical, mental, developmental, cognitive, and emotional disorders. They engage in assessment, treatment planning, case management, and advocacy to assist clients in living as independently as possible (CRCC, 2011). Core curriculum requirements emphasize individual diversity, including aging issues, and the impact of disabilities across the life span. Psychiatric and substance abuse treatment and rehabilitation as well as the implications of co-occurring disabilities are also covered (CORE, 2010).

Pastoral Counseling

Pastoral counselors incorporate religious and spiritual elements into mental health counseling (AAPC, 2012). The profession of pastoral counseling is not regulated in most states, though some pastoral counselors may qualify as an LPC (AAPC, 2009).

Occupational Therapists

Occupational therapists (OTs) work with individuals with physical, mental, developmental, and cognitive conditions to help them improve their ability to perform daily living and vocational tasks. The most common sites of employment for OTs are hospitals, outpatient settings, schools, nursing facilities, and home health care services. BLS estimates that OTs held about 100,300 jobs in 2010 (BLS, 2012g).

OTs provide a wide variety of services to older adults. According to the American Occupational Therapy Association (AOTA) Workforce Survey in 2010, over 35 percent of the workforce serves those who are 65 and older, primarily in skilled nursing facilities. OTs work with patients to improve mobility and independence in activities of daily living (ADLs), provide consultation on environmental modifications that promote safety and occupational functioning, work with a care team to address behavioral or cognitive challenges that may hinder functioning, and help patients and families with transitions home or to another facility (Washkowiak et al., 2010).

In the 2010 survey, 3 percent of respondents identified mental health as their primary work setting, including community mental health centers and outpatient psychiatric clinics (Washkowiak et al., 2010). In mental health settings, OTs may work with patients to develop coping strategies, identify and implement routines that promote wellness, and create individualized recovery and wellness plans (Champagne and Gray, 2011).

The practice of occupational therapy is regulated in all 50 states and the District of Columbia. Generally, an OT must hold a master's or doctoral degree, complete required fieldwork, and pass an examination (AOTA, 2012b). OT students are trained to understand the occupational effects of mental health conditions, and to design and implement interventions that address these effects. Accreditation standards for both degrees require that curricula prepare students for practice with a wide variety of populations, including the elderly, in areas of physical and mental health. Curricula must also include content on developmental psychology across the life span, as well as abnormal psychology. Students must complete field work in at least one setting where psychological and social factors influence occupational ability. The required duration of field experience is not specified (ACOTE, 2012). Most states also regulate occupational therapy assistants (OTAs), who have associate's degrees and provide rehabilitative services under the supervision of OTs (BLS, 2012h). OTA programs are accredited by the same body as OT programs, so curriculum standards are highly analogous, but less advanced (ACOTE, 2012).

Mental Health Certification

OTs specializing in mental health design and deliver services to patients with psychiatric conditions. Candidates for certification in mental health must demonstrate professional experience and competence in mental health across the life span, the impact of psychiatric conditions on occupational performance, and current biomedical and occupational therapy practices used to minimize the adverse effects of psychiatric conditions (AOTA, 2009). According to the AOTA, only nine OTs are certified in mental health (AOTA, 2012a).

Gerontology Certification

OTs specializing in gerontology work with older adults to minimize the impacts of disability and optimize participation in life activities. Certification in gerontology requires competence in aging-related physical, cognitive, and psychological changes, and their impact on occupational ability. There are 13 OTs certified in gerontology (AOTA, 2012a).

Direct Care Workers

Direct care workers (DCWs) are individuals who are paid to provide support to individuals with a wide range of health and human service needs. Next to family members, these workers provide the vast majority of services to elderly and younger people with disabilities. There is not a single, unified occupational title for DCWs in aging, physical disabilities, or behavioral health. Occupational titles vary within each sector and across sectors. In aging, there are generally three recognized job categories. Nursing assistants are employed in nursing homes and sometimes other residential settings such as assisted living. Home health aides are employed by Medicare- and/or Medicaid-certified home health agencies. Home care aides/personal care attendants are employed by agencies or hired directly by consumers and/or their families and are employed in a range of community-based settings, including individual homes and apartments, adult daycare centers, and residential settings. In behavioral health a broadly recognized occupational title to denote this type of work does not exist. Some are referred to as community mental health specialists; others work as psychiatric technicians or addiction counselors (non-certified). DCWs in behavioral health are employed in a range of settings, including psychiatric hospitals, outpatient clinics, small group homes, and other community-based settings.

There are currently no data on the actual number of DCWs who care for older adults with MH/SU conditions. In 2008, there were an estimated 1.47 million nursing assistants, 922,000 home health aides, and 817,000 home care/personal care aides providing services to people of all ages in institutional and community-based settings (PHI, 2011). BLS data indicate that 44,300 psychiatric aides were employed in institutional and community-based settings in 2008. The majority of nursing home residents are age 65 and over. Likewise, approximately 55 percent of those likely to receive services from a DCW in the community are age 65 and older.

Those serving the older adult population typically provide hands-on assistance with personal care and hygiene (e.g., bathing, dressing, and grooming); assistance with home skills such as meal preparation, housekeeping, and laundry; assistance with health-related tasks such as medication management; and companionship and emotional support. The direct care workforce is dominated by females. Nine out of 10 workers employed in nursing homes, home health, and home care are women. A substantial proportion of these workers are nonwhite, ranging from 51 percent in nursing homes and personal care/home care to 58 percent in home health care. Furthermore, 20 to 25 percent of nursing home, home health, and home care aides are foreign born.

DCWs in behavioral health have a slightly different profile. MH/SU-specific settings employ more male DCWs, though women still make up two-thirds of DCWs employed in psychosocial rehabilitation and 70 percent of those employed in the addictions field (Hewitt et al., 2008). Behavioral health also has a higher proportion of white DCWs, with 70 percent in psychosocial rehabilitation and 70 to 90 percent in addiction centers. DCWs employed in the behavioral health sector are more highly educated than their peers in nursing home, home health, and home care, with a much larger proportion having more than a high school education.

Requirements for training are minimal and lack consistency across settings and states. In many cases, there are no requirements. Federal requirements exist for CNAs and home health aides employed by Medicare- or Medicaid-qualified nursing homes and home health agencies. Regulation of other DCWs, including home care or personal care workers employed by assisted living facilities, home care agencies, or private consumers, is determined by the states. Staff in these settings generally receive little or no training (Stone and Urban Institute Staff, 2011).

Federal law requires CNAs working in Medicare- or Medicaid-qualified nursing homes to complete a minimum of 75 hours of training, including 16 hours of supervised clinical practice. The basic training requirements include mental health as a required topic, but the federal regulations offer little guidance on what specifically must be taught. CNAs must also pass a state-approved exam, and become listed on the state nurse's aide registry.[8] The facility employing the CNA must do an annual performance review and provide a minimum of 12 hours of in-service education per year.[9] State requirements for certification vary; many exceed the federal standards (National Clearinghouse on the Direct Care Workforce, 2004). Federal requirements for home health aides employed by Medicare- or Medicaid-qualified home health agencies are analogous to the CNA requirements.

Findings from a nationally representative sample of certified nurs-

---

[8]42 C.F.R. § 483.152 (Requirements for States and Long Term Care Facilities).

[9]42 C.F.R. § 483.75 (Requirements for States and Long Term Care Facilities).

ing assistants employed in nursing homes in 2004 found that a third felt their initial training did not prepare them well for their jobs; one in four reported that their continuing education training over the past 2 years had not been useful (Sengupta et al., 2010). A little over a fifth of the respondents indicated that they had no input into the topics that were included in their in-service training sessions. The study also identified several topics that DCWs would like in their initial training: working with abusive residents, giving dementia care, performing assistance with ADLs, communicating with coworkers, and managing time. Dementia care, communicating with residents, and working with supervisors were the most often mentioned topics to be included in continuing education. A number of studies have highlighted the lack of geriatric-specific education for these individuals (IOM, 2008b; Office of Inspector General, 2002).

DCWs may obtain voluntary credentials. The National Association for Home Care and Hospice (NAHC) offers voluntary Home Care Aide national certification, which consists of 75 hours of training, a skills demonstration assessed by an RN, and a written examination. NAHC certification has been offered since 1990.

The Direct Care Alliance (DCA) recently developed the Direct Care Alliance Personal Care and Support Credential for personal assistance workers who work with older adults (and people with disabilities) in home- and community-based settings. The DCA credential was developed with support from the Ford Foundation after extensive review of existing training programs and discussion with focus groups of direct care workers, consumers, and employers (Direct Care Alliance, 2011a). Workers earn the credential through a competency-based test. The exam covers interpersonal skills, personal care knowledge and skills, health-related knowledge and skills, and safety, but does not include MH/SU competencies (Direct Care Alliance, 2011b). The DCA began offering the exam in spring 2011 with the goal of credentialing 3,000 personal care workers by the end of the year (Direct Care Alliance, 2011b).

The National Alliance of Direct Support Professionals also offers a credentialing program, but the focus is not on an older client population (NADSP, 2011a,b). After demonstrating competence in providing specialized support to individuals with disabilities in community human services, trainees are certified as DSP-Specialists. The DSP-Specialists can obtain a specialty credential in four areas: positive behavioral support, health support, inclusion and supervision, and mentoring.

The U.S. Department of Labor registers apprenticeships in the following long-term care occupations: direct support specialist, CNA, home health aide, and health support specialist. The CNA and home health aide occupations are multilevel and allow for specialization. CNAs can advance from level 1, to advanced, to specialized CNA. Similarly, home

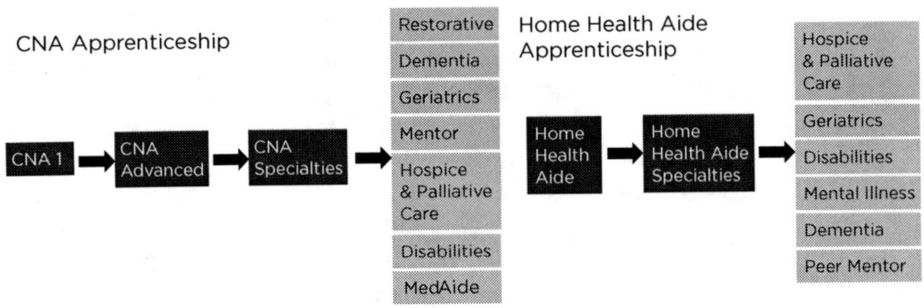

FIGURE 3-1
U.S. Department of Labor apprenticeships in long-term care occupations.

SOURCE: DOLETA Office of Apprenticeship, 2012.

health aides can advance to specialized care (Figure 3-1). CNAs and home health aides can both choose to specialize in geriatrics. Home health aides can specialize in disabilities and mental illness (DOLETA Office of Apprenticeship, 2012).

Apprenticeship programs combine workplace learning and related instruction and require DCWs to complete a specified number of hours of training and on-the-job skill implementation. In addition, apprenticeship standards require that DCWs receive a wage increase upon completion of the program. More than 50 employers have sponsored apprenticeships in the four long-term care occupations (DOLETA Office of Apprenticeship, 2012).

Peer Support Providers

In the context of mental health, a peer is someone who receives or has received MH/SU services and who self-identifies as a person with an MH/SU condition living in recovery. Peer providers may be called peer support specialists, certified peer specialists (CPSs), peer support technicians, peer counselors, peer or consumer advocates, recovery support specialists, recovery aides, client liaisons, or peer bridgers, among other titles. The variation in titles reflects the range of roles that peers may play. Peers may be employed to counsel or mentor others, provide crisis support, run drop-in centers within hospitals, create recovery-oriented programs and hobby groups, help people transition after hospital discharge, or provide other forms of support (Bluebird, 2008).

Integral to peer support is the concept of recovery, which the President's New Freedom Commission on Mental Health defines as the process in which people are able to participate fully in their communities and live fulfilling and productive lives despite disability, which may include the reduction or complete remission of symptoms (Hogan, 2003). Peer support providers are trained in a specific skill set to be role models for recovery and teach self-directed recovery tools. In a review of peer support best practices, the Defense Centers for Excellence for Psychological Health and Traumatic Brain Injury identified social support, experiential knowledge, trust, confidentiality, and easy access as the key elements that distinguish peer support (Money et al., 2011).

Peer support is increasingly being incorporated into treatment programs within mental health systems. However, analysis of the workforce in its entirety is difficult because of large variations in titles, employment status (paid versus volunteer), credentialing, work settings, and state efforts to document this workforce. No data are available on how many peer support providers work across all settings nationwide and how many provide services to older adults. The following information will discuss two groups of peer support providers for which the most data are available: those certified by state governments and those working in the Veterans Health Administration (VHA). In many settings and circumstances, peer support providers do not need state- or nationally recognized certification or training to work.

States have been able to reimburse peer support service through Medicaid since 2001. The Centers for Medicare & Medicaid Services (CMS) endorses peer support as an evidence-based model of care and issued guidance to state Medicaid directors in 2007 on Medicaid-funded peer support (CMS, 2007). Use of peer support requires supervision by a mental health professional (as defined by the state); care coordination within a comprehensive, individualized plan of care; and training and credentialing, including continuing education, that ensure providers have the competencies necessary to deliver peer support services (CMS, 2007). According to the 2010 survey of state Medicaid directors, 22 states have Medicaid reimbursement for certified peer specialist services, 8 plan to seek reimbursement in the next year, and 3 plan to establish reimbursement, but not within the next year (Daniels et al., 2011). In a 2009 survey of states with Medicaid reimbursement, 21 states reported employing a total of roughly 2,800 peer specialists (Daniels et al., 2010).

State requirements for certification vary greatly. Some states have developed their own training modules, while others have adopted well-established curricula such as the Georgia Certified Peer Specialist Training or the Recovery Opportunity Center Peer Employee Training (Johnson, 2008). In addition to didactic training, certification may require work experience. For example, Certified Recovery Support Specialists in Illinois must have 2,000 hours of paid work experience, while Pennsylvania and North Carolina require 3 months of supervised peer support work (Johnson, 2008).

BOX 3-2
Veterans Health Administration Peer Support Technician Domains of Competency

1. Recovery principles
2. Peer support principles
3. Cultural competence
4. Communications skills
5. Group facilitation skills
6. Managing stigma
7. Comprehending the illness
8. Recovery tools
9. Professional development and workplace skills
10. Managing crisis and emergency situations

SOURCE: Veterans Health Administration, 2011.

The VHA embraces a recovery model of service, and has employed peer support technicians to work in seriously mentally ill (SMI) and substance use recovery since 2005. VA facilities are required to provide access to peer support services to all veterans with SMI, whether through an onsite program or through a community provider that has similar standards of quality. Peer support technicians must pass a competency test or obtain certification as a peer provider from a state or agency, and engage in 15 hours of continuing education annually. Competency domains are listed in Box 3-2. As of 2010 there were 237 peer support technicians, and an additional 139 volunteer peer support providers, in the VA system (O'Brien-Mazza and Chinman, 2011).

Community Health Workers

Community health workers (CHWs) are members of communities who work for pay or volunteer in association with the local health care system (HRSA, 2007). CHWs offer interpretation and translation services; provide culturally appropriate health education, counseling, and guidance; assist people in navigating care; advocate for individuals and community health needs; and may provide basic direct services such as first aid and blood pressure screening. CHWs may also be referred to as community health advisors, lay health advocates, outreach educators, community health representatives, peer health promoters, or peer health educators (Goodwin and Tobler, 2008). Another common title is *promotor* or *promotora*. *Promotores* belong to and serve specific underserved minority populations. As respected members of these populations, *promotores* are in a unique position to build trust and to address unmet health needs in their communities. Programs that integrate *promotores* in their services focus on vulnerable segments of the population, such as migrant or farm worker families, or prominent health problems, such as HIV/AIDS or mental illness (Migrant Health Promotion, 2012). *Promotores* working in mental health may have roles similar to those of peer support providers, such as facilitating support groups and sharing experience in managing mental health issues (Rhett-Mariscal, 2008).

Because CHWs work under many titles, and may work for pay or as volunteers, precise estimates of the workforce are not available. In 2007 the Bureau of Health Professions completed a rigorous and comprehensive CHW workforce survey. The United States has an estimated 86,000 CHWs, with 20 percent concentrated in California and New York (HRSA, 2007). According to this survey, 27 percent of CHWs reported dealing with mental health and 29 percent worked in substance abuse.

Family Caregivers

The term "family caregiver" is broadly defined and refers to any relative, partner, friend, or neighbor who has a significant relationship with, and who provides a broad range of assistance for, an older adult or an adult with chronic or disabling condition(s). Family caregivers have been described as a "shadow workforce, acting as geriatric case managers, medical recordkeepers, paramedics, and patient advocates to fill dangerous gaps in a system that is uncoordinated, fragmented, bureaucratic, and often depersonalized" (Bookman and Harrington, 2007, p. 1005). There is no clear consensus about how large a public investment in institutional or home care is reasonable or what the true costs or benefits are of a community-based strategy that relies extensively on the time, skills, and financial resources of families. AARP's report, *Valuing the Invaluable: 2011 Update: The Contributions and Costs of Family Caregiving*, states that in 2009, about 42.1 million U.S. family caregivers provided care to an adult with ADL limitations at any given point in time, and about 61.6 million provided care at some time during the year (Feinberg et al., 2011). The estimated economic value of their unpaid contributions was approximately $450 billion in 2009.

SHORTAGE OF GERIATRIC MH/SU PROVIDERS

The committee's review of the geriatric MH/SU workforce makes apparent that the sheer number of providers entering, working in, and remaining in the fields of primary care, geriatrics, mental health, substance use, and geriatric MH/SU is disconcertingly small. Because the shortage of primary care, geriatric specialty care, and MH/SU providers has been documented and analyzed extensively in other recent IOM reports (IOM, 2001, 2006, 2008b), this chapter focuses specifically on the shortage of geriatric MH/SU specialists. In this discussion, "geriatric MH/SU specialist" refers to providers with advanced training and expertise in working with older adults with mental health and/or substance use conditions.

Geriatric MH/SU specialists are an essential part of the interdisciplinary team, as they are the most experienced and best equipped to consult and provide care for SMIs and other complex conditions. With shifting models of care and the changing roles of different professions, it is not possible to estimate with great precision how many geriatric MH/SU specialists will be necessary to serve the geriatric population. However, the rate of specialized providers entering the workforce is dwarfed by the pace at which the population is growing. One key example is geriatric psychiatry (see Figure 3-2). The number of available fellowships in geriatric psychiatry increased in the late 1990s, but has remained relatively stagnant since then. From 1996 to 2011, the number of geriatric psychiatry fellows filling these slots decreased by 50 percent. This decline, juxtaposed

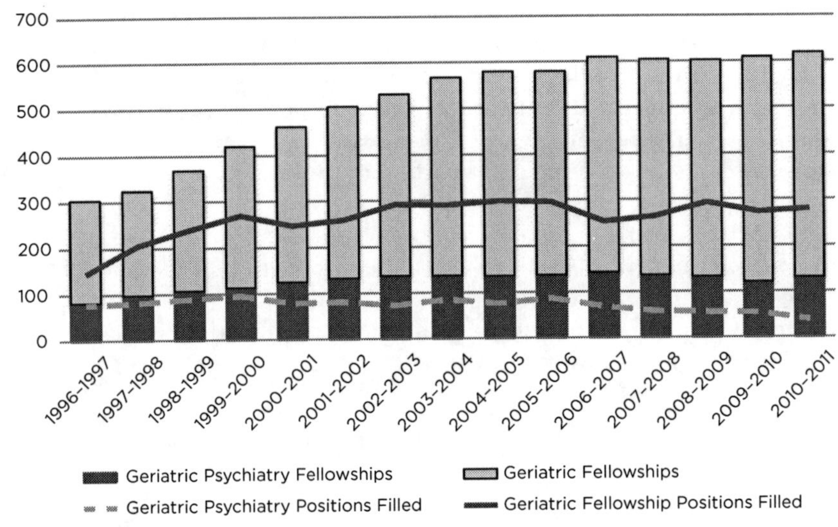

FIGURE 3-2
Comparison of geriatric fellowship and geriatric psychiatry fellowship growth.

SOURCE: Adapted from GWPSC, 2010b.

with the predicted doubling of the geriatric population in the next 20 years (AOA, 2010), will make it increasingly difficult to meet the MH/SU needs of older adults.

As discussed earlier in the chapter, assessing the precise shortage of geriatric MH/SU providers is not possible because of unclear definitions of the geriatric MH/SU workforce and because up-to-date, comprehensive data on the workforce do not exist across all professions. Estimating geriatric MH/SU specialists proves particularly difficult because only two types of mental health professionals may currently obtain specialty credentials in geriatrics: psychiatrists and clinical social workers. There are likely more providers who possess expertise in geriatric MH/SU who do not have formal credentials that indicate this. To estimate the "best case scenario," Table 3-2 tallies the number of providers specially trained in MH/SU (regardless of the age of the patient population). Of these "general" MH/SU providers, it is unknown how many possess expertise in geriatric care. However, the committee's review of professional health training and education suggests that the proportion is small.

RECRUITMENT OF GERIATRIC MH/SU SPECIALISTS

This section will describe some of the primary challenges that exist in the recruitment of potential geriatric MH/SU specialists: stigma against MH/SU and aging, lack of incentives to enter this specialty, limited opportunities for specialization, limited support and mentorship, and difficulty recruiting racial/ethnic minority students (Box 3-3). Many groups have recognized these challenges and developed and implemented various strategies to address them; their efforts will be highlighted below. Programs and initiatives highlighted in this section are meant to convey the various strategies adapted across different professions and patient populations. The list is by no means exhaustive, and inclusion in this report does not indicate a detailed review or endorsement by this committee. In some areas, many groups have taken the mantle to make improvements. Other areas have not received as much attention. The impact and potential for replication of these strategies will be discussed where evidence is available.

Stigma Associated with MH/SU and Aging

The enduring stigma associated with MH/SU and aging is a major barrier to growing the geriatric MH/SU workforce. Stigmatizing attitudes held by the general public regarding older adults and mental illness have long been recognized (HHS, 1999; IOM, 2006; World Psychiatric Association and World Health Organization, 2002). Additionally, work-

TABLE 3-2
Estimated Number of Mental Health/Substance Use Specialists, 2011

Psychiatrists	Psychologists[a]	MH/SU Social Workers	Psychiatric APRNs[b]	Substance Abuse and Behavioral Health Counselors	Mental Health Counselors	Marriage and Family Therapists
23,140	100,850	115,390	19,126	76,600	114,180	33,990
					TOTAL	483,126

[a] Psychologists include clinical, counseling, and school psychologists.
[b] Estimate for psychiatric advanced practice registered nurses (APRNs) is drawn from the 2008 National Sample Survey of Registered Nurses. All other estimates are from the U.S. Bureau of Labor Statistics.
SOURCES: BLS, 2012b,c,d,e,f,g; HRSA, 2010.

BOX 3-3
Primary Challenges in the Recruitment of Geriatric MH/SU Specialists

- Stigma against mental health and substance use (MH/SU) and aging
- Lack of financial incentives to practice in geriatric MH/SU
- Limited opportunities for specialization
- Inadequate early career support and mentorship
- Difficulty recruiting racial/ethnic minorities

ing in MH/SU carries its own stigma. A literature review by the World Psychiatric Association found that medical students widely view psychiatry as having low prestige, lacking a solid scientific foundation, and bringing low job satisfaction (Sartorius et al., 2010). Students also view careers dedicated to older adults negatively. A 2007 survey of high school students interested in pursuing nursing careers showed that 48 percent had no interest in specializing in geriatrics (Evercare, 2007). When MSW students from three large universities were asked in a 2004 survey which population they most desired to work with after graduation, the most popular answer was children, while the least popular choice was older adults (Cummings et al., 2005). As with psychiatry, students perceive working with older adults to be less glamorous and requiring less skill than working with other populations (Cummings et al., 2005). In combination, negative perceptions of mental illness and old age create a powerful barrier to recruiting more geriatric MH/SU providers.

While stigma is deeply rooted and not easily eradicated, some studies indicate that students' negative perceptions of MH/SU and old age can be reduced through education and exposure to the stigmatized populations (Cummings et al., 2005; Happell, 2008; Happell and Roper, 2003; Koder and Helmes, 2008; Wallendal et al., 2009; Wood and Wahl, 2006). Contact with individuals with mental illnesses, as opposed to instruction or factual information, appears to be the most effective way to reduce stigmatizing attitudes (Couture and Penn, 2003). Therefore, facilitating clinical experiences and personal contact with older adults and individuals with MH/SU conditions may be one effective strategy to interest students in specializing in geriatric MH/SU.

Early Exposure

Many schools give students the option to work with older adults with MH/SU conditions, but the committee did not identify any programs that require students to interact with this population before choosing a specialty area. Medicine has some programs that come close to this by requiring contact with older adults and psychiatric patients. Accredited allopathic medical schools are required to have psychiatry clerkships (Liaison Committee on Medical Education, 2011), but there is no way to know whether students interact with geriatric patients during their rotations. Some medical schools have required geriatric clerkships for fourth-year medical students that include training in MH/SU assessment skills, but as with psychiatry clerkships, it is unclear if these skills are exercised with patients who actually have MH/SU conditions. A number of medical schools have implemented senior mentor programs, where medical students are paired with volunteer mentors over age 65 to meet periodically, discuss aging experiences, and develop personal connections. Evaluations of these programs have found improvements in geriatric competencies and attitudes toward aging, but the older adults in these programs are generally healthy and active, and may or may not have MH/SU conditions (Bernard et al., 2003; Corwin et al., 2006; Eleazer et al., 2006; Hoffman et al., 2006). The committee did not identify programs in other disciplines, such as nursing or social work, that have similar requirements for interacting with older adults and MH/SU consumers.

Lack of Financial Incentives for Practicing in Geriatric MH/SU

A number of factors can influence an individual's choice to seek additional training in geriatric MH/SU. One of these factors is money, as students consider current costs of education and anticipate future returns on their training. Costs of education include tuition and other direct training costs, but most importantly the opportunity cost of the individual's time to undertake the training. For example, a psychiatry resident's opportunity cost for an extra year of geriatric fellowship is the income and experience the resident could have earned by going into practice immediately. While 1 year of practice lost does not seem like much, it is important to consider that the average amount of student debt of 2011 medical school graduates was $118,000, with nearly a third owing over $200,000 (AAMC, 2011). Enhanced competencies may make providers more effective in treating MH/SU conditions of older adults, but current health care payment systems do not recognize or reward the extra skills and knowledge. Psychiatry graduates are becoming less interested in subspecialization (Faulkner et al., 2011). Colenda and colleagues (2005) note that psychiatrists with geriatric specialty training and general psychiatrists who see a substantial proportion of older adult patients have similar compensation, suggesting there is little reason to seek specialty credentialing.

Not only do financial disincentives detract students from pursuing geriatric MH/SU, but they can also influence credentialed specialists to stop practicing in their subspecialty if they can earn more in general practice. As of 2010, fewer than half of the certificates in geriatric psychiatry earned since 1991 have been maintained (ABPN, 2010a,b). The attrition of trained geriatric providers is an ongoing threat to the general geriatric workforce (IOM, 2008b).

Loan Forgiveness and Scholarships

Providing monetary compensation through loan forgiveness or scholarships is one strategy to defray the most immediate opportunity cost of extra training. Linking training subsidies to service obligations may also potentially mitigate some attrition. South Carolina's Geriatric Loan Forgiveness Program and California's Mental Health Social Work Stipend Program are examples of how financial incentives can build and retain the geriatric MH/SU workforce to meet local needs.

In 2005 the South Carolina legislature approved the nation's first geriatric loan forgiveness program (South Carolina Lieutenant Governor's Office on Aging, 2011a). The state offers loan repayment for geriatricians or geriatric psychiatrists in exchange for a commitment to practice in South Carolina for 5 years. Physicians must become board certified in a geriatric subspecialty within the first year of the practice, agree to accept Medicare and Medicaid reimbursement, and accept patients regardless of ability to pay. The penalty for not meeting these conditions is substantial. Noncompliant participants must pay the state three times the total reimbursement plus interest at the prime rate plus 10 percent. Applicants are required to sign a statement of intent to continue working in the state after the 5-year commitment. Priority is given to South Carolina natives (those who were born in the state and continue to reside there, or those who have lived in-state for at least 15 years) and those who complete fellowships in South Carolina (South Carolina Lieutenant Governor's Office on Aging, 2011b). Since 2005, 16 physicians have received loan repayment through this program (South Carolina Lieutenant Governor's Office on Aging, 2011a), increasing the state's number of geriatric specialists from 30 to 46 (AARP South Carolina, 2010). Using South Carolina as a model, the American Geriatrics Society has created a toolkit for its other state affiliates to advocate for similar programs in their states (AGS, 2011).

California offers financial support to geriatric social work trainees in its Mental Health Social Work Stipend Program (CalSWEC-Mental

Health). MSW students at 18 participating social work schools may receive a stipend of $18,500 in their second year of training in exchange for a 1-year commitment to working in the state's community mental health system after graduation. Two of the primary goals of this program are to increase the number of social workers trained in geriatrics, and to create a more culturally competent and diverse social work workforce. From 2005 to 2010, nearly 1,000 students participated in this program; over 50 percent identified themselves as racial/ethnic minorities (CalSWEC, 2011a). Data from 2006 to 2008 show that 55 percent of the students were bilingual (Sirojudin and Jacob, 2009).

Core competencies and teaching resources in community mental health were developed for participating schools, including curricular modules on Specialized Mental Health Interventions with Older Adults, and Co-occurring Disorders (CalSWEC, 2011b). The original cohort was tracked for 2 years after completion of their commitment; 94 percent were still employed in the community mental health system (Sirojudin and Jacob, 2009). A quality-improvement study and 5-year outcomes study are in development (CalSWEC, 2011a). The program is funded by the California Mental Health Services Act of 2005, which approved a new 1 percent tax on income over $1 million to enhance community mental health services. The program has also received support from local foundations.

Limited Opportunities for Specialization in Geriatric MH/SU

The number of specially trained geriatric mental health providers is small in part because there are few ways to pursue specialization in this area. Opportunities are limited for advanced training and for recognition of expertise. As stated earlier, only two mental health professions offer certification in geriatrics: psychiatry and social work. Psychologists, psychiatric nurses, MFTs, mental health counselors, and substance use counselors do not have the option to become certified in older adult care. Though many providers without specialty credentials may have clinical expertise from working with older populations, certification and other modes of formal recognition can ensure more systematic advanced training and bring more widespread attention to the focus area.

Advanced Training Programs

As presented earlier, geriatric psychiatry fellowships have had increasingly high levels of vacancy in recent years. However, this lack of demand for advanced training is not apparent in all mental health professions. Clinical psychology programs that collect admissions data for specific concentrations report that application for the aging track outnumber available slots by a 6:1 ratio on average (Qualls et al., 2005b). Some prime training opportunities have been eliminated because of waning financial support from outside grants. HRSA's Bureau of Health Professions (BHP) Graduate Psychology Education (GPE) grants were established in 2002 to fund training for psychologists specializing in integrated care for underserved populations. In 2003, BHP added dedicated funding for geropsychology under the GPE Program. Seven awards totaling $1.8 million were granted, each for a period of 3 years. With GPE funding, psychology departments and training sites were able to create and expand geropsychology training programs. In 2006, GPE funding was cut by over 50 percent, and the geropsychology grants were discontinued (APA, 2012b). Many programs that received funds were negatively impacted when the grants were not renewed. The University of South Florida, University of Illinois at Chicago, and University of Rochester cut the geropsychology training programs they developed with the GPE grant dollars (APA, 2012a; Clay, 2006).

National Certification

Several mental health disciplines have spearheaded efforts to create geriatric certification. The counseling field identified the need for a gerontological counseling specialty beginning in the 1970s. In recognition of the dearth of counselor preparation in serving older adults, the American Counseling Association sought and received five grants from the Administration on Aging to develop aging curriculum and competencies. In the early 1990s, the Council for Accreditation of Counseling and Related Education Programs (CACREP) adopted accreditation standards for gerontological counseling programs, and the National Board of Certified Counselors began to certify gerontological counselors (Meyers, 1995). However, as noted earlier, both program accreditation and certification in gerontological counseling have been discontinued due to lack of interest and participation. In 1995, Myers predicted that without strong national leadership and advocacy, support for counseling programs through the accreditation process, and the development of continuing education opportunities, specialty gerontological counseling would not survive (Meyers, 1995).

While geropsychiatric nursing has been an active field for some time, leaders in the area are now developing a plan for a Geropsychiatric Nursing (GPN) Specialist Certificate Program which, if funded, will define the scope and preparation for specialty practice and credentialing at the graduate/postgraduate level in line with the new APRN Consensus Model (APRN Consensus Work Group and the National Council of State Boards of Nursing APRN Advisory Committee, 2008). Currently APRNs who prepared in many different fields find themselves working in areas broadly construed as "geropsych," such as dementia clinics, nursing homes, primary care settings, geropsychiatric and neurological services, acute care, home care, and so on. Over time, many of these APRNs have developed clinical expertise in a specific focus area, but few have had systematic training in GPN and, thus, have gaps in their knowledge and skill base. The proposed GPN Specialist Certificate Program will address these gaps by developing a model graduate/postgraduate certificate program in geropsychiatric nursing that can serve to further prepare graduates from a range of fields, such as psychiatric-mental health, adult gero primary and acute care, family health, and women's health, for expert mental health practice with older adults. Expected outcomes include (1) a confirmed set of core GPN competencies, (2) four to six Web-based modules covering core GPN competencies for delivery as academic credit or continuing education, (3) a design for a precepted clinical laboratory experience, (4) a gap analysis procedure to facilitate individualization of the curriculum for each learner, (5) an examination to assess learner mastery of core competencies upon completion of the program, and (6) a development plan for national certification in concert with the American Nurses Credentialing Center and/or other relevant bodies.

Lack of Support and Mentorship

Supporting students and graduates who show an interest in geriatric MH/SU early in their education and career is one strategy to develop professionals dedicated to this specialty area. In the 2011 Association of American Medical Colleges (AAMC) survey of medical school graduates, 77 percent of graduates said their role models had moderate or strong influence on their choice of specialty. Interacting and receiving individualized attention from faculty, professionals, and mentors can show students the variety of opportunities that exist in geriatric MH/SU, and guide them in succeeding in this field. Although most medical schools now have an academic geriatric program, geriatric faculty are devoted primarily to clinical practice, research, and graduate education (Warshaw et al., 2002). Less than 8 percent of geriatric faculty spent time on medical student education. Only 29 percent of baccalaureate nursing programs have a faculty member certified in geriatrics (IOM, 2011).

Early Career Support and Mentorship Programs

Initiatives such as the Geriatric Mental Health Foundation (GMHF) Scholars Fund and the Geriatric Social Work Initiative (GSWI)/John A. Hartford Foundation programs, strive to encourage students and early-career professionals who are interested in aging to orient their careers toward the older adult population by providing financial assistance and mentorship.

The American Association of Geriatric Psychiatrists (AAGP) created the GMHF Scholars Fund to attract medical students and psychiatry residents to the specialty via mentorship and education. The program provides free AAGP membership, one-on-one mentorship, a structured Scholars Program at the AAGP annual meeting, and travel expenses to attend the annual meeting. For medical students, the Scholars Program is designed to build interest in geriatric psychiatry by presenting various options for clinical and research opportunities available in medical school and residencies. Psychiatry residents go through a different program that offers more detail about the practice of geriatric psychiatry, and showcases geriatric fellowship opportunities. The Scholars Fund is supported by donations and grants. The program received over $50,000 for the 2012 cycle, $35,000 in 2011, and $18,000 in 2010 (AAGP, 2011). The current budget can support about 20 scholars. GMHF reports that nearly 75 percent of scholars go on to specialized geriatric fellowships (AAGP, 2011).

GSWI of the John A. Hartford Foundation collaborates with social work programs, organizations, and other funders around the country to prepare social workers to improve the care and well-being of older adults and their families. In 2005, the Foundation, in collaboration with the Gerontological Society of America (GSA), began a predissertation award program for doctoral students in social work. The objectives of the program were to expose students to gerontological social work research and to encourage them to advance the field of gerontological social work practice. The award provided travel expenses and registration to the GSA Annual Meeting, sessions at the GSA meeting on research and grant writing, free membership in GSA and the Association for Gerontology Education in Social Work, and networking opportunities with Hartford Doctoral Fellows and Hartford Faculty Scholars. The Hartford Foundation encouraged predissertation awardees to apply for the Hartford Doctoral Fellows program in the next phase of their academic career. The doctoral fellows program granted students up to $50,000 over 2 years to complete a dissertation related to social work and older adults, and provides additional professional development opportunities. Eighty predissertation awards were given out from 2005 to 2009 (Geriatric Social Work Initiative, 2012). The Association for Gerontology Education in Social Work adopted the program and funded 20 students from 2010 to 2011, with plans to fund 10 more in 2012 (AGESW, 2011).

Early career programs geared toward encouraging new scholars in the field of geriatric social work have also included the Doctoral Fellows Program in Geriatric Social Work and the Geriatric Social Work Scholars program, both sponsored by the John A. Hartford Foundation and GSA.

The programs fostered an intellectually stimulating, mutually supportive network of peers and colleagues involved in research and teaching in geriatric social work. Based on the integrated components of mentoring, career development, and networking, these programs have sponsored 117 faculty scholars and 104 doctoral fellows, but were recently discontinued due to financial constraints.

Difficulty Recruiting Minorities to Geriatric MH/SU

One study of medical students found that white students were three times as likely to indicate interest in geriatrics than minority peers (Voogt et al., 2008). Furthermore, fewer African American, Hispanic, and Native American students earn college and graduate degrees than their white peers (Aud et al., 2012), potentially limiting the pipeline of minority students for geriatric MH/SU specialties.

The committee did not identify any programs that specifically recruit minority students to geriatric MH/SU practice, although many initiatives recruit minority students to MH/SU professions in general. For example, in FY 2011 the Substance Abuse and Mental Health Services Administration provided $4.7 million in minority fellowship program grants to the American Nurses Association, American Psychiatric Association, American Psychological Association, Council on Social Work Education, and American Association for Marriage and Family Therapy to use over 3 years (SAMHSA, 2011b). The purpose of the minority fellowship programs is to increase the number of culturally competent and diverse MH/SU providers prepared to serve disadvantaged populations (SAMHSA, 2011a). For example, in social work the Council on Social Work Education Mental Health/Substance Abuse Fellowship Program has existed since the early 1970s, and is designed to increase the number of racial and ethnic minorities with doctoral degrees in social work education who can provide leadership in the planning and evaluation of culturally competent mental health and substance abuse programs.

One program previously existed to recruit minority researchers to this field. From 2003 to 2008, the National Institute of Mental Health operated the Institute for Research Minority Training on Mental Health and Aging to engage more minority early investigators in geriatric MH/SU research. Over 5 years, the program trained 10 participants. However, the program could not secure funding necessary to continue (Bartels et al., 2010).

INADEQUATE PREPARATION OF THE GERIATRIC MH/SU WORKFORCE

While geriatric MH/SU specialists are critical in caring for older adults with MH/SU, the more broadly defined geriatric MH/SU workforce has far greater contact with older adults who have or may be at risk for MH/SU conditions. Aside from geriatric MH/SU specialists, the remainder of the geriatric MH/SU workforce is somewhat arbitrarily defined. However, the committee believes that all professions that provide services to older adults for the assessment, diagnosis, treatment, management, or care of MH/SU conditions are part of the geriatric MH/SU workforce and should be prepared for this role.

The review of the workforce found many gaps in geriatric MH/SU training across most professions. As is evident from examining the table of required competencies in Appendix C, most providers who are not geriatric MH/SU specialists are required to have little knowledge or experiential training in mental health or substance use as related to older adults. Few students are explicitly required to understand the presentation or treatment of comorbid MH/SU conditions. Some professions barely require any learning in MH/SU or aging in general.

TRAINING THE GERIATRIC MH/SU WORKFORCE

General providers at all levels should be aware of the signs and symptoms of MH/SU conditions and be able to respond appropriately within their level of training and scope of practice. However, few professions have mandated curricular standards related to MH/SU in geriatric patients. Although curricula exist, clarity is needed in how and to what extent the concepts are applied in the classroom or in practical training. The prevalence of co-occurring conditions in the elderly and the shift toward collaborative models of care make interprofessional training essential to overall training in geriatric MH/SU care. The increasing racial, ethnic, and linguistic diversity of the geriatric population also makes cultural competence imperative. To what extent these aspects of care are being integrated into training and education is also unclear. These key areas of training are summarized in Box 3-4.

BOX 3-4
Key Areas for Improving Training

- Integrating geriatric mental health and substance use competencies into education for all health professionals
- Training for existing providers
- Training in cultural competency
- Interprofessional training

Several professional groups, schools, and other entities have developed or are working to develop tools to improve geriatric MH/SU skills and competencies in the nonspecialist workforce. These efforts are described in this section. As stated in the earlier discussion on recruitment, inclusion of an initiative in this chapter does not represent an endorsement from the committee because evidence to support the effectiveness or analyze the outcomes is often not available.

Integrating Geriatric MH/SU Competencies into Education for All Health Professionals

The development and integration of core competencies in health care education and training have increased with the recognition that critical skills, knowledge, and attitudes must be more precisely defined for more consistent advancement of the field. Significant efforts have been made to develop geriatric MH/SU competencies and to integrate these competencies into education and training programs.

The Geropsychiatric Nursing Collaborative (GPNC) started in 2008 with funding from the John A. Hartford Foundation (AAN, 2010). Its goal is to improve the quality of mental health care provided to older adults by enhancing the knowledge and skills of nurses. One of the GPNC's primary goals is to develop geropsychiatric core competencies for entry-level and advanced practice nurses. The competencies were developed to enhance current nursing curriculum for both generalist and specialist nurses. The GPNC created competency enhancements for the following audiences: entry-level nurses, gerontological clinical nurse specialists (CNSs), gerontological NPs, older adult care CNSs (CNSs who care for older adults, but are not specialized), older adult care NPs (NPs who care for older adults, but are not specialized), psychiatric mental health CNSs, and psychiatric mental health NPs. All competency enhancements cover key concepts in assessment, management, approach to older adults, and nursing roles (Box 3-5). The competency enhancements have been endorsed by 12 other nursing organizations. The GPNC posted these competency sets, along with other geriatric nursing resources, on the Portal of Online Geriatric Education (POGOe) website.[10] Deans of every school of nursing were notified about these new resources (Beck et al., 2011).

Professional geropsychology has adopted a competency-based model of training, the Pikes Peak Model for Training in Professional Geropsychology (Knight et al., 2009). It delineates attitude, knowledge, and skill competencies for geropsychology practice and acknowledges that there are multiple pathways to geropsychology competence. The Pikes Peak

[10]See http://www.pogoe.org.

BOX 3-5
Geropsychiatric Nursing Key Concepts

I. Assessment
   a. Normal aging: biopsychosocial theories
   b. Appropriate instruments/clinical evaluation tools
   c. Adapted assessment procedures
   d. Atypical presentations, co-occurring illness, psychiatric manifestations, medical conditions
   e. Common disorders
   f. Comprehensive assessments
   g. Stressors affecting mental health

II. Management
   a. Care transitions
   b. Behavioral, environmental, and pharmacological interventions and communication for behaviors
   c. Pharmacotherapeutics
   d. Referrals
   e. Influences from decisional capacity, health literacy
   f. Patient/family/peer education: mental and physical health interactions
   g. Ethical/legal and socioeconomic factors

Model builds on the APA Guidelines for Psychological Practice with Older Adults (APA, 2004) by laying out more specific goals for training. The competencies are aspirational in nature and are intended to guide entry-level psychologists with specialized practice with older adults. The Council of Professional Geropsychology Training Programs created the Pikes Peak Geropsychology Knowledge and Skill Assessment Tool for supervisors to assess trainees or for psychologists who wish to do a self-assessment (Karel et al., 2010a). The assessment tool rates the psychologist as novice, intermediate, advanced, proficient, or expert in each of the competencies outlined in the Pikes Peak Model. The tool enables supervisors and learners to identify strengths, areas for growth, and goals for training and education.

III. Approach to Older Adults

a. Age-related adaptations
b. Age/culturally appropriate interventions and communications
c. Recognition of personal and societal biases
d. Sensitivity in end-of-life care

IV. Role

a. Promotion of safety and risk factor reduction
b. Knowledge of geriatric mental health/illness
c. Lifelong learning
d. Policy/advocacy
e. Research participation/use
f. Quality-improvement initiatives
g. Interdisciplinarity
h. Delivery systems
i. Service barriers

SOURCE: POGOe, 2010.

Disseminating Training Resources

Once core competencies are identified, the challenge remains of integrating the skills and knowledge into classes and training courses. Some professions are developing and disseminating tools that instructors can use to infuse geriatric MH/SU into their curriculum. The geriatric MH/SU teaching tools from the Council on Social Work Education (CSWE) and the Hartford Institute for Geriatric Nursing are evidence based, free, and include supporting materials to simplify the use of them. The NASW also offers professional development courses on aging, substance abuse, and related topics online, including webinars, for a cost or free of charge (NASW, 2012).

The CSWE Gero-ed Center, funded by the John A. Hartford Foundation, was created with the mission of promoting gerontological competencies in social work. The Gero Innovations Grant (GIG) was one part of the

Master's Advanced Curriculum Project, which ran from 2007 to 2010 with the goal of enhancing advanced specialty training in older adult health, mental health, and substance abuse. From 2007 to 2009, the GIG provided funding to 14 MSW programs to develop and evaluate teaching tools and strategies for social work in gerontological health, mental health, and substance abuse. All but one of the grantees developed teaching modules related to mental health or substance use. The teaching modules cover diverse topics, including depression, anxiety, paranoia, mental health in older Latinos, polypharmacy, mental health in skilled nursing facilities, informal sources of mental health care in Native American traditions, and co-occurring MH/SU conditions. All of the modules are posted on the CSWE Gero-Ed Center website,[11] along with supporting materials such as lecture slides, videos, instructor scripts, course reading lists, vignettes, and case studies.

The Hartford Institute for Geriatric Nursing at the New York University College of Nursing has created a series of guides to best practices and assessment tools relevant to the care of geriatric patients. The "Try This" series has several tools related to MH/SU, including the Geriatric Depression Scale in English and Spanish, alcohol use screening and assessment, and the Horowitz Impact of Event Scale for posttraumatic stress. There are other tools that are not specifically related to MH/SU, but that are highly relevant to caring for older patients with MH/SU conditions, such as the Beers Criteria for Potentially Inappropriate Medication Use in the Elderly, the Transitional Care Model criteria for hospital discharge screening for high-risk older adults, and the Preparedness for Caregiving Scale. The assessments are intended to be simple, requiring less than 20 minutes to administer. The material is contained within a two-page brief, with background information on the issue; an explanation of the assessment's validity, strengths, and limitations; and a list of additional resources. Most assessments in the series are also accompanied by a longer "How to Try This" article from the *American Journal of Nursing* that provides case studies for more nuanced instruction, and a video that demonstrates how to administer the tool. The entire series is available for free on the Web,[12] and may be reproduced for educational purposes without fee.

Integrating Geriatric MH/SU Competencies in Education

The GeriEd Program at the Albert Einstein College of Medicine (AECOM) is one program that uses classroom and clinical lessons to

[11]See http://www.cswe.org/CentersInitiatives/GeroEdCenter.aspx.

[12]See http://www.ConsultGeriRN.org.

expose undergraduate medical students to geriatric issues, including MH/SU, before they choose a specialty. The first- and second-year curricula weave geriatric content into small-group lectures and workshops on the patient. In the first year, 15 to 20 students are assigned to a geriatric practicum to begin learning clinical interviewing skills. The geriatric program, which has been offered since 2002, focuses on the mental status exam, social and functional history, and palliative care. Students work in multidisciplinary teams across various clinical settings, including outpatient, home care, and long-term care. The clinical experiences are paired with group sessions that cover topics such as depression, dementia, and chronic illness. Students in the geriatric program can continue their learning by monitoring community-dwelling patients on an ongoing basis. In the third and fourth year, all students are required to do a 2-week clerkship in geriatrics, which includes training in assessing and managing depression. This clerkship has been required at AECOM since 1995 (Ehrlich and Jacobs, 2004).

AECOM received a $100,000 grant in 2001 from the AAMC and the Hartford Foundation to fully integrate geriatric content into relevant areas throughout undergraduate medical education. From 2006 to 2010, the Donald W. Reynolds Foundation gave AECOM nearly $2 million toward the innovative integration of geriatrics into training activities. The AAMC/Hartford Foundation and the Reynolds Foundation grant programs each gave similar awards to 39 other medical schools (AAMC, 2003; Donald W. Reynolds Foundation, 2011).

Training the Existing Health Care Workforce in Geriatric MH/SU Issues

While improving formal education is crucial to improving the workforce's competence in geriatric MH/SU, there is a large existing workforce that must be trained as well. Strengthening the geriatric MH/SU workforce requires reaching providers of all types throughout their careers. This can be done through several methods, including in-service training and continuing education.

In-Service Training

One example of geriatric mental health in-service training is a program called Training in the Assessment of Depression (TRIAD). TRIAD is a brief intervention that improves the ability of home care nurses to identify depression symptoms in older adults and make appropriate referrals. This intervention was developed by Bruce and colleagues (2007) in collaboration with three home care agencies, and tested in a randomized controlled trial with 53 home care RNs. The intervention used the depression portion of the Outcome and Assessment Information Set (OASIS) because this information is already required by Medicare and would not overburden the workload of nurses. OASIS requires nurses to document signs of depressions, but does not provide guidance on identifying symptoms. The intervention trained nurses in observing behavioral and nonverbal signs that could indicate depression, understanding conditions that can complicate depression assessment, and asking follow-up questions to determine the persistence and severity of symptoms. The training took place over two sessions, totaling 4.5 hours, and included didactic instruction, role playing, and watching demonstration videos. Bruce and colleagues found that training increased the rate of depression referrals, without increasing false-positive referrals, and that referred patients had better clinical outcomes than patients who were not referred.

To disseminate this training, TRIAD has been adapted into a Web-based learning module, called Depression Recognition and Assessment in Older Homecare Patients (Weill Medical College of Cornell University, 2004). It includes training on identifying and assessing depression, recognizing and handling suicide ideation, and making a referral. Users may also download Weill Cornell's Depression Screening Toolkit (Weill Cornell Homecare Research Partnership, 2004).

Continuing Education

Most licensed professions require practitioners to receive continuing education each year to build competency and promote professional growth. For providers who may have received little training or education in school about geriatric MH/SU, continuing education is one possible way to gain this knowledge. Boston University's Institute for Geriatric Social Work has numerous online training courses that provide continuing education credits for social workers. Topics include geriatric assessment, mental health and aging, substance abuse, compulsive hoarding, suicide prevention, among many others relevant to geriatric MH/SU. Social workers can take these online training courses to earn a certificate in Mental Health and Aging, which requires six courses (Boston University Institute for Geriatric Social Work, 2011).

University of Washington also offers several types of continuing education opportunities related to geriatric MH/SU. For example, existing providers may enroll in courses such as diagnosing and treating older adults with chronic mental illnesses, mood and thought disorders in older adults, and the psychology of aging. The courses are generally held weekly over an academic quarter, in a downtown classroom. Providers may also pursue a certificate in geriatric mental health by enrolling in a five-course program that lasts 12 to 24 months. The University of Washington geriatric MH/SU continuing education programs are geared toward an array of professionals, including social workers, mental health counselors, marriage and family therapists, and psychologists (University of Washington Professional and Continuing Education, 2012).

Training in Cultural Competency

The Stanford Geriatric Education Center (SGEC), a collaborative project from Stanford University School of Medicine, San Jose State University, Community Health Partnership, and Santa Clara County Mental Health Department, specializes in developing and providing multidisciplinary training in geriatric care for ethnic minorities. The SGEC offers training through several different media. It holds monthly webinars on clinical ethnogeriatric topics, including depression and mental health, which physicians, nurses, psychologists, social workers, or MFTs may use for continuing education credit. The SGEC also offers a 10-module curriculum for teaching culturally appropriate depression and dementia care for older adults at risk for diabetes. Instructors may download a handbook and Power Point slides for each module. The curriculum provides in-depth discussions of depression, dementia, and diabetes in African Americans, American Indians, Chinese Americans, Filipino Americans, Hmong Americans, Japanese Americans, and Mexican Americans. The SGEC and OnLok Senior Health, a local senior service organization, developed Diversity, Healing, and Health Care, a unique Web-based resource for clinicians who see older patients from diverse backgrounds. The website is a quick-reference source on ethnicity, religion, and age, so that clinicians can have a baseline context for interacting with patients. Information includes greetings and introductions in various languages, cultural attitudes about illness and disability, religious customs at time of death, and major cohort life events (see Table 3-3).

Interprofessional Training

Competencies in interdisciplinary care have been developed and endorsed by many professional education groups, including the Accreditation Council for Graduate Medical Education, American Association of Colleges of Nursing, American Geriatrics Society, American Psychological Association, American Society of Consultant Pharmacists, and Council on Social Work Education, among other professional groups. The Interprofessional Education Collaborative, a joint effort among schools of allopathic and osteopathic medicine, nursing, dentistry, pharmacy, and public health, recently published core competencies for interprofessional

TABLE 3-3
Example of a Cultural Competence Tool: Korean American Life Cohort Events

Years	Historical Events Experienced by Korean American Elders	Current Age of Older Adult			
		55-65 Years	65-75 Years	75-85 Years	85+ Years
		Life Stage at Time of Event			
1980-present	Increased fractionalization among Koreans Post–Rodney King decision focuses on Korean Americans Number of women continues to outnumber men Continued population influx: 1980 population was 354,600; 1990 population exceeded 800,000	Young adults, middle aged	Middle aged, Young-old	Young-old, old	Old
1970s	Influx of Koreans after the Immigration and Nationality Act of 1965 Women continue to outnumber men, 10:7 Educated, middle-class immigrants Stereotypes: liquor store operators and green grocers Korean towns emerge in urban areas	Adolescents, young adults	Young adults, middle aged	Middle aged, young-old	Young-old, old

1940-1960	Slow move out of Chinatowns Awareness of war brides and orphans as fallout from Korean War Population change, more women to men, 10:7 1950-1953 Korean War; war brides and war orphans	Children, adolescents	Adolescents, young adults	Young adults, middle aged	Middle aged, young-old
1920-1940	Lived in rural areas and Chinatowns Lumped with Asian groups as "Oriental" Some families, and small communities in Hawaii and California Population was 4 men for each woman 1924 Immigration Act stops picture brides	Children	Children, adolescents	Adolescents, young adults	Young adults, middle aged
1900-1920	Laborers moved to West Coast of United States 1906—beginning of picture brides Immigrants were 10 men for each woman 1902—immigration to Hawaii	—	Children	Children, adolescents	Adolescents, young adults
Pre-1900	Limited information about immigration to the United States is available; numbers of immigrants few or none	—	—	Children	Children, adolescents

SOURCE: Adapted from Stanford Geriatric Education Center, 2004.

education, delineating what this concept means in practice and what this training should accomplish (Interprofessional Education Collaborative Expert Panel, 2011).

Geropsychology training emphasizes interdisciplinary practice and competence in providing a broad range of services to older adults (Karel et al., 2010b). These include (1) assessment of psychological, intellectual, cognitive, functional, personality, emotional, and decision-making capacity; (2) psychological, psycho-educational, behavioral, cognitive rehabilitation, and pain management interventions, end-of-life care, and grief work; (3) consultation to primary care providers, long-term care settings, health and social service agencies, family members and primary caregivers, and attorneys and other legal system personnel; and (4) supervision and management of direct caregivers, interdisciplinary teams, programs, and agencies caring for the elderly.

In response to the 2008 IOM report *Retooling for an Aging America: Building the Health Care Workforce*, 21 health care provider organizations formed a coalition called the Partnership for Health in Aging (PHA). The PHA created *Multidisciplinary Competencies in the Care of Older Adults at the Completion of the Entry-Level Health Professional Degree* (Partnership for Health in Aging, 2010), which identified 23 competencies within 6 domains as essential for the following health professionals: physicians, dentists, nurses, occupational therapists, pharmacists, physical therapists, physician assistants, psychologists, and social workers. The competency domains are health promotion and safety, evaluation and assessment, care planning and coordination across the care spectrum (including end-of-life care), interdisciplinary and team care, caregiver support, and health care system and benefits. This effort did not address competency-based training for DCWs, but the domain of interdisciplinary and team care states that upon completion of the entry-level degree, health professionals should know and be able to demonstrate how to "communicate and collaborate with older adults, their caregivers, other health care professionals, and direct care workers to incorporate discipline-specific information into overall team care planning and implementation" (Partnership for Health in Aging, 2010, p. 2). The competencies are not centered on mental health in aging, but this interdisciplinary effort is a step toward improving geriatric MH/SU care because older adults with MH/SU conditions often see a constellation of providers because of other health concerns. Mental health is included in three of the six domains, in reference to health interventions, appropriate assessment, and advanced care planning.

The Geriatric Education Centers (GECs), funded through grants from HRSA, are collaborative arrangements that bring different health professionals together for training in geriatric care. To receive a grant, a GEC must offer interdisciplinary education that involves at least four health professions. The disciplines may include allopathic or osteopathic medicine, dentistry, optometry, podiatry, pharmacy, nursing, physician assistant practice, chiropractic, clinical psychology, health administration, allied health professions, professional counseling, and social work.

PROMOTING THE ROLE OF DIRECT CARE WORKERS IN GERIATRIC MH/SU CARE

DCWs are involved in the care of many older adults with MH/SU conditions. The demand for direct care services is growing with the aging population, yet the growth of this workforce is not keeping pace (Stone and Urban Institute Staff, 2011). The low professional status of DCWs and limited opportunities for growth in this field make it difficult to attract and retain a quality workforce. Most professions are recognized through credentials, such as certificates, licenses, and degrees, that verify an individual has received training and is able to perform the duties required of the profession. As discussed in the review of the direct care workforce, credentialing for direct care workers is limited. Recognition and growth of this profession will require a higher, more consistent level of training. Currently there are few advancement opportunities, or incentives to invest in such opportunities, for DCWs who excel in their work or wish to get more training in their profession. This section will discuss strategies for training DCWs and promoting their role in geriatric MH/SU care.

Training in Geriatric MH/SU

DCWs who have received special training in working with older adults and others with MH/SU disorders have been shown to provide better care for clients with these conditions. However, few direct care workers receive such training in the normal course of employment. Analysis of human capital investment, based on Becker (1962) and the stream of literature that followed this seminal work, suggests that employers do not benefit from providing general training that is transferrable to other settings because trained workers could leave for higher pay elsewhere. A result of this low investment in training is that employers do not have an incentive to increase wages or benefits in order to retain workers.

The lack of training at the organizational level is undoubtedly reinforced by the lack of national standards for this occupation. National requirements for training only exist for certain types of DCWs in specific settings, leaving a great number of DCWs for whom no consistent standards apply. Where standards exist, training requirements for DCWs tend to be minimal in hours and in content, with little included on MH/SU issues. While some groups, such as the Direct Care Alliance, the Paraprofessional Healthcare Institute (PHI), and the National Association for Home Care and Hospice, have created DCW training programs, there are few initiatives to improve older adult MH/SU care training, even though DCWs play a prominent role in long-term care and home care, where older adults are primary recipients of services.

In 2010 the state of Alaska formed a public-private collaborative to address the challenge of training DCWs. It created the Alaskan Core Competencies for Direct Care Workers in Health and Human Services, a set of competencies relevant across diverse health care sectors that include long-term care, mental health, addictions, developmental disabilities, and traumatic brain injury. The competencies can be used to develop training content for initial or continuing education, update existing curricula, or assess employee competencies. To assist organizations in using the competencies, a companion toolkit for assessing worker competencies was released in 2011. A curriculum for the competencies has been piloted with DCWs, including those from long-term care, and is scheduled for release in 2012.

This initiative has been funded by the Alaska Mental Health Trust Authority and the Alaska Department of Health and Social Services. The competencies, assessment tools, and curriculum have been developed by the Western Interstate Commission for Higher Education Mental Health Program and the Annapolis Coalition on the Behavioral Health Workforce, with oversight from a committee of Alaskans. A project description and the work products are available for review at http://www.annapoliscoalition.org/core_competencies.aspx.

The Affordable Care Act authorized, and Congress appropriated funds for a 2-year demonstration in core competency training for personal and home care aides (the Personal and Home Care Aide State Training Program or PHCAST).[13] Six states—California, Iowa, Maine, Massachusetts, Michigan, and North Carolina—were awarded funds to develop and evaluate core competencies, pilot training curricula, and certification programs for personal and home care aides. Although, the grantees are not required to include core competencies in MH/SU, Maine's program includes the development of a specialized training track to help prepare individuals to become mental health rehabilitation technicians. Michigan's program includes in-service continuing education training that focuses on critical topics, including the management of behavior issues in people with dementia.

[13]Public Law 111-148.

Professional Recognition of Competency in Geriatric MH/SU Care

As discussed in the review of the DCW workforce, there are currently few ways for DCWs to earn recognition for their skill, competency, and experience. DCWs are typically paid low entry wages that do not rise substantially with experience, either with tenure in one job or tenure in the occupation. Squillace and colleagues found "years of experience do not translate into higher wages; CNAs with 10 or more years of experience averaged just $2/hr more than aides who started working in the field less than 1 year ago" (Squillace et al., 2009, p. 185).

DCWs do not have a strong incentive to seek extra training, knowledge, or skills because their training and experience are often not certified at all. Where certification exists, it represents a very minimal standard rather than a level of achievement, such as in the case of the 75 hours of experience mandated for certified nursing assistants working in Medicare- and Medicaid-certified nursing homes. Additional training for DCWs is rarely available except through special grants and initiatives (Eaton et al., 2001; Harmuth and Konrad, 2010; Wilson et al., 2003). With basic training and recognition being so rarely obtained, recognition of competence in a specialty area such as MH/SU is even further off.

The state of California has had a well-established workforce of licensed MH/SU DCWs, called psychiatric technicians, for decades, and demonstrates a successful movement in professionalization of a historically devalued occupation. Psychiatric technicians are licensed by the Board of Vocational Nursing and Psychiatric Technicians, and are considered to be of similar skill level to LVNs. As of 2008 there are approximately 14,000 psychiatric technicians in California. They are employed by hospitals, correctional facilities, psychiatric emergency response teams, residential treatment programs, and many other settings where psychiatric services are needed. The state accredits psychiatric technician education programs and requires 576 hours of didactic learning and 954 hours of supervised clinical experience. Curriculum must include learning in gerontological nursing. Psychiatric technicians must complete 30 hours of continuing education every 2 years to maintain licensure.

The professional recognition of psychiatric technicians emerged from advocacy efforts of psychiatric "attendants" and "aides" from state mental institutions who organized into the California Society of Psychiatric Technicians in 1950. In 1951, California added psychiatric technician as a state civil service classification, which created specific minimum requirements for entry into the field. Because more psychiatric technicians were emerging in settings that were not run by the state, California created an exam that could be used to establish the eligibility of any psychiatric technician. This development eventually led the state to develop a professional license for this occupation in 1970. The California Association of

Psychiatric Technicians, which serves both as a union for state employees and as a professional organization for all psychiatric technicians, has since advocated for additional advancements in the profession. In 1989, legislation passed requiring continuing education and license renewal for psychiatric technicians. Since 1998, psychiatric technicians have been allowed to draw blood and administer hypodermic injections after receiving additional training. California is one of three states to license psychiatric technicians. The others are Colorado and Kansas. Arkansas licensed psychiatric technicians at one time, but stopped in 2009.

Several states offer DCW development initiatives, some of which include opportunities for specific training in working with older adults with MH/SU conditions. For example, the state of Iowa created a Direct Care Workforce Advisory Council that is mandated with collecting data on the DCW workforce, implementing a HRSA grant-funded pilot training and credentialing program, and making recommendations for advancing this workforce. The Council has recommended a structure of core training, advanced training, and specialty endorsement, with each level conferring an additional level of credentialing. Specialty endorsements would be created by experts in the subject area and approved by the state. Proposed areas of specialization include MH/SU-related areas, including Alzheimer's/dementia, mental health, positive behavior support, and psychiatric care. As of March 2012, Iowa is proposing legislation to license DCWs. The legislation follows the recommendations of the Advisory Council and would require the development of statewide curriculum standards and licensing requirements, with opportunities for advancement and specialization (Ozga, 2012).

EMPOWERING OLDER ADULTS AND THEIR FAMILIES

On a day-to-day basis, consumers and families carry far more responsibility for older adult MH/SU care than any professional group. Family caregiving, self-care, and peer support play a large role in the health and well-being of older adults with MH/SU conditions, whether these activities are formally organized or not. Supporting consumers in being active participants in their health is a critical aspect of patient-centered care (see Box 3-6). The President's New Freedom Commission report, the Surgeon General's report on mental health, and the IOM's *Improving the Quality of Health Care for Mental and Substance-Use Conditions* report have all called for more consumer and family involvement in the process of care in order to improve outcomes and experiences for both consumers and families (Hogan, 2003; IOM, 2006; SAMHSA, 1999).

BOX 3-6
Rules for Patient-Centered Care

Customization based on patient needs and values: The system of care should be designed to meet the most common types of needs, but have the capability to respond to individual patient choices and preferences.

The patient as the source of control: Patients should be given the necessary information and the opportunity to exercise the degree of control they choose over health care decisions that affect them. The health system should be able to accommodate differences in patient preferences and encourage shared decision making.

Shared knowledge and the free flow of information: Patients should have unfettered access to their own medical information and to clinical knowledge. Clinicians and patients should communicate effectively and share information.

The need for transparency: The health care system should make available to patients and their families information that allows them to make informed decisions when selecting a health plan, hospital, or clinical practice, or choosing among alternative treatments. This should include information describing the system's performance on safety, evidence-based practice, and patient satisfaction.

Anticipation of needs: The health system should anticipate patient needs, rather than simply reacting to events.

SOURCE: IOM, 2001.

Expanding Peer-Led Support Programs for Older Adults

The demand for more consumer-led, recovery-oriented services has increased in past decades and continues to grow, and evidence supporting the benefits of these services is emerging.[14] However, information on the availability and impact of MH/SU peer support for older adults is sparse, although some noteworthy programs provide consumer-oriented, peer-

[14]See Box 4-1 (in Chapter 4) for a description of recent trends in peer support.

led MH/SU support to older adults, including programs associated with larger establishments like Alcoholics Anonymous (AA) and the VHA.

Seniors in Sobriety (SIS) is a coalition of AA members who are concerned with spreading the message of sobriety to older adult alcoholics (SIS, 2012). SIS, originally called Sober over Sixty, began in 1990 in southeastern New York (SIS, 2012). The reach of SIS has grown, as more communities recognize the unique concerns of older adult alcoholics. According to the 2004 AA Membership Survey, 16 percent of AA members are over age 60, and 23 percent are ages 51 through 60 (Alcoholics Anonymous, 2008). Communities in Hawaii, mid-southern California, and Arizona have established standing Cooperation with the Elder Community committees to work on service and outreach to older adult alcoholics. Nearly 30 groups across 11 states and one Canadian province have started AA meetings for seniors in places of worship, senior centers, retirement homes, and other senior-oriented settings.

Vet-to-Vet is a peer-led support program for veterans with serious mental illnesses. Vet-to-Vet follows a consumer-professional partnership model, where groups are separate from formal VA medical services, but peer leaders work in close consultation with mental health professionals (Resnick et al., 2004). Many Vet-to-Vet groups are physically located at VA centers to maximize accessibility for participants and to facilitate consultation between consumer providers and mental health professionals, though the program has been adopted in non-VA community settings as well (Barber et al., 2008). A 2008 nationwide survey of Vet-to-Vet participants from 38 sites found that over 40 percent of participants were black or Latino, and 90 percent were men (Barber et al., 2008). While Vet-to-Vet is inclusive of all veterans and does not target older adults, the average age of participants is 53 (Barber et al., 2008). In a study of Vet-to-Vet attendance indicators, Resnick found that older age, more negative attitudes toward recovery, and lower levels of functioning were positively correlated with more frequent attendance, suggesting that this peer support model reaches veterans who may otherwise not typically access peer support services (Resnick, 2010).

Providing Physical, Financial, and Psychosocial Support for Families

Few family caregivers are trained to take on these roles even though the burden can be heavy. Family caregivers are at high risk for depression. A study of over 5,500 caregivers of people with dementia found that 32 percent met criteria for depression. Caregivers of people with behavioral disturbances, such as angry or aggressive behavior, and those who spent more time caregiving were more likely to experience depression (Covinsky et al., 2003). Caregiving also can cause financial strain when individuals quit their job or reduce their hours to fulfill their caregiving duties. Approximately 42 percent have less than $50,000 in household income. Caregivers also tend to have family obligations outside of tending to their sick relative. The majority are married, and more than one-third have children or grandchildren under age 18 in the household (National Alliance for Caregiving and AARP, 2009). Data on caregivers who specifically care for older adults with MH/SU conditions are limited.

Training and education for family caregivers and providing a supportive environment to talk have shown encouraging results. In a review of family psychoeducation as an intervention for serious mental illnesses, McFarlane et al. (2003) found more than 30 randomized trials with positive outcomes for patient recovery and family well-being. While more research is needed to explore the efficacy of different modes of psychoeducation delivery, McFarlane and colleagues concluded that support, information, guidance, and sharing of burden are the most critical aspects of family education. The CMS Leadership Summit on the Direct Care Workforce and Family Caregivers recommends that training for family caregivers should be flexible, optional, accessible, "just in time," self-paced, and customized to meet the needs of individual caregivers and people receiving care (Direct Service Workforce Resource Center, 2011).

Many state organizations and local affiliates of the National Alliance for Mental Illness (NAMI) have adapted programs or started other programs to meet the needs of their communities' consumers and families. NAMI New Hampshire (NAMI NH) created a program specifically for older adults with mental illness, their families and caregivers, called Side-by-Side for Independent Living (NAMI New Hampshire, 2012). Side-by-Side is an educational workshop series with nine parts: (1) meeting caregiver needs, (2) navigating the health system, (3) depression and suicide, (4) mental health issues, (5) substance abuse and misuse, (6) understanding dementia, (7) challenging behaviors, (8) legal issues, and (9) wellness and healthy living. Each session consists of 1 hour of educational material and 1 hour of discussion. NAMI NH has partnered with hospitals, senior centers, assisted living facilities, community mental health centers, and adult day programs to bring Side-by-Side to groups most likely to benefit from this information. In some communities, NAMI NH has partnered with major employers to offer workshops onsite during lunch hour to reach caregivers who may not be able to attend classes at other times. Training can be offered as a series or as individual modules to maximize flexibility and meet specific needs. In evaluations of the program, 95 percent of over 400 program participants reported being more aware of supports related to mental illness in older adults, and/or for caregiver issues (NAMI New Hampshire, 2010).

Taking time away from caregiving is critical for family caregivers.

Since 2009, the U.S. Administration on Aging has provided funding to 24 states to implement State Lifespan Respite Programs, which are designed to help families find respite providers and access respite payment resources (AoA, 2010).

Addressing the Needs of Diverse Populations

Providing culturally competent care is critical to reaching older adults with MH/SU conditions. In the case of depressive illness, older minorities with depression report higher impairment levels and are more persistently ill than non-Hispanic, white older adults (Brown et al., 1996; Williams et al., 2007), yet they also report decreased rates of mental health care (Alegria et al., 2008). For example, among Medicare beneficiaries, Latinos are approximately only half as likely as others to receive treatment for depression and are the least likely to be treated using psychotherapy (Crystal et al., 2003).

The diverse needs of the family caregiver mirror those of the consumer. Some studies have shown that caregiver depression rates may differ among racial groups. For example, African American caregivers report lower levels of burden than white caregivers (Janevic and Connell, 2001), while Hispanic caregivers experience high levels of depression and burden (Magaña et al., 2007; Pinquart and Sorensen, 2005). Differences in level of burden may be due to specific cultural values, their influences on how stress is perceived, and what coping techniques are employed, as well as issues related to perception of burden within and among subgroups of family caregivers (Adams et al., 2002; Aranda and Knight, 1997; Knight and Sayegh, 2010). Effectively reaching caregivers from diverse populations requires understanding of these specific cultural norms and developing culturally and linguistically relevant services (Aranda et al., 2003; Chadiha et al., 2006).

Engaging older consumers and families from minority populations is a unique challenge that is currently not widely addressed. One exemplary effort is from the Union of Pan Asian Communities (UPAC), a human services organization in San Diego that offers an array of support opportunities for older adults with MH/SU conditions. UPAC operates a counseling and treatment center for monolingual and limited English-proficient Asian and Pacific Islander adults and older adults with mental illness. The center focuses on helping individuals and their families to better understand the effects of posttraumatic stress, depression, and social isolation. Most clients are immigrants and refugees who face other challenges such as lack of access to health care and community resources, previous or ongoing trauma, past incarceration, and alcohol, drug, or gambling addictions. Another of UPAC's major programs, Elderly Multicultural Access and Support Services (EMASS), has helped over 800 Filipino, Latino, African American, and Somali clients learn about and discuss mental health issues through culturally tailored "Good Mental Health" forums and other activities. Focus groups run by the Health Services Research Center of the University of California, San Diego, found that EMASS participants reported an increased knowledge of prevention and early intervention for mental health problems, and a relief of mental health symptoms, including depression and anxiety (Union of Pan Asian Communities, 2011). In addition to these services, UPAC operates the East Wind Club House, which provides peer-led socialization and rehabilitation activities to approximately 180 chronically ill Southeast Asian adults and older adults with mental disabilities. It is the first program of this kind in California. UPAC also partners with other community organizations to provide multicultural peer and family support at the San Diego County Psychiatric Hospital. This program specifically staffs Older Adult Family Support Specialists (Montrose Counseling Center, 2012b).

Along with ethnic and racial minority populations, lesbian, gay, bisexual, and transgender (LGBT) older adults are also often disenfranchised as MH/SU consumers (Hunter, 2005). The Montrose Counseling Center in Houston is dedicated to providing affordable mental health services to the local LGBT community. Montrose launched the Seniors Preparing for Rainbow Years (SPRY) program in 2005 specifically to meet the needs of older adults. SPRY holds weekly men's and women's peer support groups, sponsors social activities, and provides professional counseling and case management. Montrose has launched a community campaign that encourages anyone to become an advocate for LGBT seniors. Advocates receive a 1-day training to recognize signs of depression, suicide risk, and substance abuse in LGBT seniors. Advocates are trained in QPR (Question, Persuade, and Refer) to connect older adults to SPRY services (Montrose Counseling Center, 2012a).

FINDINGS AND CONCLUSIONS

The committee's finding on the current state of the geriatric MH/SU workforce are summarized in Box 3-7. The barriers to building an adequately sized, well-trained geriatric MH/SU workforce are numerous and complex. Recent efforts to augment training show that even when provided opportunities to specialize in geriatric MH/SU, students often do not choose to pursue them. This could be because financial returns for specializing in geriatric MH/SU are relatively unfavorable. However, money does not always override negative perceptions of MH/SU and aging, or professional influences to enter more "prestigious" specialties. These observations underscore the importance of simultaneously provid-

BOX 3-7
Findings on the Geriatric Mental Health and Substance Use (MH/SU) Workforce

Defining the Geriatric MH/SU Workforce

a. The geriatric MH/SU workforce is made up of many types of providers. Workforce roles are often poorly defined and overlapping.

Estimating Workforce Supply and Demand

b. Standardized workforce data that are trended over the time required to make accurate predictions of workforce supply and demand are not available.

Shortage of Geriatric MH/SU Providers

c. The workforce prepared to care for geriatric MH/SU is inadequate in sheer numbers, with the growth of the population threatening to exacerbate this.

Recruiting Geriatric MH/SU Providers

d. Across all health professions, relatively few opportunities exist for specialization in geriatric MH/SU. There is little support or mentorship available for those who do pursue specialization.
e. Financial incentives are not in place to encourage geriatric MH/SU providers to enter and stay in this field.

Inadequate Preparation of the Geriatric MH/SU Workforce

f. Professional training in geriatric MH/SU is inconsistent and not well documented because national standards and requirements in these areas are minimal and vague. MH/SU specialists have little

ing more training opportunities, guidance, mentorship, positive experiences, and financial incentives. Building up one of these components without considering the others will not solve the workforce crisis at hand.

Training general health care professionals and direct care workers is pivotal to improving the workforce because they are the most likely to have contact with older adults with MH/SU conditions. The extent to which training and education are provided for these groups is not well documented. Relatively few standards ensure that formal training programs include competencies in addressing MH/SU conditions in older adults. Also essential to training are skills in cultural competence and interprofessional collaboration to meet the complex needs of older adults.

required training in geriatrics; geriatric specialists have little required training in MH/SU; and most general providers do not have extensive requirements in either area.

Training the Geriatric MH/SU Workforce

g. Many professions have made progress on geriatric MH/SU competency development and workforce development, though these efforts are often done in silos where their dissemination and impact are not easily measured.
h. Innovations in geriatric MH/SU workforce development are often vulnerable to grant cuts, and many promising programs end without adequate documentation or evaluation to assist future development.

Strengthening the Role of Direct Care Workers (DCWs) in Geriatric MH/SU Care

i. Complex factors, including poor working conditions, low wages, lack of training, and limited opportunities for advancement, deter the development of a stable DCW workforce.
j. DCWs have the most contact with older adult patients, yet do not have adequate training in geriatrics or MH/SU, and virtually never get trained in both.

Empowering Older Adults and Their Families

k. There is a growing emphasis on peer support and self-care, including for older adult populations.
l. Family members play a major role as caregivers, but receive little support and training for caring for older adults with any medical conditions, including MH/SU conditions.

However, the evidence base to determine what modes of training are most effective in geriatric MH/SU is largely insufficient.

Consumers and their families are often overlooked members of the workforce, though this is changing with an increasing number of initiatives to hire consumers and family members as paid providers. Even for those not formally entering the workforce, opportunities for education and support are growing. Whether these initiatives are specifically reaching older MH/SU consumers and their caregivers has not been thoroughly evaluated. The degree to which existing education and support programs are culturally sensitive and accessible to minority populations is also unknown.

REFERENCES

AACN (American Association of Colleges of Nursing). 2004. *AACN adopts a new vision for the future of nursing education and practice.* http://www.aacn.nche.edu/news/articles/2004/dnp-release (accessed October 12, 2011).

———. 2008. *The essentials of baccalaureate education for professional nursing practice.* Washington, DC: AACN.

———. 2010a. *Adult-gerontology clinical nurse specialist competencies.* http://www.aacn.nche.edu/education-resources/competencies-older-adults (accessed October 13, 2011).

———. 2010b. *Adult-gerontology primary care nurse practitioner competencies.* http://www.aacn.nche.edu/education-resources/competencies-older-adults (accessed October 13, 2011).

AACN Commission on Nurse Certification. 2011. *History of CNL certification.* http://www.aacn.nche.edu/leading-initiatives/cnl/cnl-certification/pdf/History.pdf (accessed October 13, 2011).

AACP (American Association of Colleges of Pharmacy). 2010. *Pharmacy school admission requirements, 2011-2012.* Alexandria, VA: AACP.

AAFP (American Academy of Family Physicians). 2011. *Primary care.* http://www.aafp.org/online/en/home/policy/policies/p/primarycare.html#Parsys0004 (accessed September 29, 2011).

AAGP (American Association of Geriatric Psychiatry). 2011. *Scholars fund.* http://www.aagponline.org/index.php?submenu=forstudents_submenu&src=gendocs&ref=ScholarsProgram&category=forstudents_submenu&link=ScholarsProgram (accessed April 2, 2012).

AAMC (Association of American Medical Colleges). 2003. *Geriatrics instruction in the medical school curriculum. Analysis in brief.* Washington, DC: AAMC.

———. 2008. *Physician specialty data.* https://www.aamc.org/download/47352/data/specialtydata.pdf (accessed December 5, 2011).

———. 2011. *Medical school graduate questionnaire: 2011 all schools summary report.* Washington, DC: AAMC.

AAMFT (American Association for Marriage and Family Therapy). 2006. *Medicare coverage of marriage and family therapists.* http://www.cpca.org/cpca/assets/File/Policy-and-Advocacy/Legislative/Marriage-Family-Therapists/AAMFTMedicareFactSheet.pdf (accessed March 28, 2012).

———. 2011a. *MFT licensing boards.* http://www.aamft.org/iMIS15/AAMFT/Directories/MFT_Licensing_Boards/Content/Directories/MFT_Licensing_Boards.aspx?hkey=b1033df3-6882-491e-87fd-a75c2f7be070 (accessed October 21, 2011).

———. 2011b. *Qualifications and FAQs.* http://www.aamft.org/imis15/Content/About_AAMFT/Qualifications.aspx (accessed October 20, 2011).

AAN (American Academy of Nursing). 2010. *Geropsychiatric nursing collaborative.* http://www.aannet.org/i4a/pages/index.cfm?pageid=3833 (accessed November 21, 2011).

AAPA (American Academy of Physician Assistants). 2010a. *PA facts.* Alexandria, VA: AAPA.

———. 2010b. *Physician assistant census report: Results from the 2010 AAPA census.* Alexandria, VA: AAPA.

AAPC (American Association of Pastoral Counselors). 2009. *State licensing for pastoral counselors.* http://www.aapc.org/membership/licensing.aspx (accessed March 29, 2012).

———. 2012. *About us.* http://www.aapc.org/about-us.aspx? (accessed April 12, 2012).

AARP South Carolina. 2010. *Loan forgiveness program for geriatric physicians.* http://www.aarp.org/health/doctors-hospitals/info-09-2010/loan_forgiveness_sc.html (accessed December 22, 2011).

ABFM (American Board of Family Medicine). 2011. *Diplomate statistics.* https://www.theabfm.org/about/stats.aspx (accessed October 3, 2011).

ABIM (American Board of Internal Medicine). 2011. *Candidates certified—all candidates.* Philadelphia. http://www.abim.org/pdf/data-candidates-certified/all-candidates.pdf (accessed December 5, 2011).

ABPN (American Board of Psychiatry and Neurology). 2007. *Frequently asked questions.* http://www.abpn.com/faqs.html (accessed October 3, 2011).

———. 2010a. *Initial certification statistics.* http://www.abpn.com/cert_statistics.html (accessed October 4, 2011).

———. 2010b. *Maintenance of certification statistics.* http://www.abpn.com/moc_statistics.html (accessed October 4, 2011).

ABPP (American Board of Professional Psychology). 2012. *Member specialty boards.* http://www.abpp.org/i4a/pages/index.cfm?pageid=3286 (accessed April 12, 2012).

ACA (American Counseling Association). 2012. *Licensure & certification.* http://www.counseling.org/counselors/LicensureAndCert.aspx (accessed January 23, 2012).

ACGME (Accreditation Council for Graduate Medical Education). 2003a. *ACGME program requirements for graduate medical education in addiction psychiatry.* http://www.acgme.org/acWebsite/downloads/RRC_progReq/401pr703_u105.pdf (accessed April 23, 2010).

———. 2003b. *ACGME program requirements for graduate medical education in geriatric psychiatry.* http://www.acgme.org/acWebsite/downloads/RRC_progReq/407pr703_u105.pdf (accessed April 23, 2010).

———. 2006. *ACGME program requirements for graduate medical education in geriatric medicine.* http://www.acgme.org/acWebsite/downloads/RRC_progReq/125pr0706.pdf (accessed April 23, 2010).

———. 2007. *ACGME program requirements for graduate medical education in geriatric medicine.* http://www.acgme.org/acWebsite/downloads/RRC_progReq/151pr707_ims.pdf (accessed December 5, 2011).

———. 2009. *ACGME program requirements for graduate medical education in psychiatry.* http://www.acgme.org/acWebsite/downloads/RRC_progReq/400_psychiatry_07012007_u04122008.pdf (accessed December 5, 2011).

———. 2012. *Number of accredited programs for the current academic year (2011-2012).* http://www.acgme.org/adspublic/ (accessed January 19, 2011).

ACOTE (Accreditation Council for Occupational Therapy Education). 2012. *2011 Accreditation Council for Occupational Therapy Education standards and interpretive guide.* Bethesda, MD: AOTA.

ACPE (Accreditation Council for Pharmacy Education). 2011. *Accreditation standards and guidelines for the professional program in pharmacy leading to the doctor of pharmacy degree.* Chicago: ACPE.

Adams, B. M., M. P. Aranda, B. J. Kemp, and K. Takagi. 2002. Ethnic and gender differences in appraisal, coping and social support: A comparison of white-American, African-American, Japanese-American and Mexican-American spousal caregivers of persons with dementia. *Journal of Clinical Geropsychology* 8(4):279-301.

AGESW (Association for Gerontology Education in Social Work). 2011. *Pre-dissertation initiative.* http://agesw.org/about-agesw/pre-dissertation-initiative (accessed April 6, 2012).

AGS (American Geriatrics Society). 2011. *State loan forgiveness toolkit.* http://www.americangeriatrics.org/ags_state_affiliates/state_affiliate_handbook/loan_forgiveness_toolkit/ (accessed December 22, 2011).

Alcoholics Anonymous. 2008. *Alcoholics Anonymous 2007 membership survey.* http://www.aa.org/pdf/products/p-48_07survey.pdf (accessed April 12, 2012).

Alegria, M., P. Chatterji, K. Wells, Z. Cao, C. N. Chen, D. Takeuchi, J. Jackson, and X. L. Meng. 2008. Disparity in depression treatment among racial and ethnic minority populations in the United States. *Psychiatric Services* 59(11):1264-1272.

ANA (American Nurses Association). 2011. *What is nursing?* http://www.nursingworld.org/EspeciallyForYou/StudentNurses/WhatisNursing.aspx (accessed October 6, 2011).

ANCC (American Nurses Credentialing Center). 2010a. *Gerontological nursing board certification test content outline.* http://www.nursecredentialing.org/GeroNurse-TCO2012.aspx (accessed October 12, 2011).

———. 2010b. *Psychiatric and mental health nursing board certification test content outline.* http://www.nursecredentialing.org/PsychNurse-TCO2012.aspx (accessed October 12, 2011).

———. 2012. *Renew your nursing certification.* http://www.nursecredentialing.org/Renew-Certification.aspx (accessed January 5, 2012).

AoA (Administraton on Aging). 2010. *Older Americans 2010: Key indicators of well-being.* http://www.agingstats.gov/Main_Site/Data/2010_Documents/docs/Introduction.pdf (accessed April 12, 2012).

AOA (American Osteopathic Association). 2010. *Osteopathic medical profession report.* Chicago: AOA.

———. 2011a. *Basic standards for fellowship training in addiction medicine in osteopathic family medicine and manipulative treatment.* http://www.osteopathic.org/inside-aoa/accreditation/postdoctoral-training-approval/postdoctoral-training-standards/Documents/basic-standards-for-fellowship-training-in-addiction-medicine-family-practice.pdf (accessed December 5, 2011).

———. 2011b. *Basic standards for fellowship training in geriatrics in osteopathic family medicine and manipulative treatment.* http://www.osteopathic.org/inside-aoa/accreditation/postdoctoral-training-approval/postdoctoral-training-standards/Documents/basic-standards-for-fellowship-training-in-geriatrics-osteopathic-family-practice.pdf (accessed December 5, 2011).

AOTA (American Occupational Therapy Association). 2009. *AOTA board certified in mental health candidate handbook.* Bethesda, MD: AOTA.

———. 2012a. *Board certified and specialty certified practitioners.* http://aota.org/Practitioners/ProfDev/Certification/certified.aspx (accessed March 30, 2012).

———. 2012b. *How to get a license.* http://www.aota.org/Practitioners/Licensure/HowTo.aspx (accessed March 29, 2012).

APA (American Psychiatric Association). 2000. *Diagnostic and statistical manual of mental disorders: DSM-IV-TR, 4th ed.* Washington, DC: American Psychiatric Association.

APA (American Psychological Association). 2004. Guidelines for psychological practice with older adults. *American Psychologist* 59(4):236-260.

———. 2011a. *Frequently asked questions.* http://www.apa.org/workforce/about/faq.aspx#I.6 (accessed October 13, 2011).

———. 2011b. *Public description of clinical psychology.* http://www.apa.org/ed/graduate/specialize/clinical.aspx (accessed October 14, 2011).

———. 2011c. *Public description of counseling psychology.* http://www.apa.org/ed/graduate/specialize/counseling.aspx (accessed October 14, 2011).

———. 2011d. *Recognized specialties and proficiencies in professional psychology.* http://www.apa.org/ed/graduate/specialize/recognized.aspx (accessed October 13, 2011).

———. 2012a. *Effects of cuts in funding for the graduate psychology education program in urban communities.* http://www.apa.org/about/gr/issues/gpe/urban.aspx (accessed April 5, 2012).

———. 2012b. *FY 2011 congressional appropriations request: Strengthen the graduate psychology education program.* http://www.apa.org/about/gr/education/advocacy/2010/gpe-2011.aspx (accessed April 5, 2012).

APA Commission on Accreditation. 2009. *Guidelines and principles for accreditation of programs in professional psychology.* Washington, DC: American Psychological Association.

APRN Consensus Work Group and the National Council of State Boards of Nursing APRN Advisory Committee. 2008. *Consensus model for APRN regulation: Licensure, accreditation, certification and education.* https://www.ncsbn.org/Consensus_Model_for_APRN_Regulation_July_2008.pdf (accessed April 12, 2012).

Aranda, M. P., and B. G. Knight. 1997. The influence of ethnicity and culture on the caregiver stress and coping process: A sociocultural review and analysis. *Gerontologist* 37(3):342-354.

Aranda, M. P., V. M. Villa, L. Trejo, R. Ramirez, and M. Ranney. 2003. El Portal Latino Alzheimer's Project: Model program for Latino caregivers of Alzheimer's disease-affected people. *Social Work* 48(2):259-271.

ARCEPA (Accreditation Review Commission on Education for the Physician Assistant). 2010a. *Accreditation standards for physician assistant education, 4th ed.* http://www.arc-pa.org/acc_standards/ (accessed December 5, 2011).

———. 2010b. *Accredited programs over time.* http://www.arc-pa.org/documents/AccreditedProgamsOverTimegraphasof9.2010.pdf (accessed December 5, 2011).

ASHSP (American Society of Health-System Pharmacists). 2007. *Required educational outcomes, goals, and objectives for postgraduate year two (PGY2) pharmacy residencies in psychiatry.* http://www.ashp.org/DocLibrary/Accreditation/PGY1-Goals-Objectives.aspx (accessed December 5, 2011).

———. 2011. *Online residency directory.* http://accred.ashp.org/aps/pages/directory/residencyProgramSearch.aspx#1 (accessed September 26, 2011).

ASPPB (Association of State and Provincial Psychology Boards). 2011a. *ASPPB information for EPPP candidates: Examination for Professional Practice in Psychology (EPPP).* http://www.asppb.net/files/public/IFC.pdf (accessed October 14, 2011).

———. 2011b. *Degree level requirements for licensure by jurisdiction.* http://www.asppb.org/HandbookPublic/Reports/default.aspx?ReportType=DegreeLevelLiscensure (accessed October 14, 2011).

Association of Postgraduate PA Programs. 2010. *APPAP programs by specialty.* http://www.appap.org/LinkClick.aspx?fileticket=FqFcRIQsEF4%3d&tabid=58 (accessed December 5, 2011).

ASWB (Association of Social Work Boards). 2008. *Social work laws & regulations database.* https://www.datapathdesign.com/ASWB/Laws/Prod/cgi-bin/LawWebRpts2DLL.dll/EXEC/0/0es979v0m3bmaa16a5vok02j02ck (accessed December 5, 2011).

———. 2011. *ASWB examination candidate handbook.* http://www.aswb.org/pdfs/handbook.pdf (accessed December 5, 2011).

ATTC (Addiction Technology Transfer Center). 2011. *Licensing and certification requirements.* http://www.attcnetwork.org/find/certinfo/index.asp (accessed October 20, 2011).

Aud, S., M. A. Fox, and A. Kewal Ramani. 2012. *Status and trends in the education of racial and ethnic groups.* NCES 2010-015. U.S. Department of Education, National Center for Education Statistics. Washington, DC: U.S. Government Printing Office.

Barber, J. A., R. A. Rosenheck, M. Armstrong, and S. G. Resnick. 2008. Monitoring the dissemination of peer support in the VA health care system. *Journal of Community Mental Health* 44:441-443.

Bartels, S. J., B. D. Lebowitz, C. F. Reynolds III, M. L. Bruce, M. Halpain, W. E. Faison, and P. D. Kirwin. 2010. Programs for developing the pipeline of early-career geriatric mental health researchers: Outcomes and implications for other fields. *Academic Medicine* 85(1):26-35.

Barzansky, B., and S. I. Etzel. 2001. Educational programs in U.S. medical schools, 2000-2001. *Journal of the American Medical Association* 286(9):1049-1055.

Beck, C., K. C. Buckwalter, P. M. Dudzik, and L. K. Evans. 2011. Filling the void in geriatric mental health: The Geropsychiatric Nursing Collaborative as a model for change. *Nursing Outlook* 59(4):236-241.

Becker, G. S. 1962. Investment in human capital: A theoretical analysis. *Journal of Political Economy* 70(5 Part 2):9-49.

Bernard, M. A., W. J. McAuley, J. A. Belzer, and K. S. Neal. 2003. An evaluation of a low intensity intervention to introduce medical students to healthy older people. *Journal of the American Geriatrics Society* 51(3):419-423.

BLS (U.S. Bureau of Labor Statistics). 2009a. *Occupational outlook handbook, 2010-11 edition, counselors.* http://www.bls.gov/oco/ocos067.htm (accessed March 28, 2012).

———. 2009b. *Occupational outlook handbook, social workers.* http://www.bls.gov/oco/ocos060.htm (accessed October 19, 2011).

———. 2010. *Occupational employment and wages, May 2009. 29-2061 Licensed practical and licensed vocational nurses.* http://www.bls.gov/oes/current/oes292061.htm (accessed January 19, 2012).

———. 2011. *Occupational employment and wages, May 2010. 29-2061 Licensed practical and licensed vocational nurses.* http://www.bls.gov/oes/current/oes292061.htm (accessed October 10, 2011).

———. 2012a. *Occupational employment and wages, May 2011. 19-3031 Clinical, counseling, and school psychologists.* http://www.bls.gov/oes/current/oes193031.htm (accessed April 6, 2012).

———. 2012b. *Occupational employment and wages, May 2011. 21-1011 Substance abuse and behavioral disorder counselors.* http://www.bls.gov/oes/current/oes211011.htm (accessed April 13, 2012).

———. 2012c. *Occupational employment and wages, May 2011. 21-1013 Marriage and family therapists.* http://www.bls.gov/oes/current/oes211013.htm (accessed April 13, 2012).

———. 2012d. *Occupational employment and wages, May 2011. 21-1014 Mental health counselors.* http://www.bls.gov/oes/current/oes211014.htm (accessed April 13, 2012).

———. 2012e. *Occupational employment and wages, May 2011. 21-1023 Mental health and substance abuse social workers.* http://www.bls.gov/oes/current/oes211023.htm (accessed April 13, 2012).

———. 2012f. *Occupational employment and wages, May 2011. 29-1066 Psychiatrists.* http://data.bls.gov/cgi-bin/print.pl/oes/current/oes291066.htm (accessed April 13, 2012).

———. 2012g. *Occupational employment and wages, May 2011. 29-1122 Occupational therapists.* http://www.bls.gov/oes/current/oes291122.htm (accessed March 29, 2012).

———. 2012h. *Occupational outlook handbook, occupational therapy assistants and aides.* http://www.bls.gov/ooh/Healthcare/Occupational-therapy-assistants-and-aides.htm (accessed March 29, 2012).

Bluebird, G. 2008. *Paving new ground: Peers working in inpatient settings.* Alexandria, VA: National Association of State Mental Health Program Directors.

Bobby, C. L., and R. I. Urofsky. 2008. CACREP adopts new standards. *Counseling Today* 51(2):59-60.

Bookman, A., and M. Harrington. 2007. Family caregivers: A shadow workforce in the geriatric health care system? *Journal of Health Politics, Policy and Law* 32(6):1005-1041.

Boston University Institute for Geriatric Social Work. 2011. *Online training programs.* http://www.bu.edu/igsw/online-training-programs/ (accessed June 11, 2012).

BPS (Board of Pharmacy Specialties). 2005. *Content outline for the Psychiatric Pharmacy Specialty Certification Examination.* http://www.bpsweb.org/pdfs/content_outline_psychiatric.pdf (accessed December 5, 2011)

———. 2011. *Pharmacists certified by the Board of Pharmacy Specialties.* http://www.bpsweb.org/resources/BPSInformationalSlides.pdf (accessed December 5, 2011).

Brown, C., H. C. Schulberg, and M. J. Madonia. 1996. Clinical presentations of major depression by African Americans and whites in primary medical care practice. *Journal of Affective Disorders* 41(3):181-191.

Bruce, M. L., E. L. Brown, P. J. Raue, A. E. Mlodzianowski, B. S. Meyers, A. C. Leon, M. Heo, A. L. Byers, R. L. Greenberg, and S. Rinder. 2007. A randomized trial of depression assessment intervention in home health care. *Journal of the American Geriatrics Society* 55(11):1793-1800.

Brugna, R., J. Cawley, and M. Baker. 2007. Physician assistants in geriatric medicine. *Clinical Geriatrics* 15(10):22.

CAADAC (California Association of Alcoholism and Drug Abuse Counselors). 2011. *California Certification Board of Alcohol and Drug Counselors (CCBADC) requirements for certification.* https://www.caadac.org/ladder/ (accessed October 20, 2011).

CACREP (Council for Accreditation of Counseling and Related Educational Programs). 2010. *Council for Accreditation of Counseling and Related Educational Programs 2009.* http://www.cacrep.org/doc/2009%20Standards%20with%20cover.pdf (accessed March 28, 2012).

———. 2011. *Scope of accreditation.* http://67.199.126.156/template/page.cfm?id=52 (accessed October 20, 2011).

CalSWEC (California Social Work Education Center). 2011a. *Evaluation and research.* http://calswec.berkeley.edu/CalSWEC/MH_EvalRes.html (accessed December 22, 2011).

———. 2011b. *Mental health curriculum resources.* http://calswec.berkeley.edu/CalSWEC/MHInitiative_CurricRes.html (accessed December 22, 2011).

Cates, M. E., M. R. Monk-Tutor, and S. O. Drummond. 2007. Mental health and psychiatric pharmacy instruction in U.S. colleges and schools of pharmacy. *American Journal of Pharmaceutical Education* 71(1):1-5.

CCGP (Commission for Certification in Geriatric Pharmacy). 2011. *Exam content.* http://www.ccgp.org/pharmacist/certification/disease.htm (accessed September 27, 2011).

Center to Champion Nursing in America. 2010. *Preparation and roles of nursing care providers in America.* http://championnursing.org/resources/preparation-and-roles-nursing-care-providers-america (accessed December 5, 2011).

Chadiha, L. A., E. Brown, and M. P. Aranda. 2006. Social work practice with older African Americans and other black populations. In *Handbook of social work in aging,* edited by B. Berkman. New York: Oxford University Press.

Champagne, T., and K. Gray. 2011. *Occupational therapy's role in mental health recovery.* http://www.aota.org/Practitioners/PracticeAreas/Aging/Tools/MH-Recovery.aspx?FT=.pdf (accessed April 12, 2012).

Christian, S., C. Dower, and E. O'Neil. 2007. *Chart overview of nurse practitioner scopes of practice in the United States.* San Francisco, CA: UCSF Center for the Health Professions.

Clay, R. 2006. Geropsychology grants in peril. *Monitor on Psychology* 37(4):46.

CMS (Centers for Medicare & Medicaid Services). 2007. State Medicaid Director Letter #07-011. http://downloads.cms.gov/cmsgov/archived-downloads/SMDL/downloads/SMD081507A.pdf (accessed December 13, 2011).

CNC (Commission on Nurse Certification). 2011. *Frequently asked questions about CNL® certification.* http://www.aacn.nche.edu/leading-initiatives/cnl/cnl-certification/pdf/faq.pdf (accessed October 13, 2011).

Colenda, C. C., J. E. Wilk, and J. C. West. 2005. The geriatric psychiatry workforce in 2002: Analysis from the 2002 National Survey of Psychiatric Practice. *American Journal of Geriatric Psychology* 13(9):756.

Commission for Accreditation of Marriage and Family Therapy Education. 2005. *MFT educational guidelines.* http://www.aamft.org/imis15/Documents/COAMFTE_MFT_Educational_Guidelines.pdf (accessed October 24, 2011).

CORE (Council on Rehabilitation Education). 2010. *CORE accreditation standards.* http://www.core-rehab.org/Files/Doc/PDF/COREStandards20120204.pdf (accessed March 29, 2012).

Corwin, S. J., K. Frahm, L. A. Ochs, C. E. Rheaume, and E. Roberts. 2006. Medical student and senior participants' perceptions of a mentoring program designed to enhance geriatric medical education. *Gerontology & Geriatrics Education* 26(3):47-65.

Council on Credentialing in Pharmacy. 2009. *Scope of contemporary pharmacy practice: Roles, responsibilities, and functions of pharmacists and pharmacy technicians.* Washington, DC. http://www.accp.com/docs/positions/misc/ccpwpscope_pharmacy_practice_2-2009.pdf (accessed December 5, 2011).

Couture, S., and D. Penn. 2003. Interpersonal contact and the stigma of mental illness: A review of the literature. *Journal of Mental Health* 12(3):291-305.

Covinsky, K. E., R. Newcomer, P. Fox, J. Wood, L. Sands, K. Dane, and K. Yaffe. 2003. Patient and caregiver characteristics associated with depression in caregivers of patients with dementia. *Journal of General Internal Medicine* 18(12):1006-1014.

CRCC (Commission on Rehabilitation Counselor Certification). 2011. *Rehabilitation counseling.* http://www.crccertification.com/pages/rehabilitation_counseling/30.php (accessed March 29, 2012).

Crystal, S., U. Sambamoorthi, J. T. Walkup, and A. Akincigil. 2003. Diagnosis and treatment of depression in the elderly Medicare population: Predictors, disparities, and trends. *Journal of the American Geriatrics Society* 51(12):1718-1728.

CSAT (Center for Substance Abuse Treatment). 2005. *A national review of state alcohol and drug treatment programs and certification standards for substance abuse counselors and prevention professionals.* Rockville, MD: Substance Abuse and Mental Health Services Administration.

Cummings, S. M., G. Adler, and V. A. DeCoster. 2005. Factors influencing graduate-social-work students' interest in working with elders. *Educational Gerontology* 31(8):643-655.

Daniels, A. S., E. Grant, B. Filson, I. Powell, L. Fricks, and L. Goodale. 2010. *Pillars of peer support: Transforming mental health systems of care through peer support services.* http://www.power2u.org/downloads/PillarsOfPeerSupportServiceReport.pdf (accessed December 15, 2011).

Daniels, A. S., L. Fricks, and T. P. Tunner. 2011. *Pillars of peer support-2: Expanding the role of peer support services in mental health systems of care and recovery.* www.pillarsofpeersupport.org (accessed April 12, 2011).

Direct Care Alliance. 2011a. *Direct Care Alliance personal care and support credential.* http://www.directcarealliance.org/document/docWindow.cfm?fuseaction=document.viewDocument&documentid=19&documentFormatId=21 (accessed April 12, 2012).

———. 2011b. *Direct Care Alliance personal care and support credential 2011 candidate handbook.* http://directcarealliance.org/document/docWindow.cfm?fuseaction=document.viewDocument&documentid=2&documentFormatId=2 (accessed October 10, 2011).

Direct Service Workforce Resource Center. 2011. *Building capacity and coordinating support for family caregivers and the direct service workforce: Common goals and policy recommendations emerging from the CMS leadership summit on the direct service workforce and family caregivers.* http://dswresourcecenter.org/tiki-index.php?page=Reports (accessed October 11, 2011).

DOLETA (U.S. Department of Labor Employment and Training Administration) Office of Apprenticeship. 2012. *Registered apprenticeship training in long-term care.* Washington, DC: U.S. Department of Labor.

Donald W. Reynolds Foundation. 2011. *Description of geriatrics training grants approved in June 2006.* http://www.dwreynolds.org/Programs/National/Aging/Cohort3.htm (accessed December 20, 2011).

Eaton, J. S. 2011. *An overview of U.S. accreditation.* Washington, DC: Council for Higher Education Accreditation. http://www.chea.org/pdf/Overview%20of%20US%20Accreditation%2003.2011.pdf (accessed April 9, 2012).

Eaton, S. C., C. Green, R. Wilson, and T. Osypuk. 2001. *Extended Care Career Ladder Initiative (ECCLI): Baseline report of a Massachusetts nursing initiative.* Cambridge, MA: Kennedy School of Government.

Ehrlich, A. R., and L. G. Jacobs. 2004. Albert Einstein College of Medicine of Yeshiva University. *Academic Medicine* 79(7):S3-S6.

Eleazer, G. P., D. Wieland, E. Roberts, N. Richeson, and J. T. Thornhill. 2006. Preparing medical students to care for older adults: The impact of a senior mentor program. *Academic Medicine* 81(4):393.

Evercare. 2007. *Evercare Survey of graduating high school seniors finds prospective nurses lack interest in geriatrics despite growing senior population.* http://www.businesswire.com/news/home/20070801005845/en/Evercare-Survey-Graduating-High-School-Seniors-Finds (accessed December 19, 2011).

Faulkner, L. R., D. Juul, N. N. Andrade, B. A. Brooks, C. C. Colenda, R. W. Guynn, D. A. Mrazek, V. I. Reus, B. S. Schneidman, and K. R. Shaw. 2011. Recent trends in American Board of Psychiatry and Neurology psychiatric subspecialties. *Academic Psychiatry* 35(1):35-39.

Federation of State Medical Boards of the United States, and National Board of Medical Examiners. 2011. *2011 Step 2 Clinical Knowledge (CK) content description and general information.* http://www.usmle.org/examinations/step2/ck/2011Step2CK.pdf (accessed December 5, 2011).

Feinberg, L., S. C. Reinhard, A. Houser, and R. Choula. 2011. *Valuing the invaluable: 2011 update: The growing contributions and costs of family caregiving.* http://assets.aarp.org/rgcenter/ppi/ltc/i51-caregiving.pdf (accessed April 12, 2012).

Geriatric Mental Health Foundation. 2012. *The role of the geriatric psychiatrist.* http://www.gmhfonline.org/gmhf/consumer/factsheets/geriatric_psychiatrist.html (accessed January 19, 2012).

Geriatric Social Work Initiative. 2012. *Hartford Pre-Dissertation Award Program in Geriatric Social Work.* http://www.gswi.org/programs/predissertation.html (accessed April 6, 2012).

Goodwin, K., and L. Tobler. 2008. *Community health workers: Expanding the scope of the health care delivery system.* http://www.ncsl.org/print/health/CHWBrief.pdf (accessed April 12, 2012).

GWPSC (Geriatrics Workforce Policy Studies Center). 2009a. *Figure 4.1, Required time (half days in 2002 and 2008/weeks in 2005) devoted to clinical instruction in geriatric medicine during 3-year general internal medicine residency in 2002, 2005, and 2008.* http://www.adgapstudy.uc.edu/figs_graduate.cfm (accessed December 5, 2011).

———. 2009b. *Figure 4.5, Required time (half days) devoted to clinical instruction in geriatric medicine during 3-year family medicine residency in 2001, 2004, and 2008.* http://www.adgapstudy.uc.edu/figs_graduate.cfm (accessed December 5, 2011).

———. 2009c. *Table 4.11, Required geriatric experiences in family medicine residency programs, 2004 and 2008.* http://www.adgapstudy.uc.edu/figs_graduate.cfm (accessed December 5, 2011).

———. 2010a. *Table 3.2, Geriatric medicine fellowship programs, family medicine and internal medicine 1991/92-2010/11.* http://www.adgapstudy.uc.edu/figs_graduate.cfm (accessed December 5, 2011).

———. 2010b. *Table 3.5, Geriatric psychiatry fellowship programs 1995/96-2010/11: American Geriatrics Society.* http://www.adgapstudy.uc.edu/figs_graduate.cfm (accessed December 5, 2011).

Hanrahan, N. P., and D. Hartley. 2008. Employment of advanced-practice psychiatric nurses to stem rural mental health workforce shortages. *Psychiatric Services* 59(1):109-111.

Happell, B. 2008. The importance of clinical experience for mental health nursing—Part 2: Relationships between undergraduate nursing students' attitudes, preparedness, and satisfaction. *International Journal of Mental Health Nursing* 17(5):333-340.

Happell, B., and C. Roper. 2003. The role of a mental health consumer in the education of postgraduate psychiatric nursing students: The students' evaluation. *Journal of Psychiatric and Mental Health Nursing* 10(3):343-350.

Harmuth, S., and T. R. Konrad. 2010. Strengthening the direct care workforce in North Carolina. *North Carolina Medical Journal* 71(2):158-160.

Hartigan, C. 2011. APRN regulation: The licensure-certification interface. *AACN Advanced Critical Care* 22(1):15.

Hewitt, A., S. Larson, S. Edelstein, D. Seavey, M. A. Hoge, and J. Morris. 2008. *A synthesis of direct service workforce demographics and challenges across intellectual/developmental disabilities, aging, physical disabilities, and behavioral health.* Falls Church, VA: The Lewin Group.

HHS (U.S. Department of Health and Human Services). 1999. *Mental health: A report of the Surgeon General.* Rockville, MD: HHS.

Hinrichsen, G. A. 2010. Public policy and the provision of psychological services to older adults. *Professional Psychology: Research and Practice* 41(2):97-103.

Hinrichsen, G. A., A. M. Zeiss, M. J. Karel, and V. A. Molinari. 2010. Competency-based geropsychology training in doctoral internships and postdoctoral fellowships. *Training and Education in Professional Psychology* 4(2):91.

Hoffman, K. G., P. Gray, M. C. Hosokawa, and S. C. Zweig. 2006. Evaluating the effectiveness of a senior mentor program: The University of Missouri-Columbia School of Medicine. *Gerontology & Geriatrics Education* 27(2):11.

Hogan, M. F. 2003. The President's New Freedom Commission: Recommendations to transform mental health care in America. *Psychiatric Services* 54(11):1467-1474.

Hoge, M. A., J. A. Morris, A. S. Daniels, G. W. Stuart, L. Y. Huey, N. Adams, and Annapolis Coalition on the Behavioral Health Workforce. 2007. *An action plan for behavioral health workforce development: Executive summary.* Rockville, MD: Substance Abuse and Mental Health Services Administration.

Hooker, R. S. 2006. Physician assistants and nurse practitioners: The United States experience. *Medical Journal of Australia* 185(1):4.

HRSA (Health Resources and Services Administration). 2007. Community Health Worker National Workforce Study. Rockville, MD. http://bhpr.hrsa.gov/healthworkforce/reports/chwstudy2007.pdf (accessed April 12, 2012).

———. 2010. *The registered nurse population: Findings from the 2008 National Sample Survey of Registered Nurses.* U.S. Department of Health and Human Services. http://bhpr.hrsa.gov/healthworkforce/reports/chwstudy2007.pdf (accessed April 12, 2012).

———. 2012. *Guidelines for mental health HPSA designation.* http://bhpr.hrsa.gov/shortage/hpsas/designationcriteria/mentalhealthhpsaguidelines.html (accessed March 28, 2012).

Hunter, S. 2005. *Midlife and older LGBT adults: Knowledge and affirmative practice for the social sciences.* New York: Haworth Press, Inc.

Interprofessional Education Collaborative Expert Panel. 2011. *Core competencies for Interprofessional Collaborative Practice: Report of an expert panel.* Washington, DC: Interprofessional Education Collaborative. http://www.aacn.nche.edu/education-resources/ipecreport.pdf (accessed December 5, 2011).

IOM (Institute of Medicine). 2001. *Crossing the quality chasm: A new health system for the 21st century.* Washington, DC: National Academy Press.

———. 2006. *Improving the quality of health care for mental and substance-use conditions.* Washington, DC: The National Academies Press.

———. 2008a. *Cancer Care for the Whole Patient: Meeting Psychosocial Needs.* Washington, DC: The National Academies Press.

———. 2008b. *Retooling for an aging America: Building the health care workforce.* Washington, DC: The National Academies Press.

———. 2011. *The future of nursing: Leading change, advancing health.* Washington, DC: The National Academies Press.

Janevic, M. R., and C. M. Connell. 2001. Racial, ethnic, and cultural differences in the dementia caregiving experience: Recent findings. *Gerontologist* 41(2):334-347.

Johnson, E. 2008. *Minnesota peer support implementation consultant's report.* http://www.californiaclients.org/pdf/Sue%20Watson%20Presentation%20Attachment.pdf (accessed April 12, 2012).

Karel, M. J., E. E. Emery, and V. Molinari. 2010a. Development of a tool to evaluate geropsychology knowledge and skill competencies. *International Psychogeriatrics* 22(6):886-896.

Karel, M. J., B. G. Knight, M. Duffy, G. A. Hinrichsen, and A. M. Zeiss. 2010b. Attitude, knowledge, and skill competencies for practice in professional geropsychology: Implications for training and building a geropsychology workforce. *Training and Education in Professional Psychology* 4(2):75-84.

Kennedy Malone, L., J. Penny, and M. E. Fleming. 2008. Clinical practice characteristics of gerontological nurse practitioners: A national study. *Journal of the American Academy of Nurse Practitioners* 20(1):17-27.

Knight, B. G., and P. Sayegh. 2010. Cultural values and caregiving: The updated sociocultural stress and coping model. *Journals of Gerontology Series B Psychological Sciences* 65B(1):5-13.

Knight, B. G., M. J. Karel, G. A. Hinrichsen, S. H. Qualls, and M. Duffy. 2009. Pikes Peak model for training in professional geropsychology. *American Psychologist* 64(3):205-214.

Koder, D., and E. Helmes. 2008. Predictors of interest in working with older adults: A survey of postgraduate trainee psychologists. *Gerontology & Geriatrics Education* 29(2):158.

Lafer, G., and H. Moss. 2007. *The LPN: A practical way to alleviate the nursing shortage. University of Oregon.* http://www.afscme.org/news/publications/health-care/the-lpn-a-practical-way-to-alleviate-the-nursing-shortage (accessed December 5, 2011).

Liaison Committee on Medical Education. 2011. *Functions and structure of a medical school: Standards for accreditation of medical education programs leading to the M.D. degree.* http://www.lcme.org/functions2011may.pdf (accessed December 22, 2011).

Magaña, S. M., J. I. R. García, M. G. Hernández, and R. Cortez. 2007. Psychological distress among Latino family caregivers of adults with schizophrenia: The roles of burden and stigma. *Psychiatric Services* 58(3):378-384.

Maryland Board of Nursing. 2010. *Nursing assistant certification.* http://www.mbon.org/main.php?v=norm&p=0&c=cna/cna_info.html (accessed January 25, 2012).

McFarlane, W. R., L. Dixon, E. Lukens, and A. Lucksted. 2003. Family psychoeducation and schizophrenia: A review of the literature. *Journal of Marital and Family Therapy* 29(2):223-245.

Meyers, J. E. 1995. From "forgotten and ignored" to standards and certification: Gerontological counseling comes of age. *Journal of Counseling and Development* 74(2):143-149.

Michalski, D., T. Mulvey, and J. Kohout. 2010. 2008 *APA Survey of Psychology Health Service Providers.* Washington, DC: American Psychological Association.

Midwest Pharmacy Workforce Research Consortium. 2010. 2009 *National Pharmacist Workforce Survey.* http://www.aacp.org/resources/research/pharmacymanpower/Documents/2009%20National%20Pharmacist%20Workforce%20Survey%20-%20FINAL%20REPORT.pdf (accessed December 5, 2011).

Migrant Health Promotion. 2012. *Who are promotores(as)?* http://www.migranthealth.org/index.php?option=com_content&view=article&id=41&Itemid=38 (accessed April 4, 2012).

Money, N., M. Moore, D. Brown, K. Kasper, J. Roeder, P. Bartone, and M. Bates. 2011. *Best practices identified for peer support programs.* Defense Centers for Excellence for Psychological Health and Traumatic Brain Injury. http://www.dcoe.health.mil/Content/Navigation/Documents/Best_Practices_Identified_for_Peer_Support_Programs_Jan_2011.pdf (accessed December 16, 2011).

Montrose Counseling Center. 2012a. *4Ever Family Project.* http://www.montrosecounselingcenter.org/?page_id=5634 (accessed April 11, 2012).

———. 2012b. *SPRY: Seniors Preparing for Rainbow Years.* http://www.spryhouston.org/ (accessed April 11, 2012).

Morgan, P. A., and R. S. Hooker. 2010. Choice of specialties among physician assistants in the United States. *Health Affairs* 29(5):887.

NADSP (National Alliance for Direct Support Professionals). 2011a. *15 NADSP competency areas.* https://www.nadsp.org/images/NADSP_Competency_Areas.pdf (accessed April 15, 2012).

———. 2011b. *About DSP credentialing.* https://nadsp.org/dsp-credentialing/about-dsp-credentialing.html (accessed April 15, 2012).

NAMI (National Alliance on Mental Illness) New Hampshire. 2010. *Side by side for independent living evaluation summary.* Concord, NH: NAMI NH.

———. 2012. *Side by Side.* http://www.naminh.org/side-by-side (accessed April 9, 2012).

NASW (National Association of Social Workers). 2005. *NASW standards for clinical social work in social work practice.* http://www.socialworkers.org/practice/standards/NASWClinicalSWStandards.pdf (accessed December 5, 2011).

———. 2011a. *The advanced social worker in gerontology (ASW-G).* http://www.socialworkers.org/credentials/specialty/asw-g.asp (accessed December 5, 2011).

———. 2011b. *The certified clinical alcohol, tobacco, and other drugs social worker (C-CATODSW).* http://www.socialworkers.org/credentials/specialty/c-catodsw.asp (accessed December 5, 2011).

———. 2011c. *The clinical social worker in gerontology (CSW-G).* http://www.socialworkers.org/credentials/specialty/csw-g.asp (accessed December 5, 2011).

———. 2011d. *Social work profession.* http://www.socialworkers.org/pressroom/features/general/profession.asp (accessed October 19, 2011).

———. 2011e. *The social worker in gerontology (SW-G).* http://www.socialworkers.org/credentials/specialty/sw-g.asp (accessed December 5, 2011).

———. 2012. *Continuing education for social workers.* http://www.socialworkers.org/ce/ (accessed April 10, 2012).

National Alliance for Caregiving and AARP. 2009. *Caregiving in the U.S. 2009.* http://www.caregiving.org/data/Caregiving_in_the_US_2009_full_report.pdf (accessed April 12, 2012).

National Clearinghouse on the Direct Care Workforce. 2004. *Job duties and training requirements: Nursing assistants.* http://www.directcareclearinghouse.org/dev/i_jobs_na.jsp (accessed December 12, 2011).

National Matching Services. 2011. *Summary of programs and positions offered & filled by program type for the 2011 match.* http://www.natmatch.com/ashprmp/ (accessed September 26, 2011).

NBOME (National Board of Osteopathic Medical Examiners). 2011. *COMLEX-USA bulletin of information.* http://www.nbome.org/docs/comlexBOI.pdf (accessed December 5, 2011).

NCCPA (National Commission on Certification of Physician Assistants). 2009a. *Psychiatry—content blueprint.* http://www.nccpa.net/Psychiatrycb.aspx (accessed September 27, 2011).

———. 2009b. *Psychiatry CAQ.* http://www.nccpa.net/Psychiatry.aspx (accessed September 27, 2011).

NCSBN (National Council of State Boards of Nursing). 2004. *White paper on the state of the art of approval/accreditation processes in boards of nursing.* https://www.ncsbn.org/Final_11_05_Approval_White_Paper.pdf (accessed December 5, 2011).

———. 2010a. *2010 NCLEX-RN detailed test plan.* https://www.ncsbn.org/APRN_Consensus_Model_FAQs_August_19_2010.pdf (accessed October 12, 2011)

———. 2010b. *APRN consensus model frequently-asked questions.* https://www.ncsbn.org/APRN_Consensus_Model_FAQs_August_19_2010.pdf (accessed October 12, 2011).

———. 2011a. *2011 NCLEX-PN detailed test plan.* https://www.ncsbn.org/2011_PN_Detailed TestPlan_Educator.pdf (accessed December 5, 2011).

———. 2011b. *Fact sheet: Licensure of nursing and state boards of nursing.* https://www.ncsbn.org/Fact_Sheet_Licensure_of_Nurses_and_State_Boards_of_Nursing.pdf (accessed April 9, 2012).

———. 2011c. *The consensus model for APRN regulation: Licensure, accreditation, certification, and education.* https://www.ncsbn.org/aprn.htm (accessed October 13, 2011).

North Dakota Board of Addiction Counseling Examiners. 2000. *Licensure.* http://www.ndbace.org/licensure.htm (accessed October 20, 2011).

O'Brien-Mazza, D., and M. Chinman. 2011. *Peer support implementation in DVA mental health programs; maximizing the effectiveness of mental health services in the prevention of suicide.* Paper presented at DoD/VA Suicide Prevention Conference, All the Way Home: Preventing Suicide in Service Members and Veterans, Boston, March 23.

Office of Inspector General. 2002. *State nurse aide training: Program information and data.* Report OEI-05-01-00031. HHS Region V, General Office of Evaluation and Inspections. http://www.directcareclearinghouse.org/download/OIGrpt_state_CNA_training_prgms.pdf (accessed April 15, 2012).

Ozga, M. 2012. *Iowa direct-care workers may require license.* http://phinational.org/archives/iowa-direct-care-workers-may-require-license/ (accessed April 6, 2012).

Partnership for Health in Aging. 2010. *Multidisciplinary competencies in the care of older adults at the completion of the entry-level health professional degree.* http://www.americangeriatrics.org/files/documents/pha/PHAMultidiscComps.pdf (accessed December 5, 2011).

Perry, K. M., and M. T. Boccaccini. 2009. Specialized training in APA accredited clinical psychology doctoral programs: Findings from a review of program websites. *Clinical Psychology: Science and Practice* 16(3):348-359.

PHI (Paraprofessional Health Care Institute). 2011. *Facts 3. Who are direct-care workers?* http://www.directcareclearinghouse.org/download/NCDCW%20Fact%20Sheet-1.pdf (accessed April 15, 2012).

Physician Assistant Education Association. 2009. *Twenty-fifth annual report on physician assistant educational programs in the United States.* Alexandria, VA: Physician Assistant Education Association. http://www.paeaonline.org/index.php?ht=a/GetDocumentAction/i/107753 (accessed December 5, 2011).

Pinquart, M., and S. Sorensen. 2005. Ethnic differences in stressors, resources, and psychological outcomes of family caregiving: A meta-analysis. *Gerontologist* 45(1):90-106.

POGOe (Portal of Geriatric Online Education). 2010. *Geriatric nursing key concepts.* http://www.pogoe.org/sites/default/files/Key%20concepts_GPNC.pdf (accessed December 5, 2011).

Professional Examination Service. 2011. *Information for candidates examination in marital and family therapy.* http://www.amftrb.org/PDF/info4candidate.pdf (accessed October 21, 2011).

Qualls, S. H., F. Scogin, R. Zweig, and S. K. Whitbourne. 2005a. Predoctoral training models in professional geropsychology. *Training and Education in Professional Psychology* 4(2):85.

Qualls, S. H., D. L. Segal, C. C. Benight, and M. P. Kenny. 2005b. Geropsychology training in a specialist geropsychology doctoral program. *Gerontology & Geriatrics Education* 25(4):21-40.

Resnick, S. G. 2010. Who attends Vet-to-Vet? Predictors of attendance in mental health mutual support. *Psychiatric Rehabilitation Journal* 33(4):262-268.

Resnick, S. G., M. Armstrong, M. Sperrazza, L. Harkness, and R. A. Rosenheck. 2004. A model of consumer-provider partnership: Vet-to-Vet. *Psychiatric Rehabilitation Journal* 28(2):185-187.

Rhett-Mariscal, W. 2008. *Promotores in mental health in California and the prevention and early intervention component of the MHSA.* http://www.cimh.org/LinkClick.aspx?fileticket=Qw5mqcEahTI%3d&tabid=568 (accessed April 12, 2012).

Robiner, W. N. 2006. The mental health professions: Workforce supply and demand, issues, and challenges. *Clinical Psychology Review* 26(5):600-625.

Ross, C. A., and E. M. Goldner. 2009. Stigma, negative attitudes and discrimination towards mental illness within the nursing profession: A review of the literature. *Journal of Psychiatric and Mental Health Nursing* 16(6):558-567.

SAMHSA (Substance Abuse and Mental Health Services Administration). 1999. *Mental health: A report of the Surgeon General.* http://profiles.nlm.nih.gov/ps/access/NNBBHS.pdf (accessed December 21, 2011).

———. 2011a. *FY 2011 grant request for applications (RFA): Minority Fellowship Program (short title: MFP).* http://www.samhsa.gov/Grants/2011/SM_11_005.aspx (accessed March 15, 2012).

———. 2011b. *FY 2011 SAMHSA grant awards: CMHS/SM-11-005 Minority Fellowship Program.* http://www.samhsa.gov/grants/2011/awards/sm_11_005.aspx (accessed April 6, 2012).

Sartorius, N., W. Gaebel, H. R. Cleveland, H. Stuart, T. Akiyama, J. Arboleda-Flórez, A. E. Baumann, O. Gureje, M. R. Jorge, and M. Kastrup. 2010. WPA guidance on how to combat stigmatization of psychiatry and psychiatrists. *World Psychiatry* 9(3):131.

Sengupta, M., L. D. Harris-Kojetin, and F. K. Ejaz. 2010. A national overview of the training received by certified nursing assistants working in U.S. nursing homes. *Gerontology & Geriatrics Education* 31(3):201-219.

Sirojudin, S., and A. Jacob. 2009. *Mental health social work stipend program: Three-year outcome report, 2005-2008.* University of California, Berkeley. http://calswec.berkeley.edu/CalSWEC/MH_StipendProgramReport_2009.pdf (accessed December 22, 2012).

SIS (Seniors in Sobriety). 2012. *Seniors in Sobriety (SIS): A history.* http://www.seniorsinsobriety.org/history.htm (accessed April 7, 2012).

Social Work Policy Institute. 2010. *Social work services in nursing homes: Toward quality psychosocial care.* http://www.socialworkpolicy.org/research/social-work-services-in-nursing-homes-toward-quality-psychosocial-care.html (accessed January 13, 2012).

South Carolina Lieutenant Governor's Office on Aging. 2010. *South Carolina geriatric loan forgiveness program.* Columbia, SC. http://aging.sc.gov/providers/Pages/GeriatricLoanForgivenessProgram.aspx (accessed December 22, 2011).

———. 2011a. *Geriatric loan forgiveness program.* http://aging.sc.gov/providers/Pages/GeriatricLoanForgivenessProgram.aspx (accessed December 22, 2011).

———. 2011b. *Geriatric loan forgiveness program application.* http://aging.sc.gov/SiteCollectionDocuments/G/GLFApplication.pdf (accessed December 22, 2011).

Squillace, M. R., R. E. Remsburg, L. D. Harris-Kojetin, A. Bercovitz, E. Rosenoff, and B. Han. 2009. The National Nursing Assistant Survey: Improving the evidence base for policy initiatives to strengthen the certified nursing assistant workforce. *Gerontologist* 49(2):185-197.

Stanford Geriatric Education Center. 2004. *Diversity, healing, and health care.* http://www.bonshome.org/diversity/cohort/cohort1.htm (accessed November 1, 2011).

Stone, R., and Urban Institute Staff. 2011. *Long-term care for the elderly.* Washington, DC: Urban Institute Press.

Union of Pan Asian Communities. 2011. Elder multicultural access and support services: Prevention and early intervention report. *EMASS Newsletter* 2(4):1.

University of Washington Professional and Continuing Education. 2012. *Certificate in geriatric mental health.* http://www.pce.uw.edu/certificates/geriatric-mental-health/downtown-seattle-autumn-2012/?tab=Overview (accessed June 11, 2012).

Veterans Health Administration. 2011. *Psychosocial rehabilitation and recovery services peer support.* http://www.va.gov/vhapublications/ViewPublication.asp?pub_ID=2430 (accessed April 12, 2012).

Voogt, S. J., M. Mickus, O. Santiago, and S. E. Herman. 2008. Attitudes, experiences, and interest in geriatrics of first year allopathic and osteopathic medical students. *Journal of the American Geriatrics Society* 56(2):339-344.

Wallendal, M., R. Gramann, J. Kowalsky, K. Staehler, P. S. Davis, N. Amoroso, and R. Schroeder. 2009. *Exposure to older adults influences social work student's attitudes related to working in the field of aging.* http://socialwork.nyam.org/nsw/students/journals/Exposure_to_Older_Adults_Influences_Social_Work_Students_Attitudes.pdf (accessed December 19, 2011).

Warshaw, G. A., E. J. Bragg, R. W. Shaull, and C. J. Lindsell. 2002. Academic geriatric programs in U.S. allopathic and osteopathic medical schools. *JAMA* 288(18):2313-2319.

Washkowiak, J., M. Wronski, L. K. Jones, E. Velasco, K. Schrubba, and S. J. Elliot. 2010. *Occupational therapy's role in skilled nursing facilities.* Bethesda, MD. http://www.aota.org/Consumers/Professionals/WhatIsOT/RDP/Facts/SNFs.aspx (accessed April 12, 2012).

Weill Cornell Homecare Research Partnership. 2004. *Depression screening tool kit.* Weill Medical College of Cornell University. http://www.geriu.org/uploads/applications/DepressionInHomecare/ToolKit.pdf (accessed December 5, 2011).

Weill Medical College of Cornell University. 2004. *Depression recognition and assessment in older homecare patients.* http://www.geriu.org/uploads/applications/DepressionInHomecare/DinHomecare.html (accessed November 10, 2011).

Whitaker, T., T. Weismiller, and E. Clark. 2006. *Assuring the sufficiency of a frontline workforce: A national study of licensed social workers. Special report: Social work services for older adults.* Washington, DC: National Association of Social Workers.

Williams, D. R., H. M. Gonzalez, H. Neighbors, R. Nesse, J. M. Abelson, J. Sweetman, and J. S. Jackson. 2007. Prevalence and distribution of major depressive disorder in African Americans, Caribbean blacks, and non-Hispanic whites: Results from the National Survey of American Life. *Archives of General Psychiatry* 64(3):305-315.

Wilson, R., S. C. Eaton, and A. Kamanu. 2003. *Extended Care Career Ladder Initiative (ECCLI) round 2: Evaluation report.* Cambridge, MA: Kennedy School of Government.

Wood, A. L., and O. F. Wahl. 2006. Evaluating the effectiveness of a consumer-provided mental health recovery education presentation. *Psychiatric Rehabilitation Journal* 30(1):46-53.

World Psychiatric Association and World Health Organization. 2002. *Reducing stigma and discrimination against older adults with mental disorders: A technical consensus statement.* Geneva. http://www.who.int/mental_health/media/en/499.pdf (accessed December 21, 2011).

4

Workforce Implications of Models of Care for Older Adults with Mental Health and Substance Use Conditions

Abstract: *This chapter reviews nine models of care delivery for older adults who have depression, substance use conditions, serious mental illness, or psychiatric and behavioral symptoms related to dementia. Mental health and substance use (MH/SU) care—particularly for depression and at-risk drinking—is most effective for older adults when it includes systematic outreach and diagnosis, patient and family education and self-management support, provider accountability for outcomes, and close follow-up and monitoring to prevent relapse. These elements are best obtained when care is patient-centered, in an easily accessed location (e.g., in primary care, senior centers, or individuals' homes), and coordinated by trained personnel with access to specialty consultation. These aims are not likely to be achieved, however, without significant practice redesign, critical changes in Medicare payment rules, and substantial efforts to train and retrain the workforce appropriately. Research on effective delivery of MH/SU care for individuals residing in nursing homes and other residential settings, prisoners, rurally isolated elders, and older adults with severe mental illnesses is urgently needed.*

The previous chapters described the mental health and substance use (MH/SU) needs of older adults and the available information on the health care workforce that serves them. The messages of the chapters are clear. The MH/SU needs of older adults[1] are complex, typically co-occur with other health problems, and are often inadequately addressed by today's health care system. Moreover, the health care workforce is insufficiently prepared to address the MH/SU needs of the geriatric population.

The committee agreed early in its deliberations that the effectiveness and efficiency of the geriatric mental health workforce derives not only from the skills, knowledge, and size of the workforce, but also from how care is organized and delivered. The objective of this chapter is twofold: first, to review what is known about how to optimize the capacity of the workforce to yield better outcomes, especially in light of the chronic nature of geriatric MH/SU conditions and, second, to consider the implications of such models for workforce training and deployment of health care workers.

ORGANIZATION OF THE CHAPTER

The chapter begins with a brief description of the chronic care model—the central framework for many promising innovations in MH/SU care delivery. The next section reviews nine models of care delivery for older adults who have MH/SU conditions (Table 4-1). The committee had neither the resources nor the time to conduct a systematic review of model interventions. The nine models were selected to include common geriatric MH/SU conditions as well as the important settings where older adults often receive services. The models make clear that there is indeed an evidence base demonstrating that patient outcomes can improve with reorganization of care. Thus, the committee urges that workforce planners and policy makers should move beyond dismissive summaries that "nothing works for these patients" and consider the implications of the models for workforce education, training, credentialing, and licensure.

However, the robustness of evidence does vary across care settings and older adult populations; some published evidence had to be available in order to be included in this review. Research on effective delivery of MH/SU care is particularly lacking for older adults in nursing homes, residential treatment settings, and other congregate living arrangements as well as for prisoners, rurally isolated elders, and older adults with serious mental illnesses.

For settings with several intervention models, the committee chose the model that had the most robust evidence. For example, the Prevention of Suicide in Primary Care Elderly Collaborative Trial (PROSPECT)

[1]This report uses the term "older adults" to refer to adults age 65 and older. "Mental health workforce" refers to the full range of personnel providing services to older adults with mental health and substance use conditions.

TABLE 4-1
Models Reviewed in This Chapter

Model	Target Population
Depression	
Improving Mood-Promoting Access to Collaborative Treatment (IMPACT)	Older adult population with major depression, dysthymic disorder, or both
Kaiser Nurse Telehealth Care Model	Adult population (all ages) starting antidepressant drug therapy
Program to Encourage Active and Rewarding Lives for Seniors (PEARLS)	Older, community-residing adults with minor depression and dysthymia who are receiving social services
Substance Use	
Screening, Brief Intervention, and Referral for Treatment (SBIRT)	Older adult population at risk for alcohol and substance misuse
Primary Care Research in Substance Abuse and Mental Health for the Elderly (PRISM-E)	Older primary care patients with symptoms of depression, anxiety, and at-risk drinking
Serious Mental Illness (SMI)	
Helping Older People Experience Success (HOPES)	Older adults with SMI residing in the community
Psychogeriatric Assessment and Treatment in City Housing (PATCH)	Older adults with SMI living in urban public housing
Wellness Recovery Action Planning (WRAP)	Adults (all ages) with severe and persistent mental illness
Psychiatric and Behavioral Symptoms Related to Dementia	
Providing Resources Early to Vulnerable Elders Needing Treatment (PREVENT)	Older adults with Alzheimer's and their caregivers

was an effective intervention, but did not have as large a sample size or geographic diversity as the Improving Mood-Promoting Access to Collaborative Treatment (IMPACT) trial (Bruce et al., 2004). Similarly, the Healthy IDEAS (Identifying Depression, Empowering Activities for Seniors) trial of home-based depression treatment was not a randomized controlled trial (RCT) like the PEARLS trial, although it did show some evidence of effectiveness (Casado et al., 2008; Quijano et al., 2007). The selected models include interventions for managing depression in primary care and in home care settings, for addressing substance use, for assisting older adults with severe and persistent mental illness, and for managing the psychiatric and behavioral symptoms of dementia in primary care. For additional research on models for delivering MH/SU interventions to older adults, see the following reviews: (Bruce et al., 2005; Chang-Quan et al., 2009; Eklund and Wilhelmson, 2009; Frederick et al., 2007; Skultety and Rodriguez, 2008; Skultety and Zeiss, 2006; Snowden et al., 2008; Steinman et al., 2007).

The chapter concludes with a discussion on the implications of the models for developing the workforce.

THE CHRONIC CARE MODEL

U.S. health care delivery remains in a mode of care with origins in the early 20th century, when health care problems were typically acute and life expectancy was significantly shorter than today (Grumbach and Bodenheimer, 2002; IOM, 2001; Wagner et al., 1996). However, an acute care orientation is not appropriate for much of geriatric care (IOM, 2008). For the older adult, chronic illness is the norm, not the exception—for both mental and physical health conditions. An estimated 34 million of the 38 million older adults (89 percent) in the United States in 2009 had at least one chronic health condition (Alecxih et al., 2010). As a consequence, older adults most often seek medical care for chronic conditions such as diabetes or hypertension rather than acute problems such as respiratory infections or fractures. Yet most primary care practices that care for older adults continue to be designed to respond to the needs of patients with time-limited, acute health care problems (Berenson and Horvath, 2003; Grumbach and Bodenheimer, 2002). The gap between the type of care needed and the type of care available is particularly troublesome for older persons with mental illness (WHO, 2003). Research on treatment preferences also suggests that older adults with some MH/SU conditions, such as depression, prefer to receive mental health services in a primary care setting rather than via referral to a psychiatric specialist (Gum et al., 2006). However, primary care physicians detect and adequately treat or refer only 40-50 percent of patients with MH problems (Speer and Schneider, 2003). Moreover, surveys of primary care physicians indicate that fewer than half of the patients they refer for mental health treatment actually receive services (Callahan et al., 1994; Lindley et al., 2010).

Thus the committee agreed that its assessment of how to strengthen the geriatric MH/SU workforce should assume a chronic care framework for delivering services. The committee also agreed that the Chronic Care Model (CCM), developed by Wagner and colleagues (2001), is an appropriate conceptual framework for integrating geriatric MH/SU services into primary care (Bodenheimer et al., 2002a,b; McDonald et al., 2007).

While the research on the CCM has limitations, the model has been demonstrated to lead to better outcomes across a variety of patient populations and care settings (Coleman et al., 2009; McDonald et al., 2007).[2] Moreover, the model is flexible by design so that it can vary across organizations, settings, and time. Nevertheless, successful implementation requires fundamental changes in provider behavior and practice redesign to support the longitudinal, coordinated care of populations. The committee believes that a CCM approach has far more potential to reach more older adults more effectively and efficiently than today's usual approach of referral to specialists and separation—sometimes carving out individuals' mental health concerns—from other aspects of their care.

Care Coordination

The overarching principle of the CCM is that chronic illness care is best delivered with coordinated teams of providers working in systems and within communities that support the care of populations (Coleman et al., 2009; Epping-Jordan et al., 2004; McDonald et al., 2007; Wagner, 1998; Wagner et al., 2001). Care coordination, sometimes referred to as "disease management" or "care management," is at the heart of most of the MH/SU models reviewed in this chapter. Numerous definitions of care coordination have been suggested. The committee adopted the following definition proposed by McDonald and colleagues (2007, p. 6) in a systematic review of quality-improvement strategies:

> the deliberate organization of patient care activities between two or more participants (including the patient) involved in a patient's care to

[2]For example, most of the research on chronic care management focuses on single chronic conditions in limited types of settings for only short periods of time. As a result, the findings may not be generalizable to real-world settings with more limited resources, motivation, or expertise. Evidence to support the cost-effectiveness of CCM-based interventions is also limited (Katon et al., 2005; Peikes et al., 2009). Given that most persons with chronic conditions, including those with mental illness, suffer from more than one chronic condition, there is a need for testing the broader model among populations with multiple chronic conditions. This may be particularly true for older adults who are more likely to suffer from multiple chronic conditions (Boult et al., 2010).

> facilitate the appropriate delivery of health care services. Organizing care involves the marshalling of personnel and other resources needed to carry out all required patient care activities, and is often managed by the exchange of information among participants responsible for different aspects of care.

In the context of models of care for geriatric MH/SU, the essential components of care coordination with respect to workforce roles, skills, and competencies are

- A patient-centered approach that recognizes the goals, culture, language, communication level, and needs of the individual patient or client.
- Team-based care with each team member having the appropriate skills and resources as well as understanding of his or her role on the team. The team is led by a primary care provider (e.g., generalist physician or nurse practitioner). A critical focus of the team's efforts is on engaging patients and clients in their care by helping them set goals and solve problems for improved self-management.
- Stepped care; simpler interventions are tried first, more intensive interventions are considered if a good outcome is not achieved. Inherent in the stepped-care approach is the understanding that some patients will require input, comanagement, or management by specialist physicians.
- Longitudinal tracking of the patient's care and outcomes. Continuous follow-up of care is integral to stepped care, relapse prevention, and team members' accountability for patient outcomes.
- Access to specialty care or other exceptional resources for those patients whose goals cannot be met with the earlier steps in the stepped-care approach. CCM does not eliminate the need for specialists. Rather, it seeks to improve the appropriate use of this limited resource.

These components are clearly interrelated and suggest other key resources that should be available to the care team such as an *infrastructure* to support communication with the patient and among other health care providers; the *capacity* to tailor the treatment to individual patient needs; *information technology* to allow tracking of the process and outcomes of care and decision support; and *access* to appropriately trained human resources. For most primary care practices, implementing care coordination requires system-level practice redesign and personnel retraining programs as well as electronic health records for shared access to patients' clinical data, individualized decision support, and easy communication between providers.

CARE DELIVERY MODELS FOR GERIATRIC MH/SU

This section of the chapter reviews nine models for providing MH/SU services to older adults (Table 4-1). It includes a brief review of MH/SU services in nursing home residents (despite the dearth of research on this very vulnerable population). As noted earlier, the models presented here reflect a variety of interventions (with variable levels of evidence) for depression, substance use, serious mental illness, and psychiatric and behavioral symptoms related to dementia. Several of the models began as RCTs, which yielded clinically significant results and have since been implemented in numerous sites around the country.

Models for Managing Depression

As Chapter 2 describes, depression during later life is prevalent and adversely affects many aspects of the person's life, including physical health, disability, quality of life, health services usage, and mortality (Blazer, 2003, 2009; Hybels et al., 2009).[3] Nevertheless, only a minority of older adults affected by depression receive adequate care (Garrido et al., 2011). This is despite more than two decades of research demonstrating the effectiveness of certain depression treatments such as antidepressant medications and some forms of psychotherapy for older adults (Blazer, 2009). More recent research—including well-executed RCTs—has also shown that there are effective models of care for delivering these treatments to ensure good outcomes for a variety of diverse, older adult populations (Arean et al., 2005a,b; Cavanagh et al., 2006; Ciechanowski et al., 2004; Frederick et al., 2007; Hunkeler et al., 2000, 2006; Katon et al., 2006; Proudfoot et al., 2003; Schonfeld et al., 2010; Steinman et al., 2007; Unützer et al., 2003; Williams et al., 2004). This body of evidence clearly suggests that the integration of mental health services into the primary care setting—where older adults receive the majority of their medical care—is an effective and efficient approach to improving the outcomes for older adults who have depression at the population level. Compared with usual care, these innovations have been shown to improve older adults' treatment outcomes and satisfaction with care. In addition, primary care physicians report greater satisfaction with their ability to meet the needs of patients with depression.

[3]See Chapter 2 for detailed epidemiological data.

Improving Mood-Promoting Access to Collaborative Treatment (IMPACT)

IMPACT was one of the most robust trials ever conducted to assess the effect of collaborative depression care for older adults (Unützer et al., 2002). The RCT, funded by several foundations, compared usual care with a collaborative, stepped-care treatment model for 1,801 older adults who met DSM-IV-TR criteria[4] for major depression or dysthymia. Eighteen primary care clinics in urban and semi-rural settings representing eight health care organizations in five states[5] participated in the trial (IMPACT, 2011a). The clinics included a wide variety of health care delivery systems, including several health maintenance organizations (HMOs), traditional fee-for-service clinics, an Independent Provider Association (IPA), an inner-city public health clinic, and two Veterans Affairs (VA) clinics. Following the intervention, IMPACT patients reported greater improvement in depression, greater remission rates, improved quality of life, and satisfaction with care. An analysis of study participants in two HMO settings found that the model reduced total health care costs by about $3,300 per person over a 4-year period (Unützer et al., 2008).[6]

The IMPACT model has been replicated in other trials, demonstrating its generalizability, effectiveness, and suitability for introduction into primary care practices nationwide (Ell et al., 2008, 2010; Gilmer et al., 2008; Grypma et al., 2006; Katon et al., 2004). The program has been either implemented or implementation is under way in 38 states (not all of the programs target the older adult population). Nevertheless, barriers such as Medicare payment policy, lack of infrastructure, and a dearth of trained personnel have prevented widespread implementation for older adults.

Intervention In the IMPACT model, potential patients are either referred to treatment by their primary care provider (PCP) or are identified via routine depression screening. During the initial treatment visit, a depression care manager (DCM) completes an assessment, provides education about treatments, and asks the participant about his or her preference for depression treatment: antidepressant medications or psychotherapy. The DCM is supervised by a psychiatrist. All patients are encouraged to engage in some form of behavioral activation, such as physical activity or scheduling pleasant events. The IMPACT treatment algorithm suggests an initial choice of an antidepressant medication made by the psychiatrist

[4]DSM, or DSM-IV-TR, refers to the *Diagnostic and Statistical Manual of Mental Disorders*. During the course of this study, the Fourth Edition-Text Revision (DSM-IV-TR) was in use. A fifth edition is expected in 2013 (American Psychiatric Association, 2012).

[5]The five states were California, Indiana, North Carolina, Texas, and Washington state.

[6]Cost data were not available at the other study sites.

upon review of the patient with the DCM or a course of "Problem Solving Treatment in Primary Care," a brief structured psychotherapy delivered by the DCM in the primary care office setting (Hegel and Arean, 2003).

The DCM follows up in person or by telephone approximately every 2 weeks during the intensive phase and approximately monthly for the remainder of the program. The duration of the intervention is 1 year.

Staffing Training is required to become an IMPACT DCM. The Advancing Integrated Mental Health Services Center at the University of Washington offers two training options: a 2-day in-person course or free online training (IMPACT). While most trainees have been social workers, psychologists, counselors, marriage and family therapists, psychiatrists, PCPs, nurses, and nurse practitioners, others are eligible for training. An IMPACT certificate program is under development and planned for release in 2012 (IMPACT, 2011b).

In primary care settings, IMPACT requires a partnership with a consulting psychiatrist (or other mental health specialist) who can provide regular consultation and supervision. If implemented in a mental health setting, a partnership is needed with the participant's primary care provider. The DCM works with the primary care provider and receives additional support from the psychiatrist, who focuses on difficult cases and individuals not responding as expected.

Kaiser Nurse Telehealth Model

Older adults often have difficulty getting to providers' offices because of cost, limited transportation options, or availability of services where they live (e.g., in rural areas). There is an emerging literature suggesting that telephone counseling and Internet-based programs may help overcome obstacles to accessing care and at substantially lower cost (Bee et al., 2008; Dieterich et al., 2004; Gellis et al., 2012; Hunkeler, 2011; Leach and Christensen, 2006; Pearson et al., 2003; Simon et al., 2004; Tutty et al., 2005). However, little related research specifically focuses on older adults. Patients receiving telecare must have affordable phone service with good connectivity and a private place to speak (Hunkeler, 2011). They must also hear well over the telephone, which could be a limitation for some older adults. Nurse telehealth care—including behavioral activation, supportive counseling, and monitoring of a patient's response to pharmacotherapy—has been tested in a variety of settings (Meresman et al., 2003). The Kaiser Nurse Telehealth Care Model has been implemented and evaluated in 13 unaffiliated primary care clinics in Maine (Pearson et al., 2003) with similarly positive results, although with a younger, under-65 patient population.

Intervention The Kaiser Nurse Telehealth Model was developed and evaluated in the northern California region of Kaiser Permanente as an adjunct to depression treatment (although not specifically for older adults). Hunkeler and colleagues (2000) compared usual physician care, telehealth care, and telehealth care plus peer support to evaluate two augmentations of antidepressant treatment in an unbalanced randomized trial[7] in two large primary care clinics. Participants included adults, ages 19 to 90, who were beginning antidepressant treatment for major depressive disorder or dysthymia. The patients receiving the intervention (with or without peer support) were more likely to experience improvement in depression and mental functioning compared to patients using usual Kaiser services.

Staffing Care was provided by a primary care physician and nurse and, in one arm of the trial, peer counselors (i.e., trained Kaiser members recovered from depression) as well. The nurses made 10 6-minute calls to the patients over a 4-month period. During the calls, the nurse answered patients' questions about the medication, gave advice on dealing with side effects, and reinforced the importance of continuing the medication. The nurses also offered emotional support, encouraged patients to engage in pleasurable activities, reviewed the activities of the previous week, and helped the patient plan for future activities. Peer support was provided by volunteer health plan members who had been treated successfully for depression. They received approximately 20 hours of training and were matched with individuals of similar age and sex.

Program to Encourage Active and Rewarding Lives for Seniors (PEARLS)

Depression is particularly common among older adults who are socially isolated and have medical comorbidities or physical impairments. The PEARLS (Program to Encourage Active and Rewarding Lives for Seniors) program is a home-based intervention specifically designed for homebound, frail older adults with chronic medical conditions. The PEARLS trial, funded by the Centers for Disease Control and Prevention (CDC), was one of the first studies to demonstrate the feasibility of collaborating with community service organizations to identify and effectively treat depressed, homebound older adults primarily with counseling rather than prescription drugs (Ciechanowski et al., 2004). Community service organizations in 14 states provide the PEARLS programs.[8]

[7]In an unbalanced randomized trial, more patients are put in the treatment group when there is a strong suggestion it will prove superior.

[8]See http://www.pearlsprogram.org.

The original PEARLS trial included 138 adults with minor depression or dysthymia who were recruited from community senior service agencies in Seattle, WA. The participants had an average of five chronic medical conditions. Racial and ethnic minorities made up 42 percent of the study population. More than half of the study population (58 percent) had annual incomes of less than $10,000. Patients with minor depression or dysthymia were randomized to the intervention or usual care. Intervention patients had significantly greater improvement in depression symptoms and quality of life compared to usual care patients and they showed a trend of fewer (self-reported) hospitalizations.

PEARLS has also been tested and found effective in reducing depression and suicidal ideation in adults of all ages with epilepsy (Ciechanowski et al., 2010a).

Intervention A DCM supervised by a psychiatrist provides six to eight depression management sessions in the patient's home over a 5-month period and follows up with up to six brief monthly telephone contacts. The sessions include problem-solving treatment, in which participants are taught to recognize depressive symptoms, to define problems that may contribute to their depression, and to devise steps to solve those problems; and behavioral activation such as social and physical activity planning and pleasant event scheduling.

Staffing The DCMs in the original PEARLS trial were two trained master's-level social workers and a registered nurse. In posttrial implementation, a wide selection of bachelor's-level workers, typically drawn from the staff of the community organization implementing the program, have been trained. PEARLS training includes 2 days of in-person instruction in how to deliver the problem-solving treatment, as well as techniques that encourage physical and social activation. Training is available in sites around the country (http://www.pearlsprogram.org/Training.aspx). A PEARLS toolkit is available online and an online toolkit is being developed (Ciechanowski et al., 2010b).[9]

Substance Use Models

Substance use[10] is often unappreciated as relevant to geriatric care even though, as the previous chapter reports, many older adults misuse

[9]Go to: http://www.pearlsprogram.org/LinkClick.aspx?fileticket=X-rXfpFDF0Q%3d&tabid=69.

[10]This report uses the term "substance use" to refer to misuse of alcohol and drugs (prescription, over the counter, and illicit).

prescription medications and over-the-counter drugs, engage in at-risk drinking, and, to a lesser extent, use illicit substances. Relatively few older adults are screened for substance use conditions; even fewer who need treatment receive it (Schonfeld et al., 2010). This may be due, in part, to the unique challenges in addressing geriatric substance use. Diagnosis, for example, can be difficult because older adults' chronic medical conditions and related symptoms may mimic the effects of substance misuse or be misinterpreted as normal signs of aging by both providers and older adults themselves. In addition, older adults may experience greater shame and guilt over their alcohol use and thus are less inclined to report problems. Because lower levels of drinking have dangerous health effects in older people compared to younger people, older at-risk drinkers may not perceive their alcohol use as risky (Blow, 1998).

Over the past two decades, findings from intervention studies conducted in a variety of medical and social service settings have shown that standardized screening and brief interventions can be effective in reducing nondependent substance use in adults of all ages, including older adults (Babor et al., 2007; Blow and Barry, 1999; Fleming et al., 1999; Lin et al., 2010; Moore et al., 2011; Schonfeld et al., 2010; Whitlock et al., 2004). In particular, screening and brief interventions have shown reduced alcohol consumption among older adults over an extended period of time (up to 18 months) in an array of health care and social service settings (Fleming et al., 1999; Moore et al., 2011; Schonfeld et al., 2010). One of the largest clinical studies of brief interventions in a primary care setting, the Trial for Early Alcohol Treatment (Project TrEAT), found that individuals in the intervention group had fewer hospital days and emergency department visits compared to the controls (Fleming et al., 1999). These effects were still significant after 2 years of follow-up (Fleming et al., 1999). A number of successful brief intervention studies also have been conducted in emergency department settings (Havard et al., 2008).

Because older adults receive services in a variety of settings and interact with numerous providers, there are many opportunities for screening and intervention. These include when older adults fill out new intake forms, during health care appointments, in emergency departments and urgent care clinics, during visits with home care nurses and social workers, and visits to senior centers and other social service agencies. This section describes two programs—SBIRT and PRISM-E—that use screening and brief interventions to address geriatric substance use.

Screening, Brief Intervention, and Referral for Treatment (SBIRT)

SBIRT is an early intervention and treatment model for persons who have substance use disorders. It is particularly noteworthy that Medicaid,

Medicare, and some commercial payers reimburse certain providers for providing SBIRT services in certain settings unlike other evidence-based MH/SU models (CMS, 2011; IRETA, 2010). Medicare, for example, covers SBIRT services provided by physicians, physician assistants, nurse practitioners, clinical nurse specialists, clinical psychologists, and clinical social workers for services delivered in physicians' offices and outpatient hospitals (CMS, 2011).

The SBIRT model has three parts:

- **Screening** to identify at-risk individuals, to assess the severity of misuse, and to determine the appropriate intervention.
- A **brief intervention** to increase individuals' awareness regarding substance misuse and to motivate behavioral change. In the primary care setting, brief interventions range from a brief dialogue between the provider and patient to concise counseling sessions with follow-up via telephone. For example, for the patient who engages in high-risk drinking behaviors, the provider may express concern, inform the patient that his or her current alcohol consumption levels are above recommended limits, and advise the patient to reduce or stop drinking (NIAAA, 2005).
- **Referral to treatment** to provide further assessment and care for persons with severe problems.

In 2003, in response to the state legislature's concern about substance use by the state's elderly population, the Florida Department of Children and Families Substance Abuse Program initiated a 3-year screening and brief intervention pilot program for older adults in four counties (Schonfeld et al., 2010). Schonfeld and colleagues developed the program based on Substance Abuse and Mental Health Services Administration (SAMHSA) Treatment Improvement Protocols (TIPs) and other research. TIPs are consensus-based, field-reviewed guidelines on various substance abuse treatment topics (SAMHSA, 1998). The Florida team revised the SBIRT source materials to be age appropriate and available in both English and Spanish. The objective of the pilot—referred to as Brief Intervention and Treatment for Elders or BRITE—was to identify older adults who had nondependent substance use or prescription medication problems and to provide them with effective interventions before they needed more specialized treatment.

The project's success led to a SAMHSA SBIRT grant for an additional 5-year program that eventually included 31 sites in 18 counties, including retirement communities, senior centers, general and trauma hospitals, primary care and urgent care clinics, VA medical facilities, and federally qualified health centers (Florida BRITE Project, 2009). From 2007 until the

SAMHSA grant ended in September 2011, there were more than 85,000 screenings of adults age 55 and older. An estimated 20 percent[11] of those screened later received one or more brief interventions. An evaluation of the program demonstrated significant 6-month improvements in misuse of alcohol and medications as well as depression. Future funding of BRITE is uncertain.[12]

Intervention[13] Outreach, screening, and counseling services were provided by BRITE counselors employed by four state agencies. Outreach presentations and screenings were conducted at health fairs, retirement communities, and senior housing sites. Bilingual counselors used a brief prescreening interview to identify individuals who might need further intervention. In addition, because substance misuse and depression often co-occur in older adults, individuals were also screened for depression and suicide risk. At-risk individuals were encouraged to maintain regular contact with primary care, social, aging, and other service providers.

Staffing[13] Addictions specialists, nurses, social workers, and mental health counselors completed 4 hours of training to become certified as a BRITE counselor. Certified counselors also attended annual follow-up training workshops. Training included use of screening methods, brief intervention with a "Health Promotion Workbook," and brief treatment. The counselors were instructed to initiate the brief intervention immediately after a positive screen. If the client appeared too tired, the intervention was scheduled for a follow-up visit. Individuals with severe substance use problems were referred to other agencies for detoxification or treatment.

Primary Care Research in Substance Abuse and Mental Health for the Elderly (PRISM-E)

PRISM-E was a multisite comparative trial of two models of care for treating at-risk drinking (as well as depression and anxiety) among older adults seeking primary care services in the VA health care system.[14] The study is the largest comparative trial ever conducted on MH/SU care for

[11]The 20 percent statistic is from the first 3 years (Rodriguez et al., 2010).

[12]Lawrence Schonfeld, University of South Florida, College of Behavioral and Community Sciences, personal communication, February 2, 2012.

[13]These details on the intervention and staffing are specific to BRITE because it was tailored to an older adult population.

[14]For more information on the trial's findings related to depression and anxiety, see Arean et al., 2008; Bartels et al., 2004; Gallo et al., 2004; Kaskie and Buckwalter, 2010; Krahn et al., 2006; Levkoff et al., 2004.

older adults. It was funded by a unique collaborative effort of four federal agencies: SAMHSA, the VA, the Health Resources and Services Administration, and the Centers for Medicare & Medicaid Services. Because PRISM-E was a comparative trial, response to treatment could not be assessed. The objective was to compare the clinical outcomes of an integrated care model versus "enhanced referral" to specialty care.

The PRISM-E trial included 560 primary care patients age 65 and older who screened positive for at-risk alcohol use. They were then randomized to one of two models of care: integrated MH/SU services or enhanced referral to a specialty mental health setting (Levkoff et al., 2004; Oslin et al., 2006). Men who reported more than 14 drinks per week, women who reported more than 12 drinks per week, or anyone who reported more than 3 drinks 4 or more times during the past 3 months (i.e., binge drinking) were considered at-risk drinkers. The study participants were primarily male (92 percent) and white (70 percent). Patients with both at-risk drinking and a mental disorder were treated for both disorders. Ten VA sites[15] participated, including primary care clinics and mental health specialty clinics nationwide (Levkoff et al., 2004).

Intervention In the integrated care model, services were colocated in a primary care setting where there was no apparent distinction—such as signage, clinic names, or staff—between the primary care and MH/SU care locations. At-risk drinkers received a brief, standardized treatment protocol that included three 20- to 30-minute alcohol intervention counseling sessions (Oslin et al., 2006). The protocol included a structured workbook with information on drinking cues, reasons for drinking, reasons to reduce or stop drinking, and a drinking "agreement" similar to a prescription form.

In the enhanced referral care model, MH/SU services were provided in a physically separate specialty MH/SU clinic designated by the primary care clinic. In contrast to the more typical referral process for specialty care, patients received enhanced referral support and case management. There was a clear referral process from the primary care clinic to the MH/SU specialist, transportation to the referral clinic was ensured, and an appointment was guaranteed within 4 weeks of randomization. In addition, the primary care clinic was notified if patients failed to make the first visits and patients were contacted if they missed any subsequent appointments. A process was also in place for emergency or urgent consults.

The investigators found no significant differences in at-risk alcohol

[15]Only 9 sites were included in the analysis of the trial because fewer than 10 individuals participated in the tenth site (Oslin et al., 2006).

use between the two models (Oslin et al., 2006). Participants in both treatment groups reported significantly lower average weekly drinking as well as binge drinking. The investigators concluded that older at-risk drinkers can substantially modify their drinking over time, but neither model of care was superior in achieving the result. Participating primary care clinicians, however, reported preferring the integrated care model primarily because of improved communication between themselves and mental health specialists, decreased stigma, and better coordination of mental and physical health care (Gallo et al., 2004).

Staffing In the integrated model, providers (e.g., psychiatrist, psychologist, clinical social worker, or nurse with MH/SU training) had different levels of expertise in treating substance use. They received special training and worked in collaboration with older adults' PCPs (Levkoff et al., 2004). Services in the specialty clinic were provided by licensed MH/SU clinicians, including psychiatrists, psychologists, social workers, nurses, or case managers with MH/SU training (Levkoff et al., 2004).

Models for Older Adults with Serious Mental Illness

As Chapter 2 describes, a growing number of older adults have serious mental illnesses (SMIs) such as schizophrenia, delusional disorder, bipolar disorder, and severe, recurrent, or treatment-refractory depression. Few representative data describe this particularly vulnerable population, although they are likely to have the most complex needs of any other subgroup of adults over age 65. Available studies suggest that older adults with an SMI have substantially higher rates of diabetes, lung disease, cardiovascular disease, and other comorbidities that are associated with early mortality, disability, and poor function (Bartels, 2004; Lin et al., 2011). They also have significant impairments in psychosocial functioning and are likely to experience loss of social supports as they age (Bartels and Pratt, 2009; Meeks et al., 1990b; Semke et al., 1996). Not surprisingly, older SMI patients account for disproportionately high costs and service use compared to other older adults (Borson et al., 2001). Lin and colleagues (2011) analyzed Medicare and Medicaid claims data and found that more than 40 percent of Massachusetts older adults with SMI were dually eligible for Medicare and Medicaid coverage.

In addition, lifestyle and behaviors (e.g., tobacco and alcohol use, sedentary) may put older adults with SMI at greater risk for metabolic side effects of antipsychotic medications and lead to obesity and the chronic conditions noted above (Bartels, 2004). Yet, unlike treatment interventions and services for younger persons with SMI, relatively little is known about effective service models for this population. However, evidence suggests that integration of MH/SU and primary care may lead to better outcomes for older adults with SMI (Druss et al., 2001; Mueser et al., 2010). In one RCT, for example, Druss and colleagues assessed differences in the physical and mental health outcomes for 120 middle-aged, male veterans[16] enrolled in a VA mental health clinic. The trial compared usual care to integrated mental health and primary care. In the integrated care model, the mental health clinic had clinical responsibility for individuals' primary care. A nurse practitioner, under supervision by a family practice physician, managed the patients' basic medical care. The medical clinic was located next to the mental health clinic (Druss et al., 2001). In addition to the nurse practitioner and a part-time family practice physician, staffing included a nurse case manager and administrative assistant. A provider from the integrated clinic maintained close contact via e-mail and phone and met weekly with the mental health team. The mental health providers were kept updated on patients' medical status and were encouraged to reciprocate with the integrated care team regarding patients' psychiatric status. Clinic staff made concerted efforts to coordinate medical and mental health visits and to remind patients (and family members if necessary) about appointments. The patients receiving the intervention had significant gains in health outcomes and use of primary and preventive care services compared with the control group. They also had lower costs and fewer visits to emergency departments.

Three notable models, HOPES, PATCH, and WRAP, that integrate psychiatric and medical care for older persons with SMI are described below.

Helping Older People Experience Success (HOPES)

Most older adults with SMI live in the community, although they are at high risk of costly institutionalization, especially in nursing homes (Meeks et al., 1990a; Semke et al., 1996). Social supports and age-appropriate psychosocial rehabilitation services can be key to helping older individuals with SMI to function better and to remain in the community (Meeks et al., 1990a). Although significant progress has been made in psychiatric rehabilitation for younger persons, little attention has been paid to developing psychosocial rehabilitation services for older adults with SMI (Mueser et al., 2010).

The HOPES model is an integrated psychiatric rehabilitation and

[16]Only one study participant was female. The mean age of the intervention group was 46; the mean age of the control group was 45. Most older adults with SMI live in the community, although they are at high risk of institutionalization, especially in nursing homes (Meeks et al., 1990a; Semke et al., 1996).

health management program specifically developed to improve psychosocial functioning and to reduce the medical needs of older persons with SMI (Bartels et al., 2004). The model was assessed in an RCT of 183 older adults with SMI who were age 50 and older. The study participants were recruited from three public mental health agencies in New England.

Intervention The model combines skills training (independent living skills, social skills) with management of medical care needs and promotion of preventive health care, thought to be essential for continued residence in the community. Delivered over 2 years, HOPES is designed to improve psychosocial functioning and reduce long-term medical burden for older adults with SMI. The first year uses a seven-part curriculum that focuses on intensive skills training and health management. Psychiatric nurses meet monthly with participants and manage individual's overall health care needs (Pratt et al., 2008). Rehabilitation specialists provide weekly group skills training in a variety of settings, including mental health clinics, rehabilitation centers, and senior centers. The second year is less intensive and focuses on maintenance. Participants attend skills classes, go on community practice trips, and meet with a nurse monthly. The HOPES trial demonstrated that it is feasible to engage older adults with SMI in an intensive skills training and medical management program. Compared with usual care, HOPES participants were more likely to remain in the program and to improve their social skills, psychosocial and community functioning, negative symptoms, and self-efficacy (Mueser et al., 2010).

Staffing HOPES uses community mental health nurses with training in both psychiatric and medical care. Community practice sessions and community supports (e.g., residential managers, case managers, and therapists) are integral to the HOPES model. As noted above, psychiatric nurses and rehabilitation specialists are essential members of the care team.

Psychogeriatric Assessment and Treatment in City Housing (PATCH)

Mobile outreach and treatment can be effective means of delivering MH/SU services to chronically ill, older adults with SMI who reside at home, but are unable or unwilling to access care through traditional means (e.g., community mental health or primary care centers). The roots of the PATCH program are two proactive, community-based models for adults with SMI who are experiencing serious challenges to living independently: the Assertive Community Treatment (ACT) Model (Stein and Test, 1980) and the Gatekeeper Model (Raschko, 1990).

A central concept of Gatekeeper is that lay community members, such as utility employees, bank tellers, postal carriers, and others, can be trained to identify and refer older adults who need services (Jensen, 2011). ACT is a model of community care for persons with SMI who have a recent history of psychiatric hospitalizations, criminal justice involvement, homelessness, or substance abuse (Test and Stein, 2000). The origins of ACT are in the deinstitutionalization era of the 1960s and 1970s, when mental health providers and community service agencies recognized that SMI residents of psychiatric hospitals needed help preparing for life in the community (ACTA, 2007). Both Gatekeeper and ACT have been implemented throughout the United States and internationally.

Like Gatekeeper, PATCH uses nontraditional referral sources who receive special training to learn how to identify and to refer at-risk older adults for multidisciplinary home-based mental health and community services. The model has three essential components (Robbins et al., 2000): (1) training of local workers, such as building managers, social workers, groundskeepers, and janitors, who have everyday opportunities to identify at-risk individuals; (2) referral of potential cases by these workers to a psychiatric nurse for follow-up; and (3) multidisciplinary psychiatric evaluation and treatment in residents' homes. PATCH has been operating in Baltimore public housing since 1986 (Johns Hopkins Office of Community Services, 2011).

The PATCH model originated with a prospective randomized trial, funded by the National Institute of Mental Health, to assess whether a mobile case finding and treatment program in Baltimore city public housing sites could help seriously mentally ill residents remain in their homes (Rabins et al., 2000). The trial focused on older public housing residents (average age 74) with SMI because they are at great risk of eviction or termination of lease (Barker et al., 1988; Bernstein, 1982; Rabins et al., 2000; Robbins et al., 2000). Most of the 945 study participants were African American; 78 percent were women who lived alone. The individuals who received the intervention experienced significantly greater declines in psychiatric symptoms compared with the control group. However, the intervention had no impact on tenure in the public housing site perhaps because, as the investigators suggest, some study participants were found to be living in unsafe conditions and placed into nursing homes or board and care facilities.

Intervention In PATCH, nurses meet with building managers and other personnel to describe the program and initiate a structured educational program for building staff (Robbins et al., 2000). Training is organized into seven 1-hour monthly sessions, beginning with descriptions of common mental health conditions and alcoholism and ending with two sessions on the emergency petition process and death and dying. The nurses also make presentations to building residents and tenant organizations. Upon receiving a referral, the nurse contacts the resident to schedule a home visit. The first home visit is a protocol-driven patient assessment. A team psychiatrist joins the nurse on a subsequent home visit to interview and evaluate the resident. If the team decides mental health services are needed, the nurse serves as case manager and direct care provider.

Staffing Trained "indigenous" workers, including building managers and workers, social workers, groundskeepers, and janitors who encounter older adults where they live, act as case finders. A psychiatric nurse is the primary service provider and a psychiatrist acts as supervisor and consultant.

BOX 4-1
Peer Support

With the advent of the Community Support Movement in the 1970s, there has been a growing realization of the need to re-create a therapeutic milieu "without walls" in the community. Peer services are an outgrowth of that movement; the core philosophy has been "nothing about us without us." Peer support has evolved in various forms over the decades, and only recently has it begun to be more formally incorporated into treatment programs within mental health systems. This development is in addition to the importance and use of peer support in the treatment and recovery from substance use that goes back to the early part of the past century. These peer-delivered services are based on the premise that an individual with a "lived experience" is uniquely able to contribute to the rehabilitation and recovery of a person needing services. Integral to the peer support philosophy is the concept of recovery, which refers to an ongoing process of learning to live with one's disability and gradually rebuilding a sense of purpose, agency, and meaning in life despite the limitations of the disorder.

The growth of peer support services has been impressive. A national survey published in 2006 found 7,476 peer programs nationwide, including 3,315 mutual support groups serving over 41,000 individu-

Wellness Recovery Action Planning (WRAP)

As noted earlier, self-management is a core component of chronic care management and care coordination. Self-management support—also referred to as self-care, self-help, and illness management—may include activities that are solely consumer directed; involve informal social supports such as family or friends; or include self-help activities that are guided by peers or professionals (Box 4-1). Self-management support for mental health conditions typically includes a wide variety of activities such as medication support, participation in self-directed components of psychotherapy, physical activity, recovery maintenance, relapse prevention, or vocational skills training. In the WRAP program and other peer-led support models, the peer and professionals do not assume responsibility for the individual's care. This distinction can be very important to individuals because it removes the implied hierarchy in the relationship between the professional and the person with the mental illness (Mueser et al., 2002).

als; 3,019 self-help organizations serving more than 1 million individuals; and 113 consumer-operated programs serving over half a million individuals. These numbers indicate that peer support services are becoming an important component of the health care system and the health care workforce.

Peers offer unique and distinctive skills and experiences not provided by other members of the usual care treatment team. The literature suggests that individuals can boost the recovery of their peers with serious mental illnesses, substance use disorders, or dual diagnoses. Patients report enhanced experiences when usual care is supplemented by peer-delivered services. However, research on clinical outcomes remains inconclusive.

The committee did not identify any peer support research focusing on older adults with mental health and substance use conditions. Research is clearly needed to help assess how and whether peer support services facilitate older adults' recovery. Data are also needed on the peers themselves—those who provide services as well as those who receive services. These data should include race/ethnicity and language, given the current demographic trends.

SOURCES: Barber et al., 2008; Bluebird, 2008; Castelein et al., 2008; Chinman et al., 2008; Davidson et al., 1999; Goldstrom et al., 2006; Legal Action Center and Abt Associates, 2010; Money et al., 2011; Pfeiffer et al., 2011; Resnick and Rosenheck, 2008, 2010; Resnick et al., 2004; Rogers et al., 2012; Young et al., 2005.

In the WRAP program, trained peer facilitators teach individuals with SMI the skills, attitudes, and behaviors to self-manage their condition (Cook et al., 2009, 2012). The program targets adults of all ages. The focus is on helping people manage their mental illness independent of any more formal health care services they may receive. The curriculum stresses that, with a highly individualized plan for recovery, individuals can do more than simply manage their symptoms; they can also create a meaningful life in the community. WRAP peer instructors use examples from their own lives so that participants can witness how others have benefited from the program. They are trained not to use psychiatric or medical jargon to describe individuals' needs. WRAP programs have been implemented in every state and internationally. Information on WRAP is currently available at http://copelandcenter.com/what-is-wrap/.

Cook and colleagues recently reported the results of the first randomized trial comparing the WRAP intervention to usual care (Cook et al., 2012). The 519 participants (average age 46) were recruited from a variety of mental health delivery settings in six Ohio communities, including community mental health centers, outpatient clinics, and residential programs. More than a third (37 percent) of the study participants were black, Hispanic/Latino, or another racial/ethnic minority. At 6 months, self-reports of improved symptoms, hopefulness, and quality of life were significantly higher among the WRAP participants compared to the control group.

Intervention In the WRAP RCT, the intervention included eight weekly 2.5-hour classes (Cook et al., 2012). The sessions were led by trained WRAP facilitators and included lectures, group discussions, instructional materials, and individual and group exercises. Self-guided wellness and recovery resources are available online.

Staffing Volunteer peer instructors make up the WRAP workforce. WRAP can also be solely consumer driven and self-managed. The program is managed by the Copeland Center for Wellness and Recovery in Rutland, VT. Five-day training sessions are available around the country. The fee is $1,200 to become a certified WRAP Facilitator and then be able to facilitate trainings to individuals in their community. Advanced training to become a certified Advanced-Level WRAP Facilitator costs $1,400. This training teaches those who have been WRAP Facilitators to train and certify other new facilitators.

Psychiatric and Behavioral Symptoms Related to Dementia

As Chapter 2 describes, older adults with dementia and other forms of cognitive impairment commonly exhibit disturbing behaviors and psychiatric symptoms such as delusions, agitation, verbal and physical aggression, depression, euphoria, inappropriate sexual behavior, and unsafe wandering (Chan et al., 2003; Okura et al., 2010). If left untreated, these behaviors and symptoms can compromise the health and quality of life of not only the affected individuals, but also their caregivers (Callahan et al., 2006). Evidence also shows they may lead to caregiver burnout (family members as well as paid staff), nursing home placement, and higher health costs.

The PREVENT protocol is an example of an educational intervention tested within a collaborative care management model.

Providing Resources Early to Vulnerable Elders Needing Treatment (PREVENT)

PREVENT was an Agency for Healthcare Research and Quality–funded RCT that assessed the psychiatric impact of a collaborative care management model on 153 older adults with Alzheimer's disease (and their caregivers). The trial compared a model (based on the IMPACT trial intervention) with augmented usual care at primary care practices in seven urban and racially diverse primary care practices in Indianapolis (Callahan et al., 2006). The primary care physicians treating the usual care group were free to provide any service they deemed appropriate.

Most of the study participants suffered from multiple comorbid medical conditions in addition to dementia. The program included a screening and diagnosis program to identify subjects eligible for the trial even if their primary care physicians had not yet diagnosed the dementing illness.

At 12 and 18 months after the intervention, the treatment group had significantly fewer behavioral disturbances, were more likely to receive cholinesterase inhibitors and antidepressants, and were more likely to rate their primary care as very good or excellent compared with the usual care group. There were no differences in functional decline. The intervention caregivers also reported significant improvements in distress at 12 months and sustained improvement in depression at 18 months.

The PREVENT protocol has been reengineered recently to improve its applicability and feasibility in the typical primary care practice and to facilitate its implementation in a real-world clinical practice (Boustani et al., 2011; Callahan et al., 2011). To accomplish these goals, the team developed a treatment manual with more attention to de novo implementation of the program in primary care, designed a new care model that delivers most of the intervention in the home while remaining a primary care–based service, and developed a specialty dementia clinic designed to support comanagement with primary care.

Intervention Both study groups completed a counseling visit with an advanced practice nurse who provided education about Alzheimer's disease and referral to community resources. Over the following year, intervention patients received care management by an interdisciplinary team led by a nurse practitioner (Austrom et al., 2004). Initially, the care manager met with the patient and caregiver bimonthly. Later, visits were scheduled more frequently (monthly). The intervention was carried out over 1 year.

Staffing Geriatric nurse practitioners acted as care managers. The nurse practitioner focused on the patient's behavioral symptoms and coordinated management of the patients' other chronic conditions with the primary care physician. The team used standard protocols to identify, monitor, and treat eight behavioral and psychological symptoms of dementia (primarily without prescription medications). The protocols included personal care, repetitive behavior, mobility, sleep disturbances, depression, agitation or aggression, delusions or hallucinations, and the caregiver's physical health. The intervention targeted the patient's caregiver as the primary conduit by which the patient received hands-on care.

MODELS OF MH/SU CARE FOR OLDER NURSING HOME RESIDENTS

The absence of effective models for addressing the needs of older adults who live in long-term care settings is especially worrisome. As Chapter 2 documents, a substantial proportion of older adults reside in long-term care settings. An estimated 50 percent of nursing home residents age 65 and older have depression.[17] Many nursing home residents also exhibit the behavioral symptoms associated with cognitive impairments (American Health Care Association, 2010). In contrast to the numerous RCTs on managing depression in older adults living in the community, informative research on how best to deliver MH/SU services to older adults in nursing homes is lacking. Psychiatric consultation is the most common approach to delivering specialty mental health services to nursing home residents (Bartels et al., 2002). This section provides a brief review of the evolution of consultative MH/SU services in nursing homes. Box 4-2 describes Preadmission Screening and Resident Review (PASRR) and the Minimum Data Set (MDS), two federally required pro-

[17]Shaping Long Term Care in America Project and Brown University, unpublished data provided to the IOM committee, funded in part by the National Institute on Aging (1P01AG027296), 2011.

grams that influence the delivery of MH/SU services in long-term care facilities.

Consultation Model

In the past, solo psychiatrists visited nursing homes upon request to evaluate individual residents' mental health and to make treatment recommendations if needed. By the mid-1980s, team-based consultation, with a psychiatrist at the center or in a supervising role, was common. These teams often included bachelor's- and master's-level mental health counselors, case managers, or mental health nurses. While continuing to address the needs of only the residents they were asked to see, the team had the opportunity to help nursing home staff with nonpharmacological care planning, staff education, and training. The consultative teams also provided counseling and mental health case management services to ensure that treatment recommendations were understood and followed (Conn and Silver, 1998; Loebel et al., 1991). There are too few psychiatrists, however, to support widescale implementation of this approach.

More recently, nursing homes have begun to use nurse-centered models in which a psychiatric nurse visits the nursing home to evaluate residents' mental health needs and to manage their mental health services. Typically, the nurse is supervised by a psychiatrist and acts as an "extender" of the psychiatrist's services. Although less common, the psychiatrist and nurse may come to the facility together and residents are triaged to either the nurse or psychiatrist, depending on individual need. This model might have the potential to compensate for the scarcity of psychiatrists, but fee-for-service payment arrangements are a barrier to its adoption. Medicare, for example, does not reimburse psychiatrists for supervisory services nor will Medicare pay for MH/SU services provided by nurses working in the absence of a physician (Berenson, 2003; Ostrow and Manderscheid, 2010)

Evidence on the effectiveness of any of these consultation variations is quite limited. In a 2002 review, Bartels and colleagues (2002) identified only one RCT that assessed the effectiveness of specialty consultation. The trial was at a single site and included 93 subjects. The investigators found that the majority of consultants' recommendations were not followed. They concluded that the consultative model did not show clear benefit for nursing home residents with mental health conditions.

Observational research suggests that 50 to 75 percent of residents who receive MH/SU consultation services improve in some aspect. Interdisciplinary team models are generally viewed as best practice because they allow for innovative approaches for providing ongoing care while

BOX 4-2

Two Federal Programs Concerning the Mental Health of Older Nursing Home Residents: The Preadmission Screening and Resident Review Program and the Minimum Data Set

Enacted in 1987, the Nursing Home Reform Act[a] introduced two federal programs with direct implications for the mental health status and care of nursing home residents: (1) the Preadmission Screening and Resident Review Program and (2) the Minimum Data Set. Neither program has specific requirements related to the mental health or substance use training or qualifications of nursing home staff. However, as the text below describes, both programs have largely untapped potential to identify and to facilitate the appropriate care of older nursing home residents.

Preadmission Screening and Resident Review (PASRR)

PASRR requires all individuals to be screened for mental health conditions prior to admission to a nursing home. If a mental disorder is identified, a mental health specialist must further assess the patient to determine if the nursing home admission is appropriate. If the patient is admitted, the specialist must also provide follow-up treatment recommendations for the patient's mental health care. This second-level screening is often performed by a master's-level PASRR professional whose evaluation and recommendations are reviewed by a consulting psychiatrist. However, the PASRR screener typically has neither clinical responsibility for the patient nor any ongoing relationship with the nursing home's clinical staff.

Numerous studies have demonstrated significant shortcomings in PASRR's implementation. Borson and colleagues (1997), for example, found that fewer than 10 percent of nursing home residents in King County, Washington, had received a complete PASRR evaluation. Snowden and colleagues (1998) reported very poor compliance (35 percent) with PASRR treatment recommendations for patients with mental disorders, especially for nonpharmacological interventions and for patients with depression. Molinari and coworkers (2011) recently assessed 73 randomly selected nursing home admissions and

addressing the needs of nursing homes for means to train and educate staff.

Although federal and state regulations require nursing homes to have an administrator, medical director, and director of nursing services, the rules do not require specialized mental health personnel nor do they found that although 85 percent of the patients were on a psychotropic medication, none of these patients had received the required level-2 PASRR mental health evaluation. Linkins and colleagues (2006) have documented that fewer than half of the states appear to incorporate clinically relevant PASRR information into patients' nursing home care.

Minimum Data Set (MDS)

The MDS is a mandatory nursing home patient data collection and screening instrument used to assess patients' physical and mental health status (including the behavioral symptoms of dementia). Every nursing home resident must receive an MDS assessment upon admission, every 90 days thereafter, and whenever there is a major change in the resident's status. Thus, in contrast to PASRR, the MDS provides a routine, regularly scheduled mechanism for identifying nursing home residents with mental health needs. The MDS instrument has been updated and improved since its introduction. Compared with earlier formats, MDS 3.0 (now in use) contains better validated assessments of cognition, quality of life, and depression and more resident participation and input into the assessment. However, like PASRR, the MDS assessment does not require appropriate follow-up and treatment for patients needing mental health services. Although federal rules require residents to have a repeat PASRR evaluation if their MDS assessment changes significantly, the evidence suggests that this occurs rarely.

Thus, while offering some potential as a means of providing an infrastructure for organizing and delivering mental health services, the MDS would need to be integrated into nursing home treatment protocols and quality-improvement activities to reach this potential.

[a] Public Law 100-203.

ADDITIONAL SOURCES: Borson et al., 1997; Callahan et al., 2002; CMS, 2012; Linkins et al., 2006; Molinari et al., 2011; Rahman and Applebaum, 2009; Snowden et al., 1998; Zimmerman et al., 2012.

require any nursing home staff to demonstrate minimum competence in geriatric MH/SU. Survey data indicate that about 25 percent of nursing homes report having mental health providers on staff and 24 percent use on-call providers.

IMPLICATIONS FOR THE GERIATRIC MENTAL HEALTH WORKFORCE

The research presented in this chapter has critical implications for the deployment and training of personnel who care for older adults with MH/SU conditions. The traditional and most common model for delivering MH/SU services to older adults is one in which patients are referred to a specialist who is physically located in a setting separate from the patient's usual source of care. Yet, the evidence clearly indicates that the effective delivery of MH/SU services—particularly for depression and nondependent substance use—requires a different delivery model. What works for many older adults who need MH/SU services is a patient-centered, team-based, primary care–centered model that is proactive and employs a coordinated team of personnel with specific roles and special training. Care managers are integral to the team's effectiveness. In models such as IMPACT, Kaiser Nurse Telehealth Care, PREVENT, PRISM-E, and SBIRT, the care manager has the most interaction with the patient and serves as the central care coordinator. The psychiatrist or other mental health specialist is available for consultation and supervision, but only provides direct care for a minority of the more complex patients.

See Table 4-2 for a summary of the care settings and core staff in the models reviewed in this chapter. The following section describes the key staff roles in effective MH/SU treatment models.

Care Managers

Care managers are central to the effective intervention models. Whether they are categorized as traditional mental health case managers (as in the older literature from community mental health center models) or care managers as in more recent interventions presented here, they are the workers who directly provide and/or coordinate the treatment intervention. The education and background of these individuals vary widely, especially as one moves from examination of the research effectiveness trials to examination of posteffectiveness trial dissemination and implementation research. Care managers need to have interest and empathy for the elderly, and be comfortable caring for physically ill clients. In addition, the models typically require these workers to be trained in diagnosis and triage of MH/SU conditions, cognition screening, elder abuse/neglect and self-neglect, suicidality, using standardized tools for outcome assessment/monitoring, recognizing medical decompensation, assessing and integrating cultural and linguistic issues, and effective use of supervision.

Some existing models now offer training to personnel with a variety of educational backgrounds (Ciechanowski et al., 2010b; IMPACT, 2011a,b; Kaskie and Buckwalter, 2010). Thus, programs that began as

TABLE 4-2

Care Settings and Core Staff for Selected Geriatric Mental Health (MH) and Substance Use (SU) Models

Model	Care Setting				Core Staff				
	Primary Care	Mental Health Setting[a]	Home	Other Settings[b]	Team	Primary Care Provider	Care Manager[c]	Psychiatrist or Other MH Specialist	Peers or Family Caregivers
HOPES		✔			✔		✔		
IMPACT	✔				✔	✔	✔	✔	
Kaiser Nurse Telehealth Care	✔		✔		✔	✔	✔	✔	✔[d]
PATCH			✔		✔			✔	
PEARLS			✔		✔	✔	✔	✔	
PREVENT	✔			✔	✔	✔	✔		✔
PRISM-E[e]	✔				✔	✔		✔	
SBIRT	✔			✔	✔			✔	
WRAP				✔					✔

[a] Specialty settings include private offices of psychiatrists, psychologists, social workers, and other mental health professionals and community mental health centers.

[b] Other settings include emergency departments, community senior centers, social service agencies, mobile outreach programs, health fairs, hospitals, and urgent care clinics.

[c] Care managers may be nurses, psychologists, social workers, or other depression care specialists.

[d] Peer counselors were used in one arm of the trial.

[e] PRISM-E findings refer only to the at-risk drinking intervention.

SOURCES: Austrom et al., 2004; Bartels et al., 2004; Callahan et al., 2006; Ciechanowski et al., 2004; Cook et al., 2012; Florida BRITE Project, 2009; Frederick et al., 2007; Hunkeler et al., 2000; IMPACT, 2011b; Levkoff et al., 2004; Oslin et al., 2006; Pratt et al., 2008; Rabins et al., 2000; Robbins et al., 2000; Schonfeld et al., 2010.

RCTs that used nurses or master's-level social workers as care managers are increasingly training a broader group to best fit the setting and personnel resources available. These workers are typically in much greater supply and thus become logical targets for interventionists to match the growing population of older adults. To the extent care managers can be drawn from existing aging network providers, the models can use people who have some general aging background and training and who are already "touching" the lives of the elderly population often in need of MH/SU services.

The available research does not clearly delineate the "minimum" requirements necessary to serve as an effective care manager. With adequate training and supervision as called for in the models, the advantage of flexibility and workforce availability may balance the concerns regarding possibly limited skill set and autonomy. How these workers relate to the existing certified or licensed geriatric care managers authorized to bill for services in some settings is not clear, though overlap likely exists. From the perspective of the interventions reviewed here, it is more important to view the role or function of this category of worker than the existing designation they have in the current fee-for-service environment.

Additionally, as one sees different training backgrounds in potential care managers, the models can be more flexible in the type and number of conditions to be addressed. For example, a nurse care manager can be trained to intervene in mental health conditions such as depression and primary care medical conditions such as diabetes and hypertension (Katon and Seelig, 2008). Social work training, which typically includes intensive training in care management, can easily tailor the curriculum to include older adults with MH/SU issues. However, it is not as clear that a social services agency case manager with no medical background or case management could serve as easily in a model designed for patients or clients with multiple chronic conditions.

Primary Care Providers

PCPs are key figures in several of the reviewed models. This is logical given two factors: (1) the greater abundance of primary care providers compared to MH/SU specialists; and (2) the central role primary care providers play in managing chronic conditions outside of MH/SU problems. The reviewed interventions clearly indicate that effective treatments are available for MH/SU problems for primary care patients. These models increasingly call for primary care providers to comanage patients with MH/SU providers instead of simply referring out for specialty management. For example, antidepressant prescriptions are the purview of the primary care provider in IMPACT and the Kaiser Nurse Telehealth Care

Model, and the depression care management team guides the antidepressant use via recommendations. Thus, training programs for primary care providers should require training in basic management of MH/SU problems to maximize the comfort level and skill set that primary care providers will have in team-based care.

For models based in primary care (e.g., IMPACT, Kaiser Nurse Telehealth Care, PREVENT, and PRISM-E), sharing of office space will be necessary and primary care information systems will need to incorporate identification and monitoring of MH/SU problems. The U.S. Preventive Services Task Force cautions that screening for depression in primary care settings should only be done in settings with the capacity for treatment with an intervention model like those described here. Therefore, while it may seem feasible and logical for all settings to screen and identify, the data do not support this as an effective strategy (USPSTF, 2011).

Specialists

Specialists are typically the member of the team with the highest degree of training for the MH/SU issue of interest. In some models, this is a psychiatrist (e.g., IMPACT) or geriatric psychiatrist, but could be a psychiatric nurse practitioner, general internist, or licensed clinical social worker, depending on the setting and treatment condition.

As the previous chapter described, there will never be sufficient numbers of MH/SU specialists to provide direct specialty care to older adults. This chapter shows that if the role of MH/SU specialists is redefined to one in which they serve in a supervisory and/or consultative function, care is likely to be both more efficient and more effective. There are critical barriers to changing the specialists' role:

- MH/SU specialists are often not trained in their fellowship or certification programs to manage a population of patients they never or rarely see.
- Under current rules, Medicare fee-for-service payment will not reimburse MH/SU specialists for supervisory activity.
- Practice settings must acquire the information technology systems for screening and monitoring patient-level outcomes and for communication with patients as well as other providers.
- Practice settings will often need to colocate the MH/SU providers with primary care providers. While it is clear that colocation alone is insufficient, as demonstrated in the PRISM-E trial, engagement is clearly improved via colocation versus specialty sector referral for patients who are not already involved in specialty care settings.

Patients

The models reviewed often have as a core component the education and activation of the patient (and/or caregiver) as a more engaged participant. The most promising MH/SU models include patient education and activation, with the goal of having the patient more actively participate in care choices and learn to self-manage his or her own condition. While viewed as an advantage by many of the baby boomer generation who are not as likely to simply accept the judgment of their health care provider, this may not be an attitude of some current older adults who feel it is appropriate to seek the advice and defer to the opinions of their primary care provider. Equally important, especially given the diversity of the population, is how engagement is achieved within the context of the participant's culture and language.

CONCLUSIONS

A persuasive body of evidence, drawn from two decades of research, shows that two common MH/SU disorders among older adults—depression and at-risk drinking—are most effectively addressed when care is organized to include these essential ingredients: (1) systematic outreach and diagnosis, (2) patient and family education and self-management support, (3) provider accountability for outcomes, and (4) close follow-up and monitoring to prevent relapse. Moreover, these elements are best obtained when care is patient centered (integrating patient preferences, needs, and strengths), in a location easily accessed by patients (e.g., in primary care, senior centers, or patients' homes), and coordinated by trained personnel with access to specialty consultation. There is also evidence suggesting great promise in telehealth and Web-based interventions for older adults with MH/SU conditions. Progress in these areas is not likely to be achieved, however, without practice redesign and change in Medicare payment rules. There is a fundamental mismatch between older adults' need for coordinated care and Medicare fee-for-service reimbursement that precludes payment of trained care managers and psychiatry consultation.

The committee concluded, as have many other studies, that the delivery of and payment for health care services to older adults must be reorganized to reflect the chronic nature of MH/SU and other health conditions prevalent in the 21st-century geriatric population (IOM, 2008). The workforce implications are daunting. Registered nurses are particularly well suited to coordinate MH/SU and physical health care, but they need additional training to serve in this capacity. Primary care providers, such as physicians, advanced practice registered nurses, and physician assistants are an integral component of these models, yet, many of them have not been trained in collaborative care and do not work in a practice or system supportive of comanagement, colocation, screening, and outcome monitoring.

Frontline workers within the aging provider network agencies may be a potential source of care managers. However, they will require intensive training in evidence-based program treatment as they are likely to have limited knowledge of MH/SU.

Finally, research on effective delivery of MH/SU care for certain older populations is urgently needed, especially for individuals residing in nursing homes and other residential settings, prisoners, rurally isolated elders, and older adults with severe mental illnesses.

REFERENCES

ACTA (Assertive Community Treatment Association). 2007. *ACT history and origins.* http://www.actassociation.org/origins/ (accessed February 13, 2012).

AHCA (American Health Care Association). 2010. *LTC stats: Nursing facilities patient characteristics report. June and December 2010 updates.* http://www.ahcancal.org/research_data/oscar_data/NursingFacilityPatientCharacteristics/Forms/AllItems.aspx (accessed February 21, 2012).

Alecxih, L., S. Shen, I. Chan, D. Taylor, and J. Drabek. 2010. *Individuals living in the community with chronic conditions and functional limitations: A closer look.* http://www.lewin.com/content/publications/ChartBookChronicConditions.pdf (accessed January 19, 2012).

American Psychiatric Association. 2012. *DSM-IV-TR.* http://www.dsm5.org/Pages/Default.aspx (accessed June 1, 2012).

Arean, P. A., L. Ayalon, E. Hunkeler, E. H. Lin, L. Tang, L. Harpole, H. Hendrie, J. W. Williams, Jr., and J. Unützer. 2005a. Improving depression care for older, minority patients in primary care. *Medical Care* 43(4):381-390.

Arean, P. A., A. Gum, C. E. McCulloch, A. Bostrom, D. Gallagher-Thompson, and L. Thompson. 2005b. Treatment of depression in low-income older adults. *Psychology & Aging* 20(4):601-609.

Arean, P. A., L. Ayalon, C. Jin, C. E. McCulloch, K. Linkins, H. Chen, B. McDonnell-Herr, S. Levkoff, and C. Estes. 2008. Integrated specialty mental health care among older minorities improves access but not outcomes: Results of the PRISMe study. *International Journal of Geriatric Psychiatry* 23(10):1086-1092.

Austrom, M. G., T. M. Damush, C. West Hartwell, T. Perkins, F. Unverzagt, M. Boustani, H. C. Hendrie, and C. M. Callahan. 2004. Development and implementation of non-pharmacologic protocols for the management of patients with Alzheimer's disease and their families in a multiracial primary care setting. *Gerontologist* 44(4):548-553.

Babor, T. F., B. G. McRee, P. A. Kassebaum, P. L. Grimaldi, K. Ahmed, and J. Bray. 2007. Screening, brief intervention, and referral to treatment (SBIRT): Toward a public health approach to the management of substance abuse. *Focus* 9(1):130.

Barber, J. A., R. A. Rosenheck, M. Armstrong, and S. G. Resnick. 2008. Monitoring the dissemination of peer support in the VA Health Care System. *Community Mental Health Journal* 44(6):433-441.

Barker, J. C., L. S. Mitteness, and S. J. Wood. 1988. Gate-keeping: Residential managers and elderly tenants. *Gerontologist* 28(5):610-619.

Bartels, S. J. 2004. Caring for the whole person: Integrated health care for older adults with severe mental illness and medical comorbidity. *Journal of the American Geriatrics Society* 52:S249-S257.

Bartels, S., and S. I. Pratt. 2009. Psychosocial rehabilitation and quality of life for older adults with serious mental illness: Recent findings and future research directions. *Current Opinion in Psychiatry* 22(4):381-385.

Bartels, S. J., G. S. Moak, and A. R. Dums. 2002. Models of mental health services in nursing homes: A review of the literature. *Psychiatric Services* 53(11):1390-1396.

Bartels, S. J., E. H. Coakley, C. Zubritsky, J. H. Ware, K. M. Miles, P. A. Arean, H. Chen, D. W. Oslin, M. D. Llorente, G. Costantino, L. Quijano, J. S. McIntyre, K. W. Linkins, T. E. Oxman, J. Maxwell, and S. E. Levkoff. 2004. Improving access to geriatric mental health services: A randomized trial comparing treatment engagement with integrated versus enhanced referral care for depression, anxiety, and at-risk alcohol use. *American Journal of Psychiatry* 161(8):1455-1462.

Bee, P. E., P. Bower, K. Lovell, S. Gilbody, D. Richards, L. Gask, and P. Roach. 2008. Psychotherapy mediated by remote communication technologies: A meta-analytic review. *BMC Psychiatry* 8:60.

Berenson, R. A., and J. Horvath. 2003. Confronting the barriers to chronic care management in Medicare. *Health Affairs* 22(1):37-53.

Bernstein, J. 1982. Who leaves—who stays—residency policy in housing for the elderly. *The Gerontologist* 22(3):305-313.

Blazer, D. G. 2003. Depression in late life: Review and commentary. *Journals of Gerontology, Series A: Biological Sciences and Medical Sciences* 58(3):M249-M265.

———. 2009. Depression in late life: Review and commentary. *Focus* 7(1):118-136.

Blow, F. C. 1998. *Substance abuse among older adults. Treatment Improvement Protocol (TIP) Series 26, Report No. (SMA) 98-3179.* http://www.ncbi.nlm.nih.gov/books/NBK64419/ (accessed February 1, 2012).

Blow, F., and K. Barry. 1999. Advances in alcohol screening and brief intervention with older adults. In *Advances in medical psychotherapy*, Vol. 10, edited by P. A. Lichtenberg. Dubuque, IA: Kendall Hunt.

Bluebird, G. 2008. *Paving new ground: Peers working in in-patient settings.* http://www.nasmhpd.org/general_files/publications/ntac_pubs/Bluebird%20Guidebook%20FINAL%202-08.pdf (accessed March 9, 2012).

Bodenheimer, T., E. H. Wagner, and K. Grumbach. 2002a. Improving primary care for patients with chronic illness. *JAMA* 288(14):1775-1779.

———. 2002b. Improving primary care for patients with chronic illness: The chronic care model, Part 2. *JAMA* 288(15):1909-1914.

Borson, S., J. P. Loebel, M. Kitchell, S. Domoto, and T. Hyde. 1997. Psychiatric assessments of nursing home residents under OBRA-87: Should PASRR be reformed? Pre-Admission Screening and Annual Review. *Journal of the American Geriatrics Society* 45(10):1173-1181.

Borson, S., S. J. Bartels, C. C. Colenda, G. L. Gottlieb, and B. Meyers. 2001. Geriatric mental health services research: Strategic plan for an aging population: Report of the Health Services Work Group of the American Association for Geriatric Psychiatry. *American Journal of Geriatric Psychiatry* 9(3):191-204.

Boult, C., S. R. Counsell, R. M. Leipzig, and R. A. Berenson. 2010. The urgency of preparing primary care physicians to care for older people with chronic illnesses. *Health Affairs* 29(5):811-818.

Boustani, M. A., G. A. Sachs, C. A. Alder, S. Munger, C. C. Schubert, M. Austrom, A. M. Hake, F. W. Unverzagt, M. Farlow, B. R. Matthews, A. J. Perkins, R. A. Beck, and C. M. Callahan. 2011. Implementing innovative models of dementia care: The Healthy Aging Brain Center. *Aging & Mental Health* 15(1):13-22.

Bruce, M. L., T. R. Ten Have, C. F. Reynolds, I. I. Katz, H. C. Schulberg, B. H. Mulsant, G. K. Brown, G. J. McAvay, J. L. Pearson, and G. S. Alexopoulos. 2004. Reducing suicidal ideation and depressive symptoms in depressed older primary care patients: A randomized controlled trial. *JAMA* 291(9):1081-1091.

Bruce, M. L., A. D. Van Citters, and S. J. Bartels. 2005. Evidence-based mental health services for home and community. *Psychiatric Clinics of North America* 28(4):1039-1060.

Callahan, C. M., H. C. Hendrie, R. S. Dittus, D. C. Brater, S. L. Hui, and W. M. Tierney. 1994. Improving treatment of late life depression in primary care: A randomized clinical trial. *Journal of the American Geriatrics Society* 42(8):839-846.

Callahan, C. M., F. W. Unverzagt, S. L. Hui, A. J. Perkins, and H. C. Hendrie. 2002. Six-item screener to identify cognitive impairment among potential subjects for clinical research. *Medical Care* 40(9):771-781.

Callahan, C. M., M. A. Boustani, F. W. Unverzagt, M. G. Austrom, T. M. Damush, A. J. Perkins, B. A. Fultz, S. L. Hui, S. R. Counsell, and H. C. Hendrie. 2006. Effectiveness of collaborative care for older adults with Alzheimer's disease in primary care: A randomized controlled trial. *JAMA* 295(18):2148-2157.

Callahan, C. M., M. A. Boustani, M. Weiner, R. A. Beck, L. R. Livin, J. J. Kellams, D. R. Willis, and H. C. Hendrie. 2011. Implementing dementia care models in primary care settings: The Aging Brain Care Medical Home. *Aging & Mental Health* 15(1):5-12.

Casado, B. L., L. M. Quijano, M. A. Stanley, J. A. Cully, E. H. Steinberg, and N. L. Wilson. 2008. Healthy IDEAS: Implementation of a depression program through community-based case management. *Gerontologist* 48(6):828-838.

Castelein, S., R. Bruggeman, J. T. van Busschbach, M. van der Gaag, A. D. Stant, H. Knegtering, and D. Wiersma. 2008. The effectiveness of peer support groups in psychosis: A randomized controlled trial. *Acta Psychiatrica Scandinavica* 118(1):64-72.

Cavanagh, K., D. A. Shapiro, S. Van Den Berg, S. Swain, M. Barkham, and J. Proudfoot. 2006. The effectiveness of computerized cognitive behavioural therapy in routine care. *British Journal of Clinical Psychology/British Psychological Society* 45(Pt 4):499-514.

Chan, D. C., J. D. Kasper, B. S. Black, and P. V. Rabins. 2003. Prevalence and correlates of behavioral and psychiatric symptoms in community-dwelling elders with dementia or mild cognitive impairment: The Memory and Medical Care Study. *International Journal of Geriatric Psychiatry* 18(2):174-182.

Chang-Quan, H., D. Bi-Rong, L. Zhen-Chan, Z. Yuan, P. Yu-Sheng, and L. Qing-Xiu. 2009. Collaborative care interventions for depression in the elderly: A systematic review of randomized controlled trials. *Journal of Investigative Medicine* 57(2):446-455.

Chinman, M., A. Hamilton, B. Butler, E. Knight, S. Murray, and A. Young. 2008. *Mental health consumer providers, a guide for clinical staff.* http://www.rand.org/pubs/technical_reports/2008/RAND_TR584.pdf (accessed March 9, 2012).

Ciechanowski, P., E. Wagner, K. Schmaling, S. Schwartz, B. Williams, P. Diehr, J. Kulzer, S. Gray, C. Collier, and J. LoGerfo. 2004. Community-integrated home-based depression treatment in older adults: A randomized controlled trial. *JAMA* 291(13):1569-1577.

Ciechanowski, P., N. Chaytor, J. Miller, R. Fraser, J. Russo, J. Unützer, and F. Gilliam. 2010a. PEARLS depression treatment for individuals with epilepsy: A randomized controlled trial. *Epilepsy & Behavior* 19(3):225-231.

Ciechanowski, P. S., S. Schwartz, M. Snowden, L. Steinman, C. Kaiser, P. Piering, D. Sugiyama, M. P. O'Leary, A. Yip, S. Favaro, and J. Huchital. 2010b. *Program to encourage active, rewarding lives.* http://www.pearlsprogram.org/LinkClick.aspx?fileticket=X-rXfpFDF0Q%3d&tabid=69 (accessed January 24, 2012).

CMS (Centers for Medicare & Medicaid Services). 2011. *Fact sheet: Substance (other than tobacco) abuse structured assessment and brief intervention (SBIRT) services.* https://www.cms.gov/MLNProducts/downloads/SBIRT_Factsheet_ICN904084.pdf (accessed January 31, 2012).

———. 2012. *MDS 3.0 RAI Manual.* https://www.cms.gov/Medicare/Quality-Initiatives-Patient-Assessment-Instruments/NursingHomeQualityInits/MDS30RAIManual.html (accessed March 12, 2012).

Coleman, K., B. T. Austin, C. Brach, and E. H. Wagner. 2009. Evidence on the chronic care model in the new millennium. *Health Affairs* 28(1):75-85.

Conn, D., and I. Silver. 1998. The psychiatrist's role in long-term care. *Canadian Nursing Home* 9:22-24.

Cook, J. A., M. E. Copeland, M. M. Hamilton, J. A. Jonikas, L. A. Razzano, C. B. Floyd, W. B. Hudson, R. T. Macfarlane, and D. D. Grey. 2009. Initial outcomes of a mental illness self-management program based on wellness recovery action planning. *Psychiatric Services* 60(2):246-249.

Cook, J. A., M. E. Copeland, J. A. Jonikas, M. M. Hamilton, L. A. Razzano, D. D. Grey, C. B. Floyd, W. B. Hudson, R. T. Macfarlane, T. M. Carter, and S. Boyd. 2012. Results of a randomized controlled trial of mental illness self-management using wellness recovery action planning. *Schizophrenia Bulletin* 38(4):881-891.

Davidson, L., M. Chinman, B. Kloos, R. Weingarten, D. Stayner, and J. K. Tebes. 1999. Peer support among individuals with severe mental illness: A review of the evidence. *Clinical Psychology: Science and Practice* 6(2):165-187.

Dieterich, M., C. Irving, B. Park, and M. Marshall. 2011. Intensive case management for severe mental illness. *Evidence-Based Mental Health* 14(1):29.

Druss, B. G., R. M. Rohrbaugh, C. M. Levinson, and R. A. Rosenheck. 2001. Integrated medical care for patients with serious psychiatric illness: A randomized trial. *Archives of General Psychiatry* 58(9):861-868.

Eklund, K., and K. Wilhelmson. 2009. Outcomes of coordinated and integrated interventions targeting frail elderly people: A systematic review of randomised controlled trials. *Health & Social Care in the Community* 17(5):447-458.

Ell, K., B. Xie, B. Quon, D. I. Quinn, M. Dwight-Johnson, and P. J. Lee. 2008. Randomized controlled trial of collaborative care management of depression among low-income patients with cancer. *Journal of Clinical Oncology* 26(27):4488-4496.

Ell, K., M. P. Aranda, B. Xie, P. J. Lee, and C. P. Chou. 2010. Collaborative depression treatment in older and younger adults with physical illness: Pooled comparative analysis of three randomized clinical trials. *American Journal of Geriatric Psychiatry* 18(6):520-530.

Epping-Jordan, J. E., S. D. Pruitt, R. Bengoa, and E. H. Wagner. 2004. Improving the quality of health care for chronic conditions. *Quality and Safety in Health Care* 13(4):299-305.

Fleming, M. F., L. B. Manwell, K. L. Barry, W. Adams, and E. A. Stauffacher. 1999. Brief physician advice for alcohol problems in older adults: A randomized community-based trial. *Journal of Family Practice* 48(5):378-384.

Florida BRITE Project. 2009. *Brief intervention and treatment for elders.* http://brite.fmhi.usf.edu/BRITE.htm (accessed February 2, 2012).

Frederick, J. T., L. E. Steinman, T. Prohaska, W. A. Satariano, M. Bruce, L. Bryant, P. Ciechanowski, B. DeVellis, K. Leith, K. M. Leyden, J. Sharkey, G. E. Simon, N. Wilson, J. Unützer, and M. Snowden. 2007. Community-based treatment of late life depression: An expert panel-informed literature review. *American Journal of Preventive Medicine* 33(3):222-249.

Gallo, J. J., C. Zubritsky, J. Maxwell, M. Nazar, H. R. Bogner, L. M. Quijano, H. J. Syropoulos, K. L. Cheal, H. Chen, H. Sanchez, J. Dodson, S. E. Levkoff, and the PRISM-E Investigators. 2004. Primary care clinicians evaluate integrated and referral models of behavioral health care for older adults: Results from a multisite effectiveness trial (PRISM-E). *Annals of Family Medicine* 2(4):305-309.

Garrido, M. M., R. L. Kane, M. Kaas, and R. A. Kane. 2011. Use of mental health care by community-dwelling older adults. *Journal of the American Geriatrics Society* 59(1):50-56.

Gellis, Z. D., B. Kenaley, J. McGinty, E. Bardelli, J. Davitt, and T. Ten Have. 2012. Outcomes of a telehealth intervention for homebound older adults with heart or chronic respiratory failure: A randomized controlled trial. *Gerontologist* 52(4):541-552.

Gilmer, T. P., C. Walker, E. D. Johnson, A. Philis-Tsimikas, and J. Unützer. 2008. Improving treatment of depression among Latinos with diabetes using Project Dulce and IMPACT. *Diabetes Care* 31(7):1324-1326.

Goldstrom, I. D., J. Campbell, J. A. Rogers, D. B. Lambert, B. Blacklow, M. J. Henderson, and R. W. Manderscheid. 2006. National estimates for mental health mutual support groups, self-help organizations, and consumer-operated services. *Administration and Policy in Mental Health* 33(1):92-103.

Grumbach, K., and T. Bodenheimer. 2002. A primary care home for Americans: Putting the house in order. *Journal of the American Medical Association* 288(7):889-893.

Grypma, L., R. Haverkamp, S. Little, and J. Unützer. 2006. Taking an evidence-based model of depression care from research to practice; making lemonade out of depression. *General Hospital Psychiatry* 28:101-107.

Gum, A. M., P. A. Areán, E. Hunkeler, L. Tang, W. Katon, P. Hitchcock, D. C. Steffens, J. Dickens, J. Unützer, for the IMPACT Investigators. 2006. Depression treatment preferences in older primary care patients. *Gerontologist* 46(1):14-22.

Havard, A., A. Shakeshaft, and R. Sanson-Fisher. 2008. Systematic review and meta-analyses of strategies targeting alcohol problems in emergency departments: Interventions reduce alcohol-related injuries. *Addiction* 103(3):368-378.

Hegel, M., and P. A. Arean. 2003. *Problem solving treatment in primary care (PST-PC): A treatment manual for depression.* Hanover, NH: Dartmouth College.

Hunkeler, E. 2011. *Workforce implications of telephonic and Internet-based mental health interventions (eCare for moods) for geriatric populations.* Paper presented at the June 1, 2011 Meeting of the Committee on the Geriatric Mental Health Workforce, Washington, DC.

Hunkeler, E. M., J. F. Meresman, W. A. Hargreaves, B. Fireman, W. H. Berman, A. J. Kirsch, J. Groebe, S. W. Hurt, P. Braden, M. Getzell, P. A. Feigenbaum, T. Peng, and M. Salzer. 2000. Efficacy of nurse telehealth care and peer support in augmenting treatment of depression in primary care. *Archives of Family Medicine* 9(8):700-708.

Hunkeler, E. M., W. Katon, L. Tang, J. W. Williams, Jr., K. Kroenke, E. H. B. Lin, L. H. Harpole, P. Arean, S. Levine, L. M. Grypma, W. A. Hargreaves, and J. Unützer. 2006. Long term outcomes from the IMPACT randomised trial for depressed elderly patients in primary care. *British Medical Journal* 332(7536):259-262.

Hybels, C. F., D. G. Blazer, C. F. Pieper, L. R. Landerman, and D. C. Steffens. 2009. Profiles of depressive symptoms in older adults diagnosed with major depression: Latent cluster analysis. *American Journal of Geriatric Psychiatry* 17(5):387-396.

IMPACT. 2011a. *IMPACT: Improving Mood—Promoting Access to Collaborative Treatment for Late-Life Depression.* http://impact-uw.org/files/IMPACTwebslides.pdf (accessed January 23, 2012).

———. 2011b. *Training.* http://impact-uw.org/training/ (accessed January 23, 2012).

IOM (Institute of Medicine). 2001. *Crossing the quality chasm: A new health system for the 21st century.* Washington, DC: National Academy Press.

———. 2008. *Retooling for an aging America: Building the health care workforce.* Washington, DC: The National Academies Press.

IRETA (Institute for Research, Education, and Training in Addictions). 2010. *SBIRT coding, billing and reimbursement manual.* Prepared for Wisconsin Initiative to Promote Healthy Lifestyles. sbirt.ireta.org/sbirt/pdf/SBIRTBillingManual20100217.doc (accessed February 4, 2012).

Jensen, J. 2011. *Gatekeeper model (1978): Case finding & response system.* Paper presented at Meeting of the Committee on the Geriatric Mental Health Workforce, Washington, DC, June 1.

Johns Hopkins Office of Community Services. 2011. *Community engagement inventory. Patch (psychogeriatric assessment and treatment in city housing).* https://cds.johnshopkins.edu/cei/index.cfm?fuseaction=display_program&id=173 (accessed February 10, 2012).

Kaskie, B. P., and K. C. Buckwalter. 2010. The collaborative model of mental health care for older Iowans. *Research in Gerontological Nursing* 3(3):200-208.

Katon, W. J., and M. Seelig. 2008. Population-based care of depression: Team care approaches to improving outcomes. *Journal of Occupational and Environmental Medicine* 50(4):459-467.

Katon, W. J., M. Von Korff, E. H. B. Lin, G. Simon, E. Ludman, J. Russo, P. Ciechanowski, W. Walker, and T. Bush. 2004. The Pathways Study—a randomized trial of collaborative care in patients with diabetes and depression. *Archives of General Psychiatry* 61(10):1042-1049.

Katon, W. J., M. Schoenbaum, M.-Y. Fan, C. M. Callahan, J. Williams, Jr., E. Hunkeler, L. Harpole, X.-H. A. Zhou, C. Langston, and J. Unützer. 2005. Cost-effectiveness of improving primary care treatment of late-life depression. *Archives of General Psychiatry* 62(12):1313-1320.

Katon, W., J. Unützer, M. Y. Fan, J. W. Williams, Jr., M. Schoenbaum, E. H. B. Lin, and E. M. Hunkeler. 2006. Cost-effectiveness and net benefit of enhanced treatment of depression for older adults with diabetes and depression. *Diabetes Care* 29(2):265-270.

Krahn, D. D., S. J. Bartels, E. Coakley, D. W. Oslin, H. Chen, J. McIntyre, H. Chung, J. Maxwell, J. Ware, and S. E. Levkoff. 2006. PRISM-E: Comparison of integrated care and enhanced specialty referral models in depression outcomes. *Psychiatric Services* 57(7):946-953.

Leach, L. S., and H. Christensen. 2006. A systematic review of telephone-based interventions for mental disorders. *Journal of Telemedicine & Telecare* 12(3):122-129.

Legal Action Center and Abt Associates. 2010. *Partners for recovery. Financing recovery support services: Review and analysis of funding recovery support services and policy recommendations.* http://www.friendsofrecoveryvt.org/wp-content/uploads/Partners-for-Recovery-RSS_financing_report.pdf (accessed March 9, 2012).

Levkoff, S. E., H. Chen, E. Coakley, E. C. Herr, D. W. Oslin, I. Katz, S. J. Bartels, J. Maxwell, E. Olsen, K. M. Miles, G. Constantino, and J. H. Ware. 2004. Design and sample characteristics of the PRISM-E multisite randomized trial to improve behavioral health care for the elderly. *Journal of Aging and Health* 16(1):3-27.

Lin, J. C., M. P. Karno, K. L. Barry, F. C. Blow, J. W. Davis, L. Tang, and A. A. Moore. 2010. Determinants of early reductions in drinking in older at-risk drinkers participating in the intervention arm of a trial to reduce at-risk drinking in primary care. *Journal of the American Geriatrics Society* 58(2):227-233.

Lin, W.-C., J. Zhang, G. Y. Leung, and R. E. Clark. 2011. Chronic physical conditions in older adults with mental illness and/or substance use disorders. *Journal of the American Geriatrics Society* 59(10):1913-1921.

Lindley, S., H. Cacciapaglia, D. Noronha, E. Carlson, and A. Schatzberg. 2010. Monitoring mental health treatment acceptance and initial treatment adherence in veterans: Veterans of Operations Enduring Freedom and Iraqi Freedom versus other veterans of other eras. *Annals of the New York Academy of Sciences* 1208:104-113.

Linkins, K. W., A. M. Lucca, M. Housman, and S. A. Smith. 2006. Use of PASRR programs to assess serious mental illness and service access in nursing homes. *Psychiatric Services* 57(3):325-332.

Loebel, J. P., S. Borson, T. Hyde, D. Donaldson, C. Vantuinen, T. M. Rabbitt, and E. J. Boyko. 1991. Relationships between requests for psychiatric consultations and psychiatric diagnoses in long-term-care facilities. *American Journal of Psychiatry* 148(7):898-903.

McDonald, K., V. Sundaram, D. Bravata, R. Lewis, N. Lin, S. Kraft, M. McKinnon, H. Paguntalan, and D. Owens. 2007. *Care coordination, Vol 7. Closing the quality gap: A critical analysis of quality improvement strategies.* Technical review 9. AHRQ Pub. No. 04(07)-0051-7. http://www.ahrq.gov/downloads/pub/evidence/pdf/caregap/caregap.pdf (accessed October 12, 2011).

Meeks, S., L. L. Carstensen, P. B. Stafford, L. L. Brenner, F. Weathers, R. Welch, and T. F. Oltmanns. 1990. Mental health needs of the chronically mentally ill elderly. *Psychology and Aging* 5(2):163-171.

Meresman, J. F., E. M. Hunkeler, W. A. Hargreaves, A. J. Kirsch, P. Robinson, A. Green, E. Z. Mann, M. Getzell, and P. Feigenbaum. 2003. A case report: Implementing a nurse telecare program for treating depression in primary care. *Psychiatric Quarterly* 74(1):61-73.

Molinari, V. A., D. A. Chiriboga, L. G. Branch, J. Schinka, L. Schonfeld, L. Kos, W. L. Mills, J. Krok, and K. Hyer. 2011. Reasons for psychiatric medication prescription for new nursing home residents. *Aging & Mental Health* 15(7):904-912.

Money, N., M. Moore, D. Brown, K. Kasper, J. Roeder, P. Bartone, and M. Bates. 2011. *Best practices identified for peer support programs.* http://www.dcoe.health.mil/Content/Navigation/Documents/Best_Practices_Identified_for_Peer_Support_Programs_Jan_2011.pdf (accessed March 9, 2012).

Moore, A. A., F. C. Blow, M. Hoffing, S. Welgreen, J. W. Davis, J. C. Lin, K. D. Ramirez, D. H. Liao, L. Tang, R. Gould, M. Gill, O. Chen, and K. L. Barry. 2011. Primary care-based intervention to reduce at-risk drinking in older adults: A randomized controlled trial. *Addiction* 106(1):111-120.

Mueser, K. T., P. W. Corrigan, D. W. Hilton, B. Tanzman, A. Schaub, S. Gingerich, S. M. Essock, N. Tarrier, B. Morey, S. Vogel-Scibilia, and M. I. Herz. 2002. Illness management and recovery: A review of the research. *Psychiatric Services* 53(10):1272-1284.

Mueser, K. T., S. I. Pratt, S. J. Bartels, K. Swain, B. Forester, C. Cather, and J. Feldman. 2010. Randomized trial of social rehabilitation and integrated health care for older people with severe mental illness. *Journal of Consulting & Clinical Psychology* 78(4):561-573.

NIAAA (National Institute on Alcohol Abuse and Alcoholism). 2005. *Helping patients who drink too much. A clinician's guide, updated 2005 edition.* NIH Pub. No. 07-3769 (accessed October 24, 2011).

Okura, T., B. L. Plassman, D. C. Steffens, D. J. Llewellyn, G. G. Potter, and K. M. Langa. 2010. Prevalence of neuropsychiatric symptoms and their association with functional limitations in older adults in the United States: The Aging, Demographics, and Memory Study. *Journal of the American Geriatrics Society* 58(20374406):330-337.

Oslin, D. W., S. Grantham, E. Coakley, J. Maxwell, K. Miles, J. Ware, F. C. Blow, D. D. Krahn, S. J. Bartels, C. Zubritsky, and Prism-E Group. 2006. PRISM-E: Comparison of integrated care and enhanced specialty referral in managing at-risk alcohol use. *Psychiatric Services* 57(7):954-958.

Ostrow, L., and R. Manderscheid. 2010. Medicare and mental health parity: A high potential change that is long overdue. *Journal of Behavioral Health Services & Research* 37(3):285-290.

Pearson, B., S. E. Katz, V. Soucie, E. Hunkeler, J. Meresman, T. Rooney, and B. C. Amick. 2003. Evidence-based care for depression in Maine: Dissemination of the Kaiser Permanente Nurse Telecare Program. *Psychiatric Quarterly* 74(1):91-102.

Peikes, D., A. Chen, J. Schore, and R. Brown. 2009. Effects of care coordination on hospitalization, quality of care, and health care expenditures among Medicare beneficiaries: 15 randomized trials. *JAMA* 301(6):603-618.

Pfeiffer, P. N., M. Heisler, J. D. Piette, M. A. Rogers, and M. Valenstein. 2011. Efficacy of peer support interventions for depression: A meta-analysis. *General Hospital Psychiatry* 33(1):29-36.

Pratt, S. I., S. J. Bartels, K. T. Mueser, and B. Forester. 2008. Helping older people experience success: An integrated model of psychosocial rehabilitation and health care management for older adults with serious mental illness. *American Journal of Psychiatric Rehabilitation* 11(1):41-60.

Proudfoot, J., D. Goldberg, A. Mann, B. Everitt, I. Marks, and J. A. Gray. 2003. Computerized, interactive, multimedia cognitive-behavioural program for anxiety and depression in general practice. *Psychological Medicine* 33(2):217-227.

Quijano, L. M., M. A. Stanley, N. J. Petersen, B. L. Casado, E. H. Steinberg, J. A. Cully, and N. L. Wilson. 2007. Healthy IDEAS: A depression intervention delivered by community-based case managers serving older adults. *Journal of Applied Gerontology* 26(2):139-156.

Rabins, P. V., B. S. Black, R. Roca, P. German, M. McGuire, B. Robbins, R. Rye, and L. Brant. 2000. Effectiveness of a nurse-based outreach program for identifying and treating psychiatric illness in the elderly. *JAMA* 283(21):2802-2809.

Rahman, A. N., and R. A. Applebaum. 2009. The nursing home Minimum Data Set assessment instrument: Manifest functions and unintended consequences—past, present, and future. *The Gerontologist* 49(6):727-735.

Raschko, R. 1990. The gatekeeper model for the isolated, at-risk elderly. In *Psychiatry takes to the street*, edited by N. L. Cohen. New York: Guilford. Pp. 195-209.

Resnick, S. G., and R. A. Rosenheck. 2008. Integrating peer-provided services: A quasi-experimental study of recovery orientation, confidence, and empowerment. *Psychiatric Services* 59(11):1307-1314.

———. 2010. Who attends Vet-to-Vet? Predictors of attendance in mental health mutual support. *Psychiatric Rehabilitation Journal* 33(4):262-268.

Resnick, S. G., M. Armstrong, M. Sperrazza, L. Harkness, and R. A. Rosenheck. 2004. A model of consumer-provider partnership: Vet-to-Vet. *Psychiatric Rehabilitation Journal* 28(2):185-187.

Robbins, B., R. Rye, P. S. German, M. Tlasek-Wolfson, J. Penrod, P. V. Rabins, and B. S. Black. 2000. The Psychogeriatric Assessment and Treatment in City Housing (PATCH) program for elders with mental illness in public housing: Getting through the crack in the door. *Archives of Psychiatric Nursing* 14(4):163-172.

Rodriguez, C. A., L. Schonfeld, B. King-Kallimanis, and A. M. Gum. 2010. Depressive symptoms and alcohol abuse/misuse in older adults: Results from the Florida BRITE Project. *Best Practice in Mental Health* 6(1):90-102.

Rogers, E. S., M. Farkas, W. Anthony, M. Kash, M. Maru, and Center for Psychiatric Rehabilitation. 2012. *Systematic review of peer delivered services literature 1989-2009*. http://www.bu.edu/drrk/research-syntheses/psychiatric-disabilities/peer-delivered-services/ (accessed March 9, 2012).

SAMHSA (Substance Abuse and Mental Health Services Administration). 1998. *Quick guide for clinicians: Based on TIP 26. Substance abuse among older adults*. Rockville, MD: SAMHSA.

Schonfeld, L., B. L. King-Kallimanis, D. M. Duchene, R. L. Etheridge, J. R. Herrera, K. L. Barry, and N. Lynn. 2010. Screening and brief intervention for substance misuse among older adults: The Florida BRITE project. *American Journal of Public Health* 100(1):108-114.

Semke, J., W. H. Fisher, H. H. Goldman, and A. Hirad. 1996. The evolving role of the state hospital in the care and treatment of older adults: State trends, 1984 to 1993. *Psychiatric Services* 47(10):1082-1087.

Simon, G. E., E. J. Ludman, S. Tutty, B. Operskalski, and M. Von Korff. 2004. Telephone psychotherapy and telephone care management for primary care patients starting antidepressant treatment: A randomized controlled trial. *JAMA* 292(8):935-942.

Skultety, K. M., and R. L. Rodriguez. 2008. Treating geriatric depression in primary care. *Current Psychiatry Reports* 10(1):44-50.

Skultety, K. M., and A. Zeiss. 2006. The treatment of depression in older adults in the primary care setting: An evidence-based review. *Health Psychology* 25(6):665-674.

Snowden, M., J. Piacitelli, and T. Koepsell. 1998. Compliance with PASRR recommendations for Medicaid recipients in nursing homes. Preadmission Screening and Annual Resident Review. *Journal of the American Geriatrics Society* 46(9):1132-1136.

Snowden, M., L. Steinman, and J. Frederick. 2008. Treating depression in older adults: Challenges to implementing the recommendations of an expert panel. *Preventing Chronic Disease* 5(1):1-7.

Speer, D. C., and M. G. Schneider. 2003. Mental health needs of older adults and primary care: Opportunity for interdisciplinary geriatric team practice. *Clinical Psychology: Science and Practice* 10(1):85-101.

Stein, L. I., and M. A. Test. 1980. Alternative to mental-hospital treatment. Conceptual-model, treatment program, and clinical-evaluation. *Archives of General Psychiatry* 37(4):392-397.

Steinman, L. E., J. T. Frederick, T. Prohaska, W. A. Satariano, S. Dornberg-Lee, R. Fisher, P. B. Graub, K. Leith, K. Presby, J. Sharkey, S. Snyder, D. Turner, N. Wilson, L. Yagoda, J. Unützer, M. Snowden, and Late Life Depression Special Interest Project Panelists. 2007. Recommendations for treating depression in community-based older adults. *American Journal of Preventive Medicine* 33(3):175-181.

Test, M. A., and L. I. Stein. 2000. Practical guidelines for the community treatment of markedly impaired patients. *Community Mental Health Journal* 36(1):47-60.

Tutty, S., E. J. Ludman, and G. Simon. 2005. Feasibility and acceptability of a telephone psychotherapy program for depressed adults treated in primary care. *General Hospital Psychiatry* 27(6):400-410.

Unützer, J., W. Katon, C. M. Callahan, J. W. Williams, Jr., E. Hunkeler, L. Harpole, M. Hoffing, R. D. Della Penna, P. H. Noel, E. H. Lin, P. A. Arean, M. T. Hegel, L. Tang, T. R. Belin, S. Oishi, and C. Langston. 2002. Collaborative care management of late-life depression in the primary care setting: A randomized controlled trial. *JAMA* 288(22):2836-2845.

Unützer, J., W. Katon, C. Callaban, J. Williams Jr., E. Hunkeler, L. Harpole, M. Hoffing, R. Della Penna, P. Noel, E. Lin, L. Tang, and S. Oishi. 2003. Depression treatment in a sample of 1,801 depressed older adults in primary care. *Journal of the American Geriatrics Society* 51(4):505-514.

Unützer, J., W. J. Katon, M.-Y. Fan, M. C. Schoenbaum, E. H. B. Lin, R. D. DellaPenna, and D. Powers. 2008. Long-term cost effects of collaborative care for late-life depression. *American Journal of Managed Care* 14(2):95-100.

USPSTF (U.S. Preventive Services Task Force). 2011. *Recommendations.* http://www.uspreventiveservicestaskforce.org/recommendations.htm (accessed October 12, 2011).

Wagner, E. H. 1998. Chronic disease management: What will it take to improve care for chronic illness? *Effective Clinical Practice* 1(1):2-4.

Wagner, E. H., B. T. Austin, and M. Von Korff. 1996. Organizing care for patients with chronic illness. *Milbank Quarterly* 74(4):511-543.

Wagner, E. H., B. T. Austin, C. Davis, M. Hindmarsh, J. Schaefer, and A. Bonomi. 2001. Improving chronic illness care: Translating evidence into action. *Health Affairs* 20(6):64-78.

Whitlock, E. P., M. R. Polen, C. A. Green, T. Orleans, J. Klein, and U. S. Preventive Services Task Force. 2004. Behavioral counseling interventions in primary care to reduce risky/harmful alcohol use by adults: A summary of the evidence for the U.S. Preventive Services Task Force. *Annals of Internal Medicine* 140(7):557-568.

WHO (World Health Organization). 2003. *Investing in mental health.* http://www.who.int/mental_health/en/investing_in_mnh_final.pdf (accessed January 19, 2012).

Williams, J. W., Jr., W. Katon, E. H. B. Lin, P. H. Nöel, J. Worchel, J. Cornell, L. Harpole, B. A. Fultz, E. Hunkeler, V. S. Mika, and J. Unützer. 2004. The effectiveness of depression care management on diabetes-related outcomes in older patients. *Annals of Internal Medicine* 140(12):1015-1024.

Young, A. S., M. Chinman, S. L. Forquer, E. L. Knight, H. Vogel, A. Miller, M. Rowe, and J. Mintz. 2005. Use of a consumer-led intervention to improve provider competencies. *Psychiatric Services* 56(8):967-975.

Zimmerman, S., R. Connolly, J. L. Zlotnik, M. Bern-Klug, and L. W. Cohen. 2012. Psychosocial care in nursing homes in the era of the MDS 3.0: Perspectives of the experts. *Journal of Gerontological Social Work* 55(5):444-461.

5

In Whose Hands? Recommendations for Strengthening the Mental Health and Substance Use Workforce for Older Americans

Abstract: *There is a conspicuous lack of national attention both to preparing the health care workforce to care for older adults with mental health and substance use (MH/SU) conditions and to ensuring sufficient numbers of appropriately skilled personnel. The barriers to growing and strengthening the geriatric MH/SU workforce are fundamental and entrenched in the systems and programs of numerous public and private entities. The committee recommends that both Congress and the Health and Human Services Secretary act to invigorate investment in the human capital that is the geriatric MH/SU workforce, to catalyze basic system redesign to allow for effective deployment of geriatric MH/SU personnel, and to stimulate essential research to inform the education and training of personnel and workforce planning itself.*

The dilemma of how to strengthen the nation's health care workforce to meet the needs of older adults with mental health and substance use (MH/SU) conditions reflects many of the challenges burdening U.S. health care. For decades, service providers, health care researchers, workforce experts, demographers, and others have warned policy makers that the nation's health care workforce is ill-prepared—in numbers, knowledge, and skills—to care for a rapidly aging and increasingly diverse population (IOM, 1978, 2008). In the specific disciplines of MH/SU, there have been similar warnings about serious workforce shortages, insufficient workforce diversity, and basic lack of competence and core knowledge in key areas (Hogan, 2003; Hoge et al., 2007; IOM, 2006; Jeste et al., 1999). In health care delivery overall, there is widespread concern about shortages of primary care providers, lack of coordination among health care providers, fragmentation of services, high cost, patient safety, and conflicting information technology systems.[1]

The convergence of the above issues presents unique challenges for the workforce in geriatric MH/SU care delivery. U.S. health care has always emphasized physical health over mental health (IOM, 2006). Despite some change in societal attitudes, the stigma associated with mental health and substance use conditions is persistent. Today's health care delivery system and financing arrangements both reflect these realities. For example, until recent legislation mandating parity in some (but not all) health insurance plans, coverage of MH/SU conditions has been strictly limited. The carve-out of MH/SU coverage and service delivery into separate systems is still commonplace.

As Chapter 2 reports, a substantial proportion of older adults have symptoms that warrant the attention of a provider skilled in geriatric MH/SU problems. Yet, only a minority of affected individuals receive specialty care, and the primary care they receive for MH/SU conditions is often inadequate despite the existence of evidence-based screening and treatment models (Bruce et al., 2005; Unützer et al., 2002). Moreover, a growing body of research suggests that inattention to older adults' mental health and substance use conditions is associated with higher costs and poorer health outcomes, particularly for individuals with multiple comorbidities (Counsell et al., 2007; Katon et al., 2005; Unützer et al., 1997). Available evidence, for example, indicates that older adults with untreated depression are less likely to complete prescription regimens for diabetes, hypertension, and coronary heart disease; more likely to be readmitted after a hospitalization for a medical problem; and more likely to have poor health outcomes after a cardiovascular event, compared to similar patients without mental health problems (Ciechanowski et al., 2000; Garner, 2010; Gehi et al., 2005; Gilmer et al., 2007; Jiang et al., 2001; Krousel-Wood et al., 2010; Lin et al., 2004; Williams et al., 2004).

The barriers to growing and strengthening the geriatric MH/SU workforce are fundamental and entrenched in the systems and programs of numerous public and private entities—including multiple U.S. Department of Health and Human Services (HHS) and other federal agencies, professional organizations, medical and professional training institutions, credentialing and accreditation organizations, licensing bodies, service

[1]See Chapter 1, Box 1-3, for background on the parity legislation.

systems, payers, and research institutions. The breadth and magnitude of the problem is such that no single approach, nor a few isolated changes in disparate federal agencies or programs, is going to adequately address the issue or bring about quick change.

Overcoming these challenges will require focused and coordinated action. Leadership by the HHS Secretary will be essential. Both Congress and the HHS Secretary must act to establish a locus of responsibility for geriatric MH/SU, to invigorate investment in the human capital that is the geriatric MH/SU workforce, to catalyze basic system redesign to allow for effective deployment of geriatric MH/SU personnel, and to stimulate essential research to inform the education and training of personnel and workforce planning itself.

The committee recognizes that the nation faces a broader imperative to strengthen the primary care and overall health care workforce to meet the needs of an aging and increasingly diverse population. Primary care providers, for example, are under tremendous pressure to assume an ever-expanding set of responsibilities. Nevertheless, the committee believes that policy makers must consider competence in MH/SU issues as central to improving the quality, effectiveness, and efficiency of the American health care workforce.

LOCUS OF RESPONSIBILITY

There is a conspicuous lack of national attention to preparing the health care workforce to care for older adults who have MH/SU conditions and to ensuring sufficient numbers of personnel for the rapidly growing elderly population. HHS and its many agencies, for example, have the expertise and authority to strengthen the geriatric MH/SU workforce and to improve quality of care. Yet, responsibility for geriatric MH/SU is scattered across the various HHS agencies, bureaus, and departments, including the Administration on Aging (AoA), the Agency for Healthcare Research and Quality (AHRQ), the Centers for Disease Control and Prevention, the Centers for Medicare & Medicaid Services (CMS), the Health Resources and Services Administration (HRSA), the Substance Abuse and Mental Health Services Administration (SAMHSA), and several institutes within the National Institutes of Health (NIH), including the National Institute for Mental Health (NIMH), National Institute on Aging (NIA), and the National Institute on Drug Abuse (NIDA).[2] Moreover, agencies' efforts fall far short of what is needed and appear to be dwindling. Designating a locus of responsibility is a critical first step

[2]See Table 1-3 in Chapter 1 for details on selected federal programs related to geriatric MH/SU.

toward building the nation's capacity to generate and maintain a robust and competent geriatric MH/SU workforce.

RECOMMENDATION 1: Congress should direct the Secretary of Health and Human Services (HHS) to designate a responsible entity for coordinating federal efforts to develop and strengthen the nation's geriatric MH/SU workforce.

- **The committee urges Congress to fund the already authorized National Health Care Workforce Commission to serve in this capacity. In the absence of congressional action, the Secretary of HHS should act as soon as possible to designate an alternative body.**
- **The coordinating body should have the following priorities with respect to the geriatric MH/SU workforce:**
    - **Identification, development, and refinement of methods for improving recruitment and retention of geriatric MH/SU personnel, including ways to build a workforce that reflects the increasingly diverse older adult population.**
    - **Promotion and support of widescale implementation of evidence-based models of geriatric MH/SU care that effectively deploy personnel.**
    - **Identification, development, and refinement of model curricula and curriculum development tools in geriatric MH/SU, including effective models of training for integrated rehabilitation, health promotion, health care, and social services for older adults with serious mental illness.**
    - **Identification, development, and refinement of core competencies in geriatric MH/SU for the entire spectrum of personnel who care for older adults, including direct care workers, peer support specialists, primary care physicians, nurses (at all levels), physician assistants, substance use counselors, social workers, psychologists, rehabilitation counselors, and marriage and family therapists.**
    - **Evaluation and dissemination of all of the above.**

The Role of HHS Agencies

A variety of HHS agencies and programs touch on geriatric MH/SU. These efforts, however, are minimal, lack specific focus on geriatric MH/SU, and, in some cases, are being discontinued. The following are examples.

AHRQ has initiated a noteworthy interagency effort—the Academy for Integrating Mental Health and Primary Care—to coordinate the collection, analysis, synthesis, and dissemination of research on integrating MH/SU services in primary care. The initial focus will be on developing a national integration strategy, including developing core competencies for the primary care workforce. There are also plans for work on quality measurement and a survey of small primary care practices. However, funding for the academy is quite limited (less than $0.5 million) and older adults are not a priority topic.[3]

AoA provides funding for state and local agencies to plan and deliver a wide array of health-related and social services for older adults, including those with MH/SU conditions (O'Shaunessy, 2011). Through its competitive grants programs, AoA has provided funding for several states to implement evidence-based mental health programs, such as Healthy IDEAS (Identifying Depression, Empowering Activities for Seniors) and PEARLS (Program to Encourage Active and Rewarding Lives for Seniors) (AoA, 2011). It is currently collaborating with SAMHSA to provide technical assistance, through webinars and other online materials, for states and communities that want to implement community-based mental health services for older people (AoA and SAMHSA, 2012). The 2006 reauthorization of the Older Americans Act, which funds AoA, authorized the agency to designate one staff member to be responsible for aging-related mental health services (AoA, 2010a). One full-time equivalent is currently functioning in this role. The reauthorization also identifies many aging-related mental health projects the agency is authorized, but not required, to implement, including projects intended to increase public awareness of mental health disorders, provide mental health screening, remove barriers to diagnosis and treatment, and coordinate mental health services for older adults with community health centers and other public and private organizations (AoA, 2010b). To date, AoA has not funded such projects on a wide scale, although some states are using AoA competitive grant funds for programs intended to achieve some of these objectives.

CMS, the HHS agency with perhaps the most potential to influence the delivery of geriatric MH/SU services, has a substantial range of projects under way to evaluate new approaches to improving the quality and effectiveness of services provided to Medicare and Medicaid beneficiaries (Box 5-1).

CMS payment policy, limited in part by statutory restrictions, is particularly problematic.[4] A plethora of evidence shows that current Medi-

[3]C. Mullican, Senior Advisor for Mental Health Research, AHRQ, personal communication, October 24, 2011, and April 18, 2012.

[4]More comprehensive reviews of MH/SU financing are available elsewhere (Barry et al., 2010; Fisher et al., 2009; Goldman and Grob, 2006; Levit et al., 2008; MedPAC, 2010; Sarata, 2010; Shirk, 2008; Slade et al., 2005; Unützer et al., 2006).

BOX 5-1
Research and Demonstrations at the Centers for Medicare & Medicaid Services (CMS)

CMS is sponsoring an ambitious range of demonstration projects to stimulate innovation and improve the quality and efficiency of health care delivery. Because the details of these initiatives were evolving during the committee's deliberations, it was unclear whether older adults with mental health and substance use conditions would be a primary focus of any of the demonstration projects. However, it appears that the innovation grants have the potential to stimulate workforce improvements. Some key elements of selected innovation grants are described below.

Accountable Care Organization (ACO) Initiatives

- *Medicare Shared Savings Program (MSSP).* This program will reward ACOs that reduce their growth in costs while meeting standards for quality care. The quality standards include depression screening and follow-up. Grant applicants must identify how their care model would transform the workforce and update the skills of existing health professionals, identify and train new types of workers to enhance care delivery, and/or expand the use of team-based care.
- *Advance Payment.* Open to MSSP awardees, this demonstration will test whether advance payments of future shared savings facilitate participation in the shared savings program. The advances will be

care and Medicaid payment policies act to deter rather than to facilitate access to effective and efficient MH/SU services (Unützer et al., 2006). Some of the models of service delivery described in Chapter 4 have been demonstrated to be efficacious and possibly cost saving. However, Medicare limitations on which types of personnel can be reimbursed for providing essential elements of the models precludes key providers from offering needed services. For example, although care managers are integral to effective management of depression, they cannot be paid by Medicare.

Medicaid and Medicare pay for most nursing home care, and thus CMS plays a central role in the oversight of the services, including MH/SU services, provided to older adults residing in nursing homes. As Chapter 4 describes, two Medicaid programs are particularly important to older available to participating physician-owned and rural providers who make new investments to improve care and to generate Medicare savings—including investments in hiring new nurse care coordinators to expand care management.

Health Care Innovation Challenge

Under the auspices of the Center for Medicare & Medicaid Innovation, these challenge grants have multiple objectives, including testing new roles and skills for existing health professionals, using new types of workers to support care transformation, and employing team-based models to better use the mix of health providers. Grant applicants must focus on high-cost/high-risk populations including those with multiple chronic conditions, mental health or substance use conditions, the frail elderly, and others.

Independence at Home Demonstration

This demonstration adds extensive primary care services to existing Medicare home care benefits for patients with multiple chronic illnesses (including mental health conditions). Medical practices that meet the program's quality standards and generate savings may receive incentive payments. To participate in the demonstration, medical practices must be led by physicians or nurse practitioners with experience providing home-based primary care.

SOURCES: CMMI, 2011a,b.

adults with mental health conditions: the Pre-Admission Screening and Resident Review Program (PASRR) and the Minimum Data Set (MDS). Both programs provide an infrastructure with the potential to organize, deliver, and promote quality mental health services to older nursing home residents. However, the available evidence suggests that Medicaid oversight and enforcement of both programs has been inadequate.

HRSA is the central HHS agency tasked with promoting the production and training of key health personnel. The Bureau of Health Professions oversees a variety of programs, described in Box 5-2, that have the potential to expand expertise in geriatric MH/SU. However, MH/SU is not a mandatory requirement in the bureau's geriatric programs.

Several **NIH** institutes have missions related to aging and mental health or substance use. For example, Congress has charged the **NIA** with

BOX 5-2
HRSA Geriatric Training Programs

The Health Resources and Services Administration (HRSA) programs described below provided training and education in mental health (88 percent) and substance use (22 percent) to 93,616 individuals from 2007 to 2010. Participants represented a wide range of disciplines, including nursing (24 percent), medicine (15 percent), social work (12 percent), and others (49 percent).

Geriatric Training for Physicians, Dentists, and Behavioral and Mental Health Professionals

Supports awards to schools of medicine and osteopathic medicine, teaching hospitals, and graduate medical education programs for geriatric training projects to train physicians, dentists, and behavioral and mental health professionals who plan to teach geriatric medicine, geriatric dentistry, or geriatric behavioral or mental health. Applicants must propose projects that support interprofessional training in geriatrics through one or both of the following training options: (1) a 1-year faculty retraining program in geriatrics, and/or (2) a 2-year internal medicine or family medicine fellowship program providing emphasis in clinical geriatrics and geriatrics research. The program requires participating institutions to sponsor applicants in the medical, dental, and mental health arenas. The Patient Protection and Affordable Care Act (ACA) expanded the types of behavioral health professionals eligible to participate in the 1-year faculty retraining option to include those with a graduate or postgraduate degree from an accredited institution of higher education in psychiatry, psychology, psychiatric nursing, social work, substance abuse disorder prevention and treatment, marriage and family counseling, or professional counseling.

Geriatric Academic Career Awards (GACAs)

Five-year grants to promote the career development of junior, nontenured faculty as academic geriatric specialists. Awardees must provide training in clinical geriatrics, including the training of interprofessional teams of health care professionals. Geriatrics mental health professionals are eligible to apply for the grants. The ACA authorized an expansion of the GACA program to include a wider scope of disciplines, including allopathic medicine, osteopathic medicine, nursing, social work, psychology, dentistry, pharmacy, and allied health. The ACA also authorized that payment be made to accredited schools of allopathic medicine, osteopathic medicine, nursing, social work, psychology, dentistry, pharmacy, or allied health.

Geriatric Education Centers (GECs)

Institutional awards to schools of the health professions to (1) improve the interprofessional education and training of health professionals in geriatrics; (2) develop and disseminate curricula relating to the treatment of health problems of elderly individuals; (3) provide faculty training in geriatrics; (4) provide continuing education to health professionals to provide geriatric care; and (5) provide students with clinical training in geriatrics in nursing homes, chronic and acute disease hospitals, ambulatory care centers, and senior centers. Like the GACA program, the provision of interprofessional education and training in the identification and treatment of mental health and substance use disorders is optional. Currently funded GEC grantees were required to select one of five evidence-based practice areas to link their education and training activities to participant practice improvement. The five areas are delirium, depression, diabetes mellitus, fall prevention, and pain care. Of the 45 grantees, 6 grantees are addressing delirium and 6 are addressing depression.

Comprehensive Geriatric Education Program

Institutional awards to an accredited school of nursing, health care facility, program leading to certified nurse assistant certification, a partnership between a school of nursing and a health care facility, or a partnership between a school of nursing and a program leading to certification as a certified nursing assistant. The grants may be used to provide training to individuals who provide geriatric care for the elderly; to develop and disseminate curricula relating to the treatment of health problems of elderly individuals; to train faculty members in geriatrics; to provide continuing education to individuals who provide geriatric care; or to establish traineeships for individuals who are preparing for advanced education nursing degrees in geriatric nursing, long-term care, geropsychiatric nursing, or other nursing areas that specialize in geriatrics.

SOURCES: HRSA, 2010a,b,c, 2012.

providing leadership in aging research, training, health information dissemination, and other programs relevant to aging and older people, particularly related to Alzheimer's disease. Nevertheless, geriatric MH/SU is not a focus of the institute's activities. In the past, the **NIMH** funded important research to inform the effective delivery of MH/SU services to older adults. At present, the institute is scaling back grant support for interventions and services research in favor of research in basic translational neuroscience.

SAMHSA is the lead federal agency charged by Congress to direct services and resources to people with MH/SU conditions, yet it has consistently devoted only a small fraction of its budget to older adults. It is particularly disconcerting that the agency is reducing its activities related to geriatric MH/SU. For example, SAMHSA has eliminated future funding for its Older Adults Targeted Capacity Expansion grants program. It has also discontinued support for a successful adaptation of the Screening, Brief Intervention, and Referral to Treatment for older adults who have nondependent substance use or prescription medication problems (known as the Brief Intervention and Treatment for Elders).

RECOMMENDATION 2: The Secretary of HHS should ensure that its agencies—including the Administration on Aging (AoA), Agency for Healthcare Research and Quality (AHRQ), Centers for Medicare & Medicaid Services (CMS), Health Resources and Services Administration (HRSA), National Institute of Mental Health (NIMH), National Institute on Drug Abuse (NIDA), and Substance Abuse and Mental Health Services Administration (SAMHSA)—assume responsibility for building the capacity and facilitating the deployment of the MH/SU workforce for older Americans:

- **CMS**
  - **CMS should evaluate alternative methods for funding primary care and other personnel who provide evidence-based models of care to older adults with MH/SU conditions. This should include reimbursing care managers as well as the psychiatrists and other mental health specialists providing supervision of their work.**
  - **CMS should evaluate alternative payment methods to encourage effective deployment of the workforce to provide integrated primary care, chronic disease self-management, and health promotion for older adults receiving care in community mental health centers and other specialty mental health settings.**

o CMS should explore approaches and strategies for improving care delivery to older adults with MH/SU conditions through its contracts with quality-improvement organizations.

o CMS should enforce and monitor implementation of the Pre-Admission Screening and Resident Review (PASRR) and Minimum Data Set (MDS) nursing home requirements regarding residents' mental health. The agency should also ensure that PASRR and MDS mental health assessments inform residents' care plans and that nursing home personnel implement the care plans accordingly.

- **HRSA**
  - **The HRSA Administrator should ensure that the National Center for Health Care Workforce Analysis devotes sufficient attention to geriatric MH/SU with guidance from the national coordinating body described below.**
  - **The HRSA Administrator should ensure that the Geriatric Academic Career Awards career development grants include awards to geriatric MH/SU specialists if they commit to working with older adults in acute or long-term care settings.**
  - **The HRSA Administrator should ensure that the Geriatric Education Centers and the Comprehensive Geriatric Education Program institutional awards fund programs that train individuals in geriatric MH/SU care.**
- **NIMH**
  - **The Director of NIMH should ensure that the institute conducts research on methods for increasing the capacity of the mental health workforce to provide competent and effective care for older adults who reside in the community or in nursing homes or other congregate residential settings.**
- **SAMHSA**
  - **The SAMHSA Administrator should ensure that the agency devotes sufficient attention to the capacity of the behavioral health workforce to provide both geriatric mental health and geriatric substance use services.**
  - **The SAMHSA Administrator should ensure that the agency restores funding of the Older Adult Mental Health Targeted Capacity Expansion Grant program.**
  - **The SAMHSA Administrator should require states that receive MH/SU block grants to document and to report how the funds are used to support local capacity to serve older adults.**

INVESTMENT IN HUMAN CAPITAL

The capacity of the geriatric MH/SU workforce derives from the competence that is embodied in the individual personnel (human capital), the group's overall productive potential, and the organizational and policy contexts that facilitate its growth and competence. Support or accountability for training, recruitment, and retention of key geriatric MH/SU personnel—public or private—is wholly inadequate. Chapter 3 shows that the educational, training, and certification and licensure requirements for the workforce that cares for older adults with geriatric MH/SU conditions are vague, inconsistent, and minimal at best. For individuals pursuing specialty training in mental health or substance use, few specific standards exist for competence in geriatrics. For individuals pursuing specialty training in geriatrics, few, if any, training requirements are related to mental health or substance use. For the large group of individuals who will have the most contact with older adults—trainees in primary care—there are few requirements related to geriatric mental health and substance use.

Workforce Competence in Geriatric MH/SU

The concept of "core competencies" is not new to health care workforce education and training. Many expert groups, individually and in collaboration (including geriatrics, social work, family medicine, geriatric nursing, geropsychology, direct care workers, and others) have identified or are developing sets of essential skills, knowledge, and attitudes that are central to their specific discipline or are common across professions (Canadian Centre on Substance Abuse, 2010; Council of Professional Geropsychology Training Programs, 2011; Geropsychiatric Nursing Collaborative, 2010a,b,c; Heflin et al., 2011; Hoge and McFaul, 2010; Karel et al., 2010; Leipzig et al., 2009; Partnership for Health in Aging, 2008; University of Minnesota Research and Training Center on Community Living, 2011).

The United States needs a workforce that is able to address the complex health care needs of older adults, with basic knowledge of geriatric MH/SU; expertise in team-based, collaborative care; cultural competence; and multilingual skills. The previous chapters make clear that the broad spectrum of the geriatric MH/SU workforce—from the most entry-level caregiving positions to advanced practice nursing to physicians—should be aware of the signs and symptoms of MH/SU conditions in older adults as well as potential abuse and neglect situations. All these individuals should be able to respond appropriately within their level of training, scope of practice, and the range of care settings in which they encounter older adults such as primary care, home care, hospitals, nursing homes, and other congregate living settings.

Chapter 4 presents compelling evidence that team skills are also essential to effective geriatric MH/SU care.[5] All team members should possess the skills to work in collaboration with staff at different levels. Team-based care is more than the sum of each team member's technical proficiency; it is about being "on the same page," checking in with one another, and knowing when to delegate and when to consult more senior staff.

Credentialing and accreditation are important inducements for obtaining specific knowledge and skills. Yet, as Chapter 3 describes, the committee found only indirect and vague references to the subject of geriatric MH/SU in published standards. Most private-sector organizations that educate, train, accredit, and certify the various workforce sectors demonstrate little or no focus on ensuring providers' competence in geriatric MH/SU. A special concern is that current curricula—across nearly all the relevant disciplines—largely ignore the topic of geriatric MH/SU (see Appendix C). There is little evidence of dedicated geriatric curricula in training programs for MH/SU specialists (e.g., psychiatrists, psychologists, psychiatric nurses, social workers, substance use counselors) or dedicated geriatric MH/SU curricula in training programs for primary care providers (e.g., general medical internists, family medicine physicians, geriatricians, physician assistants, advanced practice registered nurses).

RECOMMENDATION 3: Organizations responsible for accreditation, certification, and professional examination, as well as state licensing boards, should modify their standards, curriculum requirements, and credentialing procedures to require professional competence in geriatric MH/SU for all levels of personnel that care for the diversity of older adults.

- **These efforts should include requirements for recredentialing and professional development for already licensed and certified personnel.**

Dearth of Support or Incentives for Training, Recruitment, and Retention in Geriatric MH/SU

Chapter 3 also makes clear that few opportunities or financial incentives are available for individuals to pursue specialized geriatric MH/SU training, for employers to invest in improving their staff's competence in

[5]See Chapter 4, Table 4-2.

geriatric MH/SU care, or for personnel to enter and stay in the field. The Patient Protection and Affordable Care Act (ACA)[6] workforce provisions present an important opportunity for increasing the numbers of geriatric MH/SU specialists across several disciplines as well as improving the competency of nonspecialists in identifying, managing, and referring older adults for MH/SU services.[7] Although these programs do not specifically target geriatric MH/SU, they do not preclude investment in this area. However, nearly all are unfunded (Baumrucker et al., 2011; Heisler and Sarata, 2011; Redhead et al., 2011b).The committee urges Congress to appropriate the funds for these programs with the proviso that the responsible funding agency—HRSA—direct a share of the monies to specifically support training and education in geriatric MH/SU. These supports should be applied across the workforce spectrum, from the direct care workers who care for older adults in their homes or in nursing facilities to the most highly trained specialists. The following describes examples of relevant workforce planning and training in the legislation.

Workforce Planning

- **National Health Care Workforce Commission.** Establishes a commission to review workforce supply/demand and recommend priorities and goals for nursing, mental health, allied and public health, and emergency medicine; to oversee and report on state health care workforce development grants; to evaluate ways to finance health care education and training; and to assess reports from the National Center for Health Care Workforce Analysis.
- **State health care workforce development grants.** Establishes a grants program to enable state- and local-level partnerships to develop strategies for health care workforce development.

Workforce Pipeline and Training to Increase Competence in Geriatrics

- **Geriatric education and training.** Expands eligibility for geriatric education center grants to new types of entities, individuals, and professions, including allied health, medicine, advanced practice nursing, clinical psychology, clinical social work, marriage and family therapy, counseling, and physician assistant programs. Grants/contracts are for short-term intensive courses on geriatrics, chronic care management, and long-term care (LTC) for medical

[6]Public Law 111-148.

[7]For a complete summary of the ACA workforce provisions, see *Discretionary Funding in the Patient Protection and Affordable Care Act* (Redhead et al., 2011a).

school faculty and other health profession schools—in return for teaching or practicing in geriatrics, LTC, or chronic care management for at least 5 years. Grantees must offer family caregiver and direct care provider training (at no or nominal cost to enrollees).

- **Nursing workforce.** Modifies and reauthorizes several existing nursing education programs to support nursing workforce development, including grants and scholarship programs for graduate and undergraduate nursing education in cultural competency, workforce diversity, nurse faculty members, advanced education nurses, and geriatric nursing. Includes an increase in the maximum loan amount.
- **Medicare Graduate Nurse Education Demonstration Program.** Establishes a Medicare demonstration program for up to five eligible hospitals to receive reimbursement for providing advanced practice nurses with clinical training in primary care, preventive care, transitional care, and chronic care management.
- **Demonstration projects to address health professions workforce needs.** Establishes two demonstration grants to provide low-income individuals with opportunities for education, training, and career advancement. Offers financial aid and other supportive services to states, Indian tribes, institutions of higher education, and local workforce investment boards to help low-income individuals obtain education and training in health care jobs that pay well and are in high demand. Also includes grants to states developing core training competencies and certification programs for personal and home care aides.
- **Training opportunities for direct care workers.** Establishes a grant program for educational institutions who partner with LTC providers to provide new training opportunities (i.e., tuition and fee assistance) for direct care workers in LTC settings, including nursing homes, assisted living facilities, skilled nursing facilities, and home- and community-based settings.

RECOMMENDATION 4: Congress should appropriate funds for the Patient Protection and Affordable Care Act (ACA) workforce provisions that authorize training, scholarship, and loan forgiveness for individuals who work with or are preparing to work with older adults who have MH/SU conditions. This funding should be targeted to programs with curricula in geriatric MH/SU and directed specifically to the following types of workers who make a commitment to caring for older adults who have MH/SU conditions:

- **Psychiatrists, psychologists, psychiatric nurses, social workers, MH/SU counselors, and other specialists who require skills and knowledge of both geriatrics and MH/SU.**
- **Primary care providers, including geriatricians and other physicians, registered nurses (RNs), advanced practice registered nurses (APRNs), and physician assistants.**
- **Potential care managers for older adults who have MH/SU conditions, including RNs, APRNs, social workers, physician assistants, and others.**
- **Faculty in medicine, nursing, social work, psychology, substance use counseling, and other specialties.**
- **Direct care workers and other frontline employees in home health agencies, nursing homes, and assisted living facilities (including personal care attendants not employed by an agency).**
- **Family caregivers of older adults with MH/SU conditions.**

BUILDING BLOCKS OF INFORMED WORKFORCE PLANNING

The dearth of even the most basic data is a significant barrier to workforce planning in the United States, especially in geriatric MH/SU. As Chapters 2 and 3 indicate, little is known about the clinical and demographic characteristics of older adults with MH/SU conditions, the existing skills and makeup of the workforce that serves them, or the educational establishment that trains the workforce. There is a particular void of information on the older adults with MH/SU conditions who reside in nursing homes and other residential settings, prisoners, rurally isolated elders, and those with severe mental illnesses.

Recommendation 1 (above) describes the importance of investing in ongoing research on recruitment and retention methods, evidence-based models of geriatric MH/SU care, curriculum development, and core competencies. The committee also recommends that HHS build an information infrastructure that ensures routine collection, dissemination, and analysis of data on the older adult population with MH/SU conditions and the workforce that serves them.

RECOMMENDATION 5: HHS should direct a responsible entity (as described above) to develop and coordinate implementation of a data collection and reporting strategy for geriatric MH/SU workforce planning. Data collection and reporting should include the following:

- **Prevalence data for *Diagnostic and Statistical Manual of Mental Disorders* (DSM)-defined disorders and other MH/SU conditions, including data on comorbidity of these conditions. Representative data on the following subgroups are essential:**

- **Age within the 65+ population (65-74, 75-84, and 85 and older)**
- **Gender**
- **Race and ethnicity (including non–English speakers)**
- **Veteran status**
- **Living situation (private household, public housing or senior housing facility, group home, assisted living or other residential care facility, and nursing home)**
- **Coexisting physical health conditions**
- **Coexisting cognitive and functional impairments**
- **Geographic area**

- **Use of MH/SU services for the above subgroups**
- **Comprehensive and comparable information on the full range of geriatric MH/SU personnel with sufficient detail to assess the workforce supply by race and ethnicity, language skills, geographic location and distribution, qualifications, training and certification, areas of practice, and hours spent in the care of older adults.**

REFERENCES

AoA (Administration on Aging). 2010a. *National Aging Network.* http://www.aoa.gov/AoA Root/AoA_Programs/OAA/Aging_Network/Index.aspx (accessed April 14, 2011).

———. 2010b. *Unofficial compilation of the Older Americans Act of 1965 as amended in 2006* (Public Law 109-365). http://www.aoa.gov/AoA_programs/OAA/oaa_full.asp (accessed June 4, 2012).

———. 2011. *Health, Prevention, and Wellness Program.* http://www.aoa.gov/AoARoot/AoA_Programs/HCLTC/Evidence_Based/index.aspx (accessed November 13, 2011).

AoA and SAMHSA (Substance Abuse and Mental Health Services Administration). 2012. *Older Americans behavioral health issue brief: Series overview.* http://www.nasuad.org/documentation/nasuad_materials/OA_Issue_BriefSeriesOverview.pdf (accessed June 4, 2012).

Barry, C. L., H. A. Huskamp, and H. H. Goldman. 2010. A political history of federal mental health and addiction insurance parity. *Milbank Quarterly* 88(3):404-433.

Baumrucker, E. P., C. Binder, K. Colello, P. A. Davis, A. Corby-Edwards, S. A. Lister, A. K. Sarata, and S. R. Talaga. 2011. *CRS memorandum: Deadline for the HHS secretary and other federal entities in the Patient Protection and Affordable Care Act: Addendum to CRS congressional distribution memorandum dated April 5, 2011.* Washington, DC: Congressional Research Service. Bruce, M. L., A. D. Van Citters, and S. J. Bartels. 2005. Evidence-based mental health services for home and community. *Psychiatric Clinics of North America* 28(4):1039-1060.

Canadian Centre on Substance Abuse. 2010. *Competencies for Canada's substance abuse workforce: Section VI technical competencies (v.1).* Ottawa, ON.

Ciechanowski, P. S., W. J. Katon, and J. E. Russo. 2000. Depression and diabetes: Impact of depressive symptoms on adherence, function, and costs. *Archives of Internal Medicine* 160(21):3278-3285.

CMMI (Center for Medicare and Medicaid Innovation). 2011a. *Advance payment solicitation.* http://innovations.cms.gov/documents/payment-care/APACO_Solicitation_10_20_11_Compliant1.pdf (accessed January 8, 2012).

———. 2011b. *Health care innovation challenge. Cooperative agreement. Initial announcement.* http://innovations.cms.gov/documents/pdf/innovation-challenge-foa.pdf (accessed January 9, 2012).

Council of Professional Geropsychology Training Programs. 2011. *Recommended resources associated with the Pikes Peak Model competencies.* http://copgtp.org/uploads/documents/CoPGTP_Resources.pdf (accessed April 24, 2012).

Counsell, S. R., C. M. Callahan, D. O. Clark, W. Tu, A. B. Buttar, T. E. Stump, and G. D. Ricketts. 2007. Geriatric care management for low-income seniors: A randomized controlled trial. *JAMA* 298(22):2623-2633.

Fisher, W. H., J. L. Geller, and J. A. Pandiani. 2009. The changing role of the state psychiatric hospital. *Health Affairs* 28(3):676-684.

Garner, J. B. 2010. Problems of nonadherence in cardiology and proposals to improve outcomes. *American Journal of Cardiology* 105(10):1495-1501.

Gehi, A., D. Haas, S. Pipkin, and M. A. Whooley. 2005. Depression and medication adherence in outpatients with coronary heart disease: Findings from the Heart and Soul Study. *Archives of Internal Medicine* 165(21):2508-2513.

Geropsychiatric Nursing Collaborative. 2010a. *Recommended geropsychiatric competency enhancements for entry level professional nurses.* www.aannet.org/GPNCresources (accessed April 24, 2012).

———. 2010b. *Recommended geropsychiatric competency enhancements for gerontological nurse practioners.* www.aannet.org/GPNCresources (accessed April 24, 2012).

———. 2010c. *Recommended geropsychiatric competency enhancements for psychiatric mental health clinical nurse specialists.* www.aannet.org/GPNCresources (accessed April 24, 2012).

Gilmer, T. P., S. Roze, W. J. Valentine, K. Emy-Albrecht, J. A. Ray, D. Cobden, L. Nicklasson, A. Philis-Tsimikas, and A. J. Palmer. 2007. Cost-effectiveness of diabetes case management for low-income populations. *Health Services Research* 42(5):1943-1959.

Goldman, H. H., and G. N. Grob. 2006. Defining mental illness in mental health policy. *Health Affairs* 25(3):737-749.

Heflin, M., E. Bragg, H. Fernandez, C. Christmas, D. Osterweil, K. Sauvigne, G. Warshaw, H. J. Cohen, R. M. Leipzig, D. B. Reuben, and S. C. Durson. 2011. The Donald W. Reynolds Consortium for Faculty Development to Advance Geriatrics Education (FD~AGE): A model for dissemination of subspecialty educational expertise. *Academic Medicine* 87(5):1-9.

Heisler, E. J., and A. K. Sarata. 2011. *Physician supply and the Patient Protection and Affordable Care Act.* Report No. R42029. Washington, DC: Congressional Research Service.

Hogan, M. F. 2003. The President's New Freedom Commission: Recommendations to transform mental health care in America. *Psychiatric Services* 54(11):1467-1474.

Hoge, M. A., and M. McFaul, eds. 2010. *Alaskan core competencies for direct care workers in health and human services version 1.0.* Vol. 2010. Anchorage: The Alaska Mental Health Trust Authority.

Hoge, M. A., J. A. Morris, A. S. Daniels, G. W. Stuart, L. Y. Huey, N. Adams, and Annapolis Coalition on the Behavioral Health Workforce. 2007. *An action plan for behavioral health workforce development: Executive summary.* Washington, DC: Substance Abuse and Mental Health Services Administration.

HRSA (Health Resources and Services Administration). 2010a. *Geriatric academic career award funding announcement.* https://grants.hrsa.gov/webexternal/FundingOppDetails.asp?FundingCycleId=DB2BCDEB-2269-405D-B518-C907C6FF027A&ViewMode=EU&GoBack=&PrintMode=&OnlineAvailabilityFlag=False&pageNumber=4 (accessed November 13, 2011).

———. 2010b. *Geriatric education centers funding announcement.* https://grants.hrsa.gov/webExternal/FundingOppDetails.asp?FundingCycleId=F218CA5E-FBC6-46BC-BDA7-D94028370E55&ViewMode=EU&GoBack=&PrintMode=&OnlineAvailabilityFlag=True&pageNumber=2&Popup= (accessed November 13, 2011).

———. 2010c. *Geriatric training program for physicians, dentists, and behavioral and mental health professionals announcement.* https://grants.hrsa.gov/webexternal/FundingOppDetails.asp?FundingCycleId=63A7E2B1-2A30-47D9-9D5A-180E5ABA45BA&ViewMode=EU&GoBack=&PrintMode=&OnlineAvailabilityFlag=True&pageNumber=4 (accessed November 13, 2011).

———. 2012. *Funding opportunities: Comprehensive geriatric education program.* https://grants.hrsa.gov/webExternal/FundingOppDetails.asp?FundingCycleId=62B7BE7C-D0F0-483D-BF85-C675766F87A0&ViewMode=EU&GoBack=&PrintMode=&OnlineAvailabilityFlag=&pageNumber=&version=&NC=&Popup= (accessed April 3, 2012).

IOM (Institute of Medicine). 1978. *Aging and medical education.* Washington, DC: National Academy Press.

———. 2006. *Improving the quality of health care for mental and substance-use conditions.* Washington, DC: The National Academies Press.

———. 2008. *Retooling for an aging America: Building the health care workforce.* Washington, DC: The National Academies Press.

Jeste, D. V., G. S. Alexopoulos, S. J. Bartels, J. L. Cummings, J. J. Gallo, G. L. Gottlieb, M. C. Halpain, B. W. Palmer, T. L. Patterson, C. F. Reynolds, and B. D. Lebowitz. 1999. Consensus statement on the upcoming crisis in geriatric mental health—research agenda for the next 2 decades. *Archives of General Psychiatry* 56(9):848-853.

Jiang, W., J. Alexander, E. Christopher, M. Kuchibhatla, L. H. Gaulden, M. S. Cuffe, M. A. Blazing, C. Davenport, R. M. Califf, R. R. Krishnan, and C. M. O'Connor. 2001. Relationship of depression to increased risk of mortality and rehospitalization in patients with congestive heart failure. *Archives of Internal Medicine* 161(15):1849-1856.

Karel, M. J., B. G. Knight, M. Duffy, G. A. Hinrichsen, and A. M. Zeiss. 2010. Attitude, knowledge, and skill competencies for practice in professional geropsychology: Implications for training and building a geropsychology workforce. *Training and Education in Professional Psychology* 4(2):75-84.

Katon, W. J., M. Schoenbaum, M.-Y. Fan, C. M. Callahan, J. Williams, Jr., E. Hunkeler, L. Harpole, X.-H. A. Zhou, C. Langston, and J. Unützer. 2005. Cost-effectiveness of improving primary care treatment of late-life depression. *Archives of General Psychiatry* 62(12):1313-1320.

Krousel-Wood, M., T. Islam, P. Muntner, E. Holt, C. Joyce, D. E. Morisky, L. S. Webber, and E. D. Frohlich. 2010. Association of depression with antihypertensive medication adherence in older adults: Cross-sectional and longitudinal findings from CoSMO. *Annals of Behavioral Medicine* 40(3):248-257.

Leipzig, R. M., L. Granville, D. Simpson, M. B. Anderson, K. Sauvigné, and R. P. Soriano. 2009. Keeping granny safe on July 1: A consensus on minimum geriatrics competencies for graduating medical students. *Academic Medicine* 84(5):604.

Levit, K. R., C. A. Kassed, R. M. Coffey, T. L. Mark, E. M. Stranges, J. A. Buck, and R. Vandivort-Warren. 2008. Future funding for mental health and substance abuse: Increasing burdens for the public sector. *Health Affairs* 27(6):W513-W522.

Lin, E. H. B., W. Katon, M. Von Korff, C. Rutter, G. E. Simon, M. Oliver, P. Ciechanowski, E. J. Ludman, T. Bush, and B. Young. 2004. Relationship of depression and diabetes self-care, medication adherence, and preventive care. *Diabetes Care* 27(9):2154-2160.

MedPAC (Medicare Payment Advisory Commission). 2010. Chapter 6. Inpatient psychiatric care in medicare: Trends and issues. In *Aligning incentives in Medicare*. Washington, DC: MedPAC.

O'Shaunessy, C. V. 2011. The aging services network: Serving a vulnerable and growing elderly population in tough economic times. Washington, DC: National Health Policy Forum.

Partnership for Health in Aging. 2008. *Multidisciplinary competencies in the care of older adults at the completion of the entry-level health professional degree.* http://www.americangeriatrics.org/about_us/partnership_for_health_in_aging/multidisciplinary_competencies/multidisciplinary_competencies/multidisciplinary_competencies778926 (accessed January 1, 2012).

Redhead, C. S., K. Colello, E. J. Heisler, S. A. Lister, and A. K. Sarata. 2011a. *Discretionary funding in the Patient Protection and Affordable Care Act (ACA).* http://www.cq.com/pdf/crsreports-4006435 (accessed January 8, 2012).

———. 2011b. *Discretionary funding in the Patient Protection and Affordable Care Act (ACA).* Report No. R41390. http://www.cq.com/pdf/crsreports-3998017 (accessed December 13, 2011).

Sarata, A. K. 2010. *Mental health parity and the Patient Protection and Affordable Care Act of 2010.* CRS Report for Congress. Washington, DC: Congressional Research Service.

Shirk, C. 2008. *Medicaid and mental health services.* Washington, DC: National Health Policy Forum.

Slade, E. P., D. S. Salkever, R. Rosenheck, J. Swanson, M. Swartz, D. Shern, G. Gallucci, C. Harding, L. Palmer, and P. Russo. 2005. Cost-sharing requirements and access to mental health care among Medicare enrollees with schizophrenia. *Psychiatric Services* 56(8):960-966.

University of Minnesota Research and Training Center on Community Living. 2011. *Road map of core competencies for the direct service workforce, phase I: Direct service worker competency inventory* (draft). Minneapolis, MN: Research and Training Center on Community Living.

Unützer, J., D. L. Patrick, G. Simon, D. Grembowski, E. Walker, C. Rutter, and W. Katon. 1997. Depressive symptoms and the cost of health services in HMO patients aged 65 years and older. A 4-year prospective study. *JAMA* 277(20):1618-1623.

Unützer, J., M. L. Bruce, and N. A. D. Workgroup. 2002. The elderly. *Mental Health Services Research* 4(4):245-247.

Unützer, J., M. Schoenbaum, B. G. Druss, and W. J. Katon. 2006. Transforming mental health care at the interface with general medicine: Report for the President's Commission. *Psychiatric Services* 57(1):37-47.

Williams, J. W., Jr., W. Katon, E. H. B. Lin, P. H. Nöel, J. Worchel, J. Cornell, L. Harpole, B. A. Fultz, E. Hunkeler, V. S. Mika, and J. Unützer. 2004. The effectiveness of depression care management on diabetes-related outcomes in older patients. *Annals of Internal Medicine* 140(12):1015-1024.

Appendix A

Abbreviations and Acronyms

AA	Alcoholics Anonymous
AAGP	American Association of Geriatric Psychiatrists
AAMC	Association of American Medical Colleges
ACA	Patient Protection and Affordable Care Act
ACO	accountable care organization
ACT	Assertive Community Treatment Model
ADAMS	Aging, Demographics, and Memory Study
ADLs	activities of daily living
AECOM	Albert Einstein College of Medicine
AHRQ	Agency for Healthcare Research and Quality
AIMS	Advancing Integrated Mental Health Services Center at the University of Washington
AoA	Administration on Aging
APA	American Psychological Association
APPIC	Association of Psychology Postdoctoral and Internship Centers
APRN	advanced practice registered nurse
ASPE	Office of the Assistant Secretary for Planning and Evaluation
ASWB	Association of Social Work Boards
ATOD	Certified Clinical Alcohol, Tobacco, and Other Drug Social Worker

BHP	Bureau of Health Professions, HRSA
BLS	Bureau of Labor Statistics
BRFSS	Behavioral Risk Factors Surveillance System
BRITE	Brief Intervention and Treatment for Elders
CACREP	Council for Accreditation of Counseling and Related Educational Programs
CalSWEC	California Social Work Education Center
CAPT	California Association of Psychiatric Technicians
CCM	Chronic Care Model
CDC	Centers for Disease Control and Prevention
CGEP	Comprehensive Geriatric Education Program
CHW	community health worker
CMMI	Center for Medicare and Medicaid Innovation, CMS
CMS	Centers for Medicare & Medicaid Services
CNA	certified nursing assistant
CNL	clinical nurse leader
CPES	Collaborative Psychiatric Epidemiological Studies
CPS	certified peer specialist
CRCC	Council on Rehabilitation Counselor Certification
CSWE	Council on Social Work Education
DAWN	Drug Abuse Warning Network
DCA	Direct Care Alliance
DCM	depression care manager
DCW	direct care worker
DOL	U.S. Department of Labor
DSM	*Diagnostic and Statistical Manual of Mental Disorders*
ECA	Epidemiologic Catchment Area survey
EMASS	Elderly Multicultural Access and Support Services
GACA	Geriatric Academic Career Award
GDS	Geriatric Depression Scale
GEC	Geriatric Education Center
GIG	Gero Innovations Grant
GMHF	Geriatric Mental Health Foundation
GPE	Graduate Psychology Education
GPN	geropsychiatric nursing
GPNC	Geropsychiatric Nursing Collaborative
GSA	Gerontological Society of America
GSWI	Geriatric Social Work Initiative
GTPD	Geriatric Training for Physicians, Dentists and Behavioral and Mental Health Professionals

HCC	HealthCare for Communities household study
Healthy IDEAS	Identifying Depression, Empowering Activities for Seniors
HHS	U.S. Department of Health and Human Services
HIGN	Hartford Institute for Geriatric Nursing
HOPES	Helping Older People Experience Success
HRS	Health and Retirement Study surveys
HRSA	Health Resources and Services Administration
HSRC	Health Services Research Center of the University of California, San Diego
IMPACT	Improving Mood-Promoting Access to Collaborative Treatment
IPA	Independent Provider Association
IPEC	Interprofessional Education Collaborative
LGBT	lesbian, gay, bisexual, transgender
LPC	licensed professional counselor
LPN	licensed practical nurse
LTC	long-term care
LVN	licensed vocational nurse (see LPN)
MAC	Master's Advanced Curriculum
MDS	Minimum Data Set
MEPS	Medical Expenditure Panel Survey
MFT	marriage and family therapist
MH/SU	mental health and substance use
MHSAP	CSWE Mental Health/Substance Abuse Fellowship Program
MIDUS	Midlife Development in the United States
MSSP	Medicare Shared Savings Program
MSW	master's in social work
NAHC	National Association for Home Care and Hospice
NAMI	National Alliance on Mental Illness
NAMI NH	NAMI New Hampshire
NASMHPD	National Association of State Mental Health Program Directors
NASW	National Association of Social Workers
NCS-R	National Comorbidity Survey-Replication
NESARC	National Epidemiological Survey of Alcohol and Related Conditions

NESARC 1	National Epidemiological Survey of Alcohol and Related Conditions Wave 1
NESARC 2	National Epidemiological Survey of Alcohol and Related Conditions Wave 2
NHIS	National Health Interview Survey
NIA	National Institute on Aging
NIAA	National Institute on Alcohol Abuse and Alcoholism
NIDA	National Institute on Drug Abuse
NIH	National Institutes of Health
NIMH	National Institute of Mental Health
NLAAS	National Latino and Asian American Study
NSAL	National Study of American Life
NSDUH	National Survey of Drug Use and Health
OASIS	Outcome and Assessment Information Set
OT	occupational therapist
PA	physician assistant
PASRR	Pre-Admission Screening and Resident Review
PATCH	Psychogeriatric Assessment and Treatment in City Housing
PCP	primary care provider
PEARLS	Program to Encourage Active and Rewarding Lives for Seniors
PHA	Partnership for Health in Aging
PharmD	doctor of pharmacy
POGOe	Portal of Online Geriatric Education
PREVENT	Providing Resources Early to Vulnerable Elders Needing Treatment
PRISM-E	Primary Care Research in Substance Abuse and Mental Health for the Elderly
Project TrEAT	Trial for Early Alcohol Treatment
PTSD	posttraumatic stress disorder
QIO	quality-improvement organization
QPR	Question, Persuade, and Refer
RCT	randomized controlled trial
RN	registered nurse
SAMHSA	Substance Abuse and Mental Health Services Administration

SBIRT	Screening, Brief Intervention, and Referral for Treatment
SGEC	Stanford Geriatric Education Center
SIS	Seniors in Sobriety
SMI	serious mental illness
SPRY	Seniors Preparing for Rainbow Years
TAC	technical assistance center
TCE	Older Adults Targeted Capacity Expansion Grants
TIP	SAMHSA Treatment Improvement Protocol
TRIAD	Training in the Assessment of Depression
UPAC	Union of Pan Asian Communities
VA	Department of Veterans Affairs
VHA	Veterans Health Administration
WMH-CIDI	World Mental Health Composite International Diagnostic Interview
WPA	World Psychiatric Association
WRAP	Wellness Recovery Action Planning

Appendix B

Public Workshop Agenda

SELECTED PERSPECTIVES ON THE MENTAL HEALTH AND SUBSTANCE USE WORKFORCE FOR THE GERIATRIC POPULATION: FILLING IN THE GAPS

JUNE 1, 2011

Keck Center
500 Fifth Street, NW
Room 100
Washington, DC

9:00 Welcome and Introductory Remarks
Dan Blazer, *Chair, Institute of Medicine Committee*

9:05 PANEL #1—CONSUMERS, FAMILIES, AND CAREGIVERS

Objective: *To learn about successful models for consumer, family, and caregiver participation in mental health and substance use care and the related implications for workforce training.*

Moderator: Octavio Martinez, MD, MPH, MBA, *Executive Director, Hogg Foundation for Mental Health*

Panelists:
- Mary Ellen Copeland, *Wellness Recovery Action Planning (WRAP)*
- Marian Scheinholtz, *Public Health Advisor, Community Support Programs Branch, Substance Abuse and Mental Health Services Administration*
- Bernadette Seifert, *Coordinator of Older Adult Services, National Alliance on Mental Illness, New Hampshire*
- Moe Armstrong, *Founder, Vet-to-Vet*

Q & A/Open Discussion

10:25 PANEL #2—CROSS-COMPETENCIES IN AGING, MENTAL HEALTH, AND SUBSTANCE USE IN SELECTED SETTINGS

Objective: *To learn about selected approaches to ensuring cross-competencies among professionals and nonprofessionals who work with older adults with mental health and substance use conditions in a variety of settings.*

Moderator: Michael Hoge, *Professor of Psychiatry (in Psychology), Yale University School of Medicine and Director of Yale Behavioral Health*

Panelists:
- Patrick J. Raue, *Associate Professor of Psychology in Psychiatry, Weill Cornell Medical College—Home Care Nurses*
- Kathy Kuhn, *Director of Workforce Development, Institute for Geriatric Social Work, Boston University—Social Workers, Case Managers, and Outreach Workers*
- Carol Colleran, *Retired Director of Public Policy and National Affairs, Hanley Center—Addiction Counselors*

Q & A/Open Discussion

11:45 LUNCH

12:30 PANEL #3—WORKFORCE IMPLICATIONS OF SELECTED MODELS OF CARE

Objective: *To learn about the workforce implications of various evidence-based models of mental health and substance use care for older people.*

Moderator: Mark Snowden, *Associate Professor, University of Washington School of Medicine, Department of Psychiatry and Behavioral Sciences*

Panelists:
- Michael Schoenbaum, *Senior Advisor for Mental Health Services, Epidemiology, and Economics, Office of the Director, National Institute of Mental Health—Providing Depression Care in a Primary Care Setting—IMPACT*
- Julie Jensen, *Program Manager, Older Adult Services, HEROS Program, Good Samaritan Behavioral Health, Puyallup, WA—Gatekeeper Model*
- Stephen Ferrante, *Director, Aging Academy, Florida Atlantic University—Screening, Brief Intervention, and Referral to Treatment (SBIRT) Model for Older Adults with Substance Use Problems*
- Enid Hunkeler, *Senior Scientist and Codirector, Inter-Divisional Depression Initiative, Kaiser Permanente Northern California Division of Research*

Q & A/Open Discussion

2:00 PANEL #4—POLICY OPPORTUNITIES FOR GROWING AND IMPROVING THE GERIATRIC MENTAL HEALTH WORKFORCE

Objectives: *(1) To learn about current policy directions that may affect the geriatric mental health and substance use care workforce, and (2) to hear the recommendations of key thought leaders on how to grow and strengthen the geriatric mental health and substance use care workforce.*

Moderator: Steve Bartels, *Professor of Psychiatry and Community & Family Medicine, Dartmouth Medical School and Director, Dartmouth-New England Geriatric Education Center*

Panelists:
- Tim Engelhardt, *Director, Demonstration Program, CMS Federal Coordinated Health Care Office (Duals Office)*
- Dan Timmel, *Medicaid Long Term Care Policy Analyst, CMS Disabled and Elderly Health Programs Group*

- Robyn Golden, *Director of Older Adult Programs, Rush University Medical Center*
- Harold Pincus, *Codirector, Irving Institute of Clinical and Translational Research, and Professor, Department of Psychiatry, Columbia University*
- Jurgen Unützer, *Professor, University of Washington Department of Psychiatry*

Q & A/Open Discussion

3:30 ADJOURN

Appendix C

Required Knowledge, Skills, and Training for Mental Health, Substance Use, and Geriatric Care Providers

CONTENTS

GENERAL POPULATION		
Mental Health (MH)	**Substance Use (SU)**	**Co-occurring MH and SU**
I. PHYSICIANS		
Allopathic Physicians (MD)[a]		
Early identification and intervention of mental disorders (e.g., suicide potential, depression, alcohol/substance abuse, family involvement in schizophrenia); biologic markers of mental disorders and mental retardation syndromes; intended/unintended effects of therapeutic interventions for mental disorders, including effects of drugs on neurotransmitters; diagnosis of mental disorders usually first diagnosed in infancy, childhood, or adolescence, schizophrenia and other psychotic disorders, mood disorders, anxiety disorders, somatoform disorders, other disorders/conditions; principles of mental disorder management (Pharmacotherapy only, Management decision, Treatment only).	Diagnosis of substance-related disorders (e.g., alcohol and other substances).	None
Family Medicine (MD)[b]		
Responsibility for the total health care of the individual and family, taking into account behavioral dimensions; Family-oriented comprehensive care experience, including individual behavioral counseling and family counseling; knowledge and skills in human behavior and mental health should be acquired through a program in which behavioral science and psychiatry are integrated with all disciplines throughout the total educational experience; skills in the diagnosis and management of psychiatric disorders in children and adults, emotional aspects of nonpsychiatric disorders, psychopharmacology, the physician-patient relationship, patient interviewing skills, and counseling skills.	Must have instruction and development of skills in the diagnosis and management of alcoholism and other substance abuse.	None

GERIATRIC POPULATION			
General Care	Mental Health (MH)	Substance Use (SU)	Co-occurring MH and SU
General principles of senescence (normal physical and mental changes associated with aging); medical ethics and jurisprudence regarding death and dying (e.g., diagnosing death, organ donation, euthanasia, physician-assisted suicide) and palliative care (e.g., hospice, pain management, family counseling, psychosocial and spiritual issues, fear, and loneliness).	None	None	None
Resident panels must include continuity experience for patients requiring home care and care in long-term care facilities; nursing home experience must consist of at least two patients as a continuity experience over a minimum of 24 consecutive months, in addition to rotation; must perform at least two home visits with at least one being for an older adult continuity patient; educational experiences must be in both common and complex clinical problems of older patients; training must include the appropriate preventive modalities, functional assessment, and the physiologic and psychologic aspects of senescence; supervised clinical experiences dealing with common acute and chronic diseases of aging; learn about, and practically apply, a multidisciplinary approach to the care of older patients in the hospital, the family medicine center (FMC),	Training must include the psychologic aspects of senescence.	None	None

GENERAL POPULATION		
Mental Health (MH)	Substance Use (SU)	Co-occurring MH and SU
Geriatric Family Medicine (MD)[c]		
N/A	N/A	N/A

GERIATRIC POPULATION			
General Care	Mental Health (MH)	Substance Use (SU)	Co-occurring MH and SU
the long-term care facility, and the home; competence in preventive health care, promotion of independent living, and maximizing function and quality of life; competency in assessing and meeting the health care needs of declining elders, episodic, illness-related care, delivery of health care in the home, FMC, hospital, and long-term facility, and end-of-life care.			
Primary specialty.	Ambulatory care experience must be designed to provide care, in a geriatric clinic or family medicine center, to elderly patients who may require the services of multiple medical disciplines, including psychiatry and social work; experience in relevant ambulatory specialty and subspecialty clinics (e.g., geriatric psychiatry and neurology) strongly recommended; identifiable structured didactic and clinical experiences in geriatric psychiatry must be included in the program of each fellow; formal instruction in physical and mental examination, topics of special interest to geriatric medicine, including, but not limited to, cognitive impairment, depression and related disorders, psychosocial aspects of aging, including interpersonal and family relationships, living situations, adjustment disorders, depression, bereavement, and anxiety, and behavioral sciences such as psychology/social work.	None	None

GENERAL POPULATION		
Mental Health (MH)	Substance Use (SU)	Co-occurring MH and SU
Internal Medicine (MD)[d]		
Clinical experience must include opportunities for experience in psychiatry.	None	None
Geriatric Internal Medicine (MD)[e]		
N/A	N/A	N/A

GERIATRIC POPULATION			
General Care	Mental Health (MH)	Substance Use (SU)	Co-occurring MH and SU
Institution must have patients of a broad age range, including geriatric patients; clinical experience must include an assignment in geriatric medicine; clinical experience in outpatient chronic disease management, preventive health, patient counseling, and common acute ambulatory problems with a diversity of ages.	None	None	None
Primary specialty.	Formal instruction in physical and mental examination, topics of special interest to geriatric medicine, including, but not limited to, cognitive impairment, depression and related disorders, psychosocial aspects of aging, including interpersonal and family relationships, living situations, adjustment disorders, depression, bereavement, and anxiety, and behavioral sciences such as psychology/social work; ambulatory care experience must be designed to provide care in a geriatric clinic or internal medicine center to elderly patients who may require the services of multiple medical disciplines, including psychiatry and social work; experience in relevant ambulatory specialty and subspecialty clinics (e.g., geriatric psychiatry and neurology) strongly recommended; Fellows must develop clinical competence in assessment of cognitive status and affective states; clinical experience in the	None	None

GENERAL POPULATION		
Mental Health (MH)	**Substance Use (SU)**	**Co-occurring MH and SU**
Psychiatry (MD)[f]		
Primary specialty.	One month full-time equivalent organized experience focused on the evaluation and clinical management of patients with substance abuse/ dependence problems, including dual diagnosis.	Evaluation and clinical management of patients with substance abuse/ dependence problems, including dual diagnosis.
Geriatric Psychiatry (MD)[g]		
N/A	N/A	N/A
Addiction Psychiatry (MD)[h]		
Primary specialty.	Primary specialty.	Primary specialty.
Osteopathic Physicians (DO)[i,j,k]		
Take a comprehensive history (including symptoms, psychological factors, and social factors); perform a standard history and physical examination, including mini-mental and basic neurologic examinations; understand the concepts and principles of social and behavioral sciences and apply these to the understanding, management, and treatment of patient presentations.	Population health concepts and patients with presentations related to health promotion, chronic disease management, and human development, including detection and monitoring of	None

GERIATRIC POPULATION			
General Care	Mental Health (MH)	Substance Use (SU)	Co-occurring MH and SU
	management of elderly patients must include understanding of the behavioral aspects of illness; identifiable structured didactic and clinical experiences in geriatric psychiatry must be included in the program of each Fellow.		
N/A	One month full-time equivalent organized experience focused on the specific competencies in areas that are unique to the care of the elderly.	None	None
N/A	Primary specialty.	Epidemiology, diagnosis, and treatment of all major psychiatric disorders seen in the elderly, seen alone and in combination, including substance-related disorders.	Epidemiology, diagnosis, and treatment of all major psychiatric disorders seen in the elderly, seen alone and in combination, including substance-related disorders.
N/A	Clinical experience must include the opportunity to evaluate and follow a variety of patients of both sexes, including geriatric age groups spanning a broad range of diagnoses.	Clinical experience must include the opportunity to evaluate and follow a variety of patients of both sexes, including geriatric age groups spanning a broad range of diagnoses.	Clinical experience must include the opportunity to evaluate and follow a variety of patients of both sexes, including geriatric age groups spanning a broad range of diagnoses.
Determine and monitor the nature of a patient's concern or problem using a patient-centered approach that is appropriate to the age of the patient; provide effective patient care in the outpatient, inpatient, and home	COMLEX-USA covers patients with presentations related to trauma, including elder abuse.	None	None

GENERAL POPULATION		
Mental Health (MH)	**Substance Use (SU)**	**Co-occurring MH and SU**
COMLEX-USA covers patients with presentations related to cognition and behavior, including anxiety, behavioral disturbances, confusion/disorientation, dementia, depression, eating disorders, learning difficulties, life adjustment, suicidal ideation; psychosocial management.	substance abuse. COMLEX-USA covers patients with presentations related to substance abuse, including alcohol abuse, controlled substance abuse, non-controlled drug abuse, and tobacco abuse.	
Family Medicine (DO)[l]		
Must maintain current knowledge of behavioral medicine that reflects the majority of patient care issues that present to osteopathic family practice settings; training in behavioral science, which at a minimum shall include psychiatric and psychological diagnoses common to family practice, didactic instruction and clinical experiences, interviewing skills, counseling skills, psychopharmacology, and physician well-being; 50 hours or 2 weeks of documented training in community medicine, which may include time spent in occupational health, mental health agencies, community-based screening programs, public health agencies, community health centers, free clinics, or homeless shelters.	Program must include training in behavioral science, which at a minimum shall include the treatment of substance abuse; 50 hours or 2 weeks of documented training in community medicine, which may include time spent in drug and alcohol treatment centers.	
Geriatrics in Family Medicine (DO)[m]		
N/A	N/A	N/A

GERIATRIC POPULATION			
General Care	**Mental Health (MH)**	**Substance Use (SU)**	**Co-occurring MH and SU**
care settings, and across the lifecycle; recognize patient presentation of symptoms and disorders of human development; explore a patient's beliefs, concerns, expectations, and literacy about health and illness, and provide care appropriate for contextual factors such as a patient's age. COMLEX-USA covers population health concepts and patients with presentations related to health promotion, chronic disease management, and human development, including aging physiology; end-of-life management.			
At least 100 hours or 1 month of training in the care of the geriatric patient, in addition to training that occurs in the continuity of care site or general internal medicine rotations, which at a minimum shall include physiological changes of aging, pharmacokinetics in the elderly, functional assessment of the elderly, extended care facility management, hospice, home care; competencies in providing acute care, chronic care, and preventive care across the full spectrum of ages and genders; awareness and proper attention to issues of age; patient population of the continuity of care site must include a variety of patients in terms of age.			
Primary specialty.	Maintain current knowledge of behavioral medicine that reflects	None	None

GENERAL POPULATION		
Mental Health (MH)	Substance Use (SU)	Co-occurring MH and SU
Addiction in Family Medicine[n]		
Scope of training must include additional training in all branches of psychiatry that are of special concern in the addicted patient.	Primary specialty.	None
Internal Medicine (DO)[o]		
None	None	None
Geriatric Internal Medicine (DO)[p]		
N/A	N/A	N/A
General Psychiatry (DO)[q]		
Primary specialty.	Must be experienced with patients with substance abuse	None

GERIATRIC POPULATION			
General Care	Mental Health (MH)	Substance Use (SU)	Co-occurring MH and SU
	the majority of patient care issues present in geriatric settings; programs must include didactic presentations on psychology of aging, and mental health concerns including loss of a spouse, death and dying, depression, dependency, caregiver burden, and sexuality in the elderly; programs must include clinical training in psychiatric and psychological needs and evaluation of the geriatrics patient.		
N/A	None	None	None
None	None	None	None
Primary specialty.	Base institution or an affiliate must have rehabilitation and psychiatry services; biopsychosocial components of aging, including normal physiological age changes, psychological models of late-life development and sexuality; assessment of older patients' health status, including cognitive/ neuropsychologic status; preventive geriatric medicine, including the relationship between physical health/mental health status; common geriatric syndromes including dementia, delirium, depression, and elder abuse.	Mental health disorders, including substance disorders and the appropriate treatment options.	None
N/A	Must be exposed to adequate numbers of patients of various ages;	None	None

GENERAL POPULATION		
Mental Health (MH)	Substance Use (SU)	Co-occurring MH and SU
	problems, including experience with detoxification and management as well as an understanding of community resources.	
Geriatric Psychiatry (DO)[r]		
N/A	N/A	N/A
Addiction Psychiatry (DO)[s]		
Primary specialty.	Primary specialty.	Must be fully trained in the techniques required in the treatment of the larger group of patients with the dual diagnosis of addictive disorders abuse.

GERIATRIC POPULATION			
General Care	Mental Health (MH)	Substance Use (SU)	Co-occurring MH and SU
	must be experienced with geriatric patients with various psychiatric disorders in which residents have primary responsibility for diagnosis and treatment; didactic curriculum must include major theories of development through adulthood and old age.		
N/A	Primary specialty.	Diagnosis, treatment, and epidemiology of all major psychiatric disorders seen in the elderly, including substance abuse disorders.	Diagnosis, treatment, and epidemiology of all major psychiatric disorders seen in the elderly, typically including but not limited to affective disorders, dementia, delirium, late-onset psychoses, medical presentations of psychiatric disorders, iatrogenesis, adjustment disorders, anxiety disorders, sleep disorders, sexual disorders, substance abuse disorders, personality disorders, and continuation of psychiatric illnesses that began earlier in life. These disorders can present either singularly or in combination.
N/A	Clinical experience must include the opportunity to evaluate and follow a variety of patients of both sexes, including geriatric age groups spanning a broad range of diagnoses; number	None	None

GENERAL POPULATION		
Mental Health (MH)	Substance Use (SU)	Co-occurring MH and SU
		and other psychiatric disorders; clinical experience must include evaluation, consultation, and treatment of psychiatric inpatients and outpatients with chemical dependencies and comorbid psychopathology, to include a broad range of psychiatric diagnoses; curriculum should emphasize functional assessment, signs and symptoms of neuropsychiatric impairment associated with substance abuse; knowledge of the signs and symptoms of the social and psychological problems as well as the medical and psychiatric disorders that often accompany the chronic use and abuse of the major categories of drugs; experience in the use of psychoactive medications in the treatment of psychiatric disorders often accompanying the major categories of substance.
II. PHYSICIAN ASSISTANTS[f]		
Instruction in the social and behavioral sciences as well as normal and abnormal development across the life span, including psychiatric/behavioral conditions; supervised clinical practice experiences must provide sufficient patient exposure to care for behavioral and mental health conditions; supervised clinical practice experiences should occur with preceptors practicing in behavioral and mental health care.	Instruction in the social and behavioral sciences as well as normal and abnormal development across the life span, including detection and treatment of substance abuse.	None

GERIATRIC POPULATION			
General Care	Mental Health (MH)	Substance Use (SU)	Co-occurring MH and SU
	and variety of new and follow-up patients spanning the lifecycle from adolescence to old age must be sufficient to ensure an adequate outpatient and inpatient experience.		
Instruction in the provision of clinical medical care across the life span, including preventive, emergent, acute, chronic, rehabilitative, palliative, and end-of-life care relevant to adult and elderly populations; supervised clinical practice experiences must provide sufficient patient exposure to medical care across the life span, including the elderly.	Instruction in the social and behavioral sciences as well as normal and abnormal development across the life span, including psychiatric/behavioral conditions.	Instruction in the social and behavioral sciences as well as normal and abnormal development across the life span, including detection and treatment of substance abuse.	None

GENERAL POPULATION		
Mental Health (MH)	**Substance Use (SU)**	**Co-occurring MH and SU**
III. NURSES		
Licensed Practical Nurses/Licensed Vocational Nurses[u]		
Identify client risk factors for abusing or neglecting others; identify signs and symptoms of physical, psychological, or financial abuse in client; recognize risk factors for domestic, child and/or elder abuse/neglect and sexual abuse; monitor client appearance, mood, and psychomotor behavior and observe for changes; assist client with achieving self-control of behavior; assist client in using behavioral strategies to decrease anxiety; assist in or reinforce education of caregivers/family on ways to manage client with behavioral disorders; participate in behavior management program by recognizing environmental stressors and/or providing therapeutic environment; participate in reminiscence therapy, validation therapy, or reality orientation; participate in client group session; reinforce client participation in therapy; use behavioral management techniques when caring for a client; evaluate client response to behavioral management interventions; collect data regarding client psychosocial functioning; identify client use of effective and ineffective coping mechanisms; use therapeutic techniques to assist client with coping ability; identify client in crisis; identify client risk for self-injury and/or violence; use crisis intervention techniques to assist client in coping; provide opportunities for client to understand why the crisis occurred; guide client to resources for recovery from crisis; reinforce client teaching on suicide/violence prevention; report changes in client behavior (indicating a developing crisis) to supervisor; recognize cultural issues that may impact client understanding/acceptance of psychiatric diagnosis; identify client reaction to loss; provide client with resources to adjust to loss/bereavement (e.g., individual counseling, support groups); identify expected behaviors of client with independent or dependent personality; identify client symptoms of acute or chronic mental illness (e.g., schizophrenia, depression, bipolar disorder); recognize change in client mental status; recognize client symptoms of relapse; explore why client is refusing or not following treatment plan; identify client emotional problems related to religious/spiritual beliefs; use therapeutic communication techniques with client.	Identify signs and symptoms of substance abuse/chemical dependency, withdrawal or toxicity; plan and provide care to client experiencing substance-related withdrawal or toxicity (e.g., nicotine, opioid, sedative); reinforce provided information on substance abuse diagnosis and treatment plan to client; encourage client participation in support groups (e.g., Alcoholics Anonymous, Narcotics Anonymous); monitor client response to treatment plan and contribute to revision of plan as needed.	None

GERIATRIC POPULATION			
General Care	Mental Health (MH)	Substance Use (SU)	Co-occurring MH and SU
Identify client knowledge on aging process and assist in reinforcing teaching on expected changes related to aging; provide care that meets the special needs of adults ages 65 to 85; provide care that meets the special needs of adults greater than age 85; assist client with expected life transition (e.g., retirement); modify approaches to care in accordance with client development stage; identify client end-of-life needs; identify client ability to cope with end-of-life interventions; provide care or support for client/family at end of life; assist client in resolution of end-of-life issues.	Recognize risk factors for elder abuse/neglect.	None	None

GENERAL POPULATION		
Mental Health (MH)	Substance Use (SU)	Co-occurring MH and SU
Registered Nurse (Diploma, Associate's, and Baccalaureate)[v]		
Recognize client who is socially or environmentally isolated; assess client for potential or actual abuse/neglect and intervene when appropriate; identify risk factors for domestic, child, elder abuse/neglect and sexual abuse; plan interventions for victims/suspected victims of abuse; counsel victims/suspected victims of abuse and their families on coping strategies; assess client appearance, mood, and psychomotor behavior and identify/respond to inappropriate/abnormal behavior; assist client with achieving and maintaining self-control of behavior; assist client to develop and use strategies to decrease anxiety; orient client to reality; participate in group sessions; incorporate behavioral management techniques when caring for a client; evaluate client response to treatment plan; assess client reaction to diagnosis of acute or chronic mental illness; provide information to client on stress management techniques; assess the potential for violence and initiate/maintain safety precautions; identify client in crisis; use crisis intervention techniques to assist client in coping; apply knowledge of client psychopathology to crisis intervention; guide client to resources for recovery from crisis; recognize cultural issues that may impact client understanding/acceptance of psychiatric diagnosis; encourage client participation in group/family therapy; provide client with resources to adjust to loss/bereavement (e.g., individual counseling, support groups); evaluate client coping and fears related to grief and loss; recognize signs and symptoms of acute and chronic mental illness (e.g., schizophrenia, depression, bipolar disorder); explore why client is refusing/not following treatment plan; assess client for alterations in mood, judgment, cognition, and reasoning; apply knowledge of client psychopathology to mental health concepts applied in individual/group/family therapy; provide care and education for acute and chronic behavioral health issues (e.g., anxiety, depression, dementia, eating disorders); evaluate client ability to adhere to treatment plan; identify the emotional problems of client or client needs that are related to religious/spiritual beliefs; recognize nonverbal cues to physical and/or psychological stressors; use therapeutic communication techniques to provide support to client; provide a therapeutic environment for clients with emotional/behavioral issues.	Assess client reactions to the diagnosis/treatment of substance-related disorder; assess client for drug-/alcohol-related dependencies, withdrawal, or toxicities and intervene when appropriate; plan and provide care to client experiencing substance-related withdrawal or toxicity (e.g., nicotine, opioid, sedative); provide information on substance abuse diagnosis and treatment plan to client; encourage client to participate in support groups (e.g., Alcoholics Anonymous, Narcotics Anonymous); evaluate client response to treatment plan and revise as needed.	None

GERIATRIC POPULATION			
General Care	Mental Health (MH)	Substance Use (SU)	Co-occurring MH and SU
Assess client reactions to expected age-related changes; provide care and education that meets the special needs of adults ages 65 to 85; provide care and education that meets the special needs of adults greater than age 85; identify expected physical, cognitive, and psychosocial stages of development; identify expected body image changes associated with client developmental age (e.g., aging); compare client development to expected age/developmental stage and report any deviations; assist client in coping with life transition (e.g., retirement); modify approaches to care in accordance with client developmental stage (use age-appropriate explanations of procedures and treatments); provide education to client/staff members about expected age-related changes and age-specific growth and development; assess client ability to cope with end-of-life interventions; identify end-of-life needs of client; recognize need for and provide psychosocial support to family/caregiver; assist client in resolution of end-of-life issues; provide end-of-life care and education to clients (e.g., hospice).	Identify risk factors for elder abuse/neglect; evaluate client abnormal response to the aging process (e.g., depression).	None	None

GENERAL POPULATION		
Mental Health (MH)	Substance Use (SU)	Co-occurring MH and SU
Gerontological Nurses[w]		
N/A	N/A	N/A
Psychiatric and Mental Health Nurses[x]		
Primary specialty.	None	None
Advanced Practice Registered Nurses (Master's[y] **and Doctoral**[z]**)**		
Assumes mastery of baccalaureate essentials; advanced health/physical assessment, including psychological assessment; knowledge and skills to identify signs and symptoms of common emotional illnesses.	None	None
Acute Care Nurse Practitioners[aa]		
Performs evaluations for substance use, violence, neglect, and abuse; assesses the impact of an acute, critical, and/or chronic illness or injury on the individual's	Diagnoses common substance use or addictive disorder/ disease, such as	Diagnoses common mental health and substance use or addictive disorder/

GERIATRIC POPULATION			
General Care	Mental Health (MH)	Substance Use (SU)	Co-occurring MH and SU
Primary specialty.	Evidence-based tools and techniques for history taking used with older adults (e.g., psychological); evidence-based tools and techniques for physical exams and psychosocial assessments used with older adults in many settings (e.g., mental status exam); pathophysiology and diagnostic tests (e.g., geriatric depression scale); identifying risk factors (e.g., abuse and neglect, suicide behavior, self-harm); norms and variances (e.g., psychosocial assessment, psychological); coordinating with others to implement the plan of care (e.g., occupational therapy, social work, spiritual care, family).	Identifying risk factors (e.g., addiction).	None
N/A	Normal and abnormal mental changes across the life span; using age-appropriate, system-specific, evidence-based assessment instruments, tools, and techniques.	None	None
Assumes mastery of baccalaureate essentials; knowledge and skills to compare and contrast physiologic changes over the life span and analyze the relationship between normal physiology and pathological phenomena produced by altered states across the life span.	Assumes mastery of baccalaureate essentials.	None	None
Distinguishes between normal and abnormal developmental and age-related physiologic and	None	None	None

GENERAL POPULATION		
Mental Health (MH)	**Substance Use (SU)**	**Co-occurring MH and SU**
health status (physical and mental); provides for the promotion of health and protection from disease by assessing for risks associated with care of complex acute, critical, and chronically ill patients, such as psychological risk, including, but not limited to, impaired sleep and communication, and crisis related to threat to life, self-image, finances, medication side effects, home and educational environment, and altered family dynamics; diagnoses common mental health disorder/disease, such as anxiety and depression, in the presence of complex acute, critical, and chronic illness.	alcohol and drug use, in the presence of complex acute, critical, and chronic illness; demonstrates effective communication skills in addressing sensitive topics with patients and families such as substance use.	disease, such as anxiety, depression, and alcohol and drug use, in the presence of complex acute, critical, and chronic illness.
Adult Psychiatric-Mental Health Nurse Practitioners[bb]		
Primary specialty.	Because substance-related disorders are one of the DSM-IV-TR Axis I diagnoses, they have been included as a psychiatric disorder in these standards.	None
Adult-Gerontology Primary Care Nurse Practitioners[cc]		
N/A	N/A	N/A
Adult-Gerontology Clinical Nurse Specialists[dd]		
N/A	N/A	N/A

GERIATRIC POPULATION			
General Care	Mental Health (MH)	Substance Use (SU)	Co-occurring MH and SU
behavioral changes in complex acute, critical, and chronic illness; implements palliative and end-of-life care in collaboration with the family, patient (when possible), and other members of the multidisciplinary health care team; provides anticipatory guidance that is age and developmentally appropriate within the context of complex acute, critical, chronic illness.			
N/A	Orders age-appropriate tests and other procedures that provide data that contribute to the treatment plan; detects and minimizes adverse drug reactions with knowledge of pharmacokinetics and dynamics with special attention to vulnerable populations such as older adults.	Because substance-related disorders are one of the DSM-IV-TR Axis I diagnoses, they have been included as a psychiatric disorder in these standards.	None
Primary specialty.	Assesses mental health status using age, gender, and culturally appropriate standardized assessment instruments or processes; assesses for syndromes that may be manifestations of other common health problems (e.g., risk-taking behaviors, self-injury, stress, delirium, or depression); acute and chronic physical and mental illnesses; treats and manages geriatric syndromes such as delirium, depression, and dementia.	Fosters a trusting relationship that facilitates discussion of sensitive issues with the individual, family, and other caregivers such as substance use/abuse.	Assesses individuals with complex health issues and comorbidities, including the interaction with acute and chronic physical and mental health problems.
Primary specialty.	Assesses the interaction between acute and chronic physical and mental health problems;	Evaluates for common mental health disorders such	None

GENERAL POPULATION		
Mental Health (MH)	Substance Use (SU)	Co-occurring MH and SU
IV. PSYCHOLOGISTS[ee]		
Primary specialty.	Behavioral genetics, transmission and expression of genetic information and its modification and the role of this information in understanding diseases and disorders (e.g., substance abuse disorders) with consideration of comorbidities and	Behavioral genetics, transmission and expression of genetic information and its modification and the role of this information in understanding diseases and disorders (e.g., substance abuse disorders), with consideration of comorbidities and

GERIATRIC POPULATION			
General Care	Mental Health (MH)	Substance Use (SU)	Co-occurring MH and SU
	uses reliable and valid age-appropriate assessment instruments to assess acute and chronic health concerns, including mental status, delirium, dementia, and pain; evaluates for common mental health disorders such as depression, dementia, anxiety, or substance-related disorders; manages or appropriately refers the patient with signs and symptoms of mental health disorders; uses behavioral, communication, and environmental-modification strategies with individuals who have cognitive and psychiatric impairments; advises patients, families, and caregivers on how to address sensitive issues such as suicide prevention, substance use, potential for abuse, and end-of-life concerns; modifies health information, patient education programs, and interventions for patients with mental illness limitations; provides education to patients, families, caregivers, and the community, including the interaction between physical and mental health.	as depression, dementia, anxiety, or substance-related disorders; advises patients, families, and caregivers on how to address sensitive issues such as substance use.	
N/A	Influence of psychosocial factors (e.g., life span development) on beliefs/cognitions and behaviors; normal growth and development across the full life span; family development and functioning and its impact on the individual across the full life span; normative and nonnormative life	None	Comorbidity of mental illness with substance abuse, comorbidity rates, age ranges affected.

GENERAL POPULATION		
Mental Health (MH)	Substance Use (SU)	Co-occurring MH and SU
	population differences in genetic information.	population differences in genetic information; comorbidity of mental illness with substance abuse, comorbidity rates, age ranges affected.
Clinical Psychology[ff]		
Primary specialty.	None	None
Counseling Psychology[gg]		
Primary specialty.	None	None
Couple and Family Psychology[hh]		
Primary specialty.	None	None

GERIATRIC POPULATION			
General Care	Mental Health (MH)	Substance Use (SU)	Co-occurring MH and SU
	event changes (e.g., retirement) that can influence the normal course of development; disorders/diseases that impact expected course of development over the full life span.		
N/A	Sensitivity to and skills in dealing with multicultural/diverse populations, including broad scope of age; conducts assessments of cases from any developmental level across the life span; performs interventions that may take the form of any modality of psychotherapy or environmental modification in cases from any developmental level across the life span.	None	None
N/A	Sensitivity to and skills in dealing with multicultural/ diverse populations, including broad scope of age; perform interventions that may reflect any modality of psychotherapy or environmental modification and may come from any developmental level across the life span.	None	None
N/A	Knowledge in life span human development; assessment procedures should be appropriate for the client's developmental age and stage of lifecycle; use of instruments that have normative data from age-appropriate samples; interpretations and conclusions take into account couple/ family/identified patient uniqueness (developmental age and stage of lifecycle).	None	None

GENERAL POPULATION		
Mental Health (MH)	**Substance Use (SU)**	**Co-occurring MH and SU**
Rehabilitation Psychology[ii]		
Primary specialty.	Appropriate selection, administration, modification (where indicated), and interpretation of standardized tests, behavioral observations, and/or clinical interviews, given the needs of the patient/client, upon which recommendations are made and communicated to promote useful outcomes in the assessment of substance use/abuse identification; effective consultation with other professionals appropriate to the needs of the client in ways that will promote useful outcomes for the patient/client in substance abuse identification and management.	None
V. LICENSED COUNSELORS		
Rehabilitation Counseling[jj]		
Recognize individuals with a disability who demonstrate psychological or mental health-related problems and make appropriate referrals when appropriate; analyze diagnostic and assessment information (e.g., vocational and educational tests, records, and psychological and medical data) and communicate this information to the consumer; explain and use standard diagnostic classification systems for mental health conditions within the limits of the role and responsibilities of the rehabilitation counselor; recognize and communicate a basic understanding of how to assess individuals, groups, and families who exhibit suicide ideation, psychological and emotional crisis; identify and recommend treatment options that facilitate recovery and successful psychiatric rehabilitation outcomes.	Describe different recovery models that apply to substance abuse treatment and rehabilitation; identify and recommend treatment options that facilitate recovery and successful rehabilitation outcomes.	None

GERIATRIC POPULATION			
General Care	Mental Health (MH)	Substance Use (SU)	Co-occurring MH and SU
N/A	Sensitivity to and skills in dealing with multicultural/diverse populations, including broad scope of age; an awareness of science-based theories and research on individual and cultural diversity (i.e., age).	None	None
Identify the influences of aging differences and integrate this knowledge into practice; articulate a working knowledge of human development and the needs of individuals with disabilities across the life span.	None	None	None

GENERAL POPULATION		
Mental Health (MH)	Substance Use (SU)	Co-occurring MH and SU
Addiction Counseling[kk]		
Primary specialty.	Primary specialty.	Recognize the potential for addictive disorders to mimic a variety of medical and psychological disorders and the potential for medical and psychological disorders to coexist with addiction and substance abuse; provide appropriate counseling strategies when working with clients with addiction and co-occurring disorders; screen for co-occurring mental and/or addictive disorders; knowledge of the impact of co-occurring addictive disorders on medical and psychological disorders; demonstrate appropriate use of diagnostic tools, including the current edition of the DSM-IV-TR, to describe the symptoms and clinical presentation of clients with addictive disorders and mental and emotional impairments.
Clinical Mental Health Counseling		
Primary specialty.	Core curricula for all counselors should include theories and etiology of addictions and addictive behaviors, including strategies for prevention, intervention, and treatment. In addition, identifies standard screening and assessment instruments for substance use disorders and process addictions.	Recognizes the potential for substance use disorders to mimic and coexist with a variety of medical and psychological disorders; knows the disease concept and etiology of addiction and co-occurring disorders; provides appropriate counseling strategies when working with clients with addiction and co-occurring disorders; screens for addiction, as well as co-occurring

GERIATRIC POPULATION			
General Care	Mental Health (MH)	Substance Use (SU)	Co-occurring MH and SU
N/A	None	Core curricula for all counselors should include theories of individual and family development and transitions across the life span; theories for facilitating optimal development and wellness over the life span.	None
N/A	Core curricula for all counselors should include theories of individual and family development and transitions across the life span; theories for facilitating optimal development and wellness over the life span.	None	None

GENERAL POPULATION		
Mental Health (MH)	Substance Use (SU)	Co-occurring MH and SU
		mental disorders; knows the impact of co-occurring substance use disorders on medical and psychological disorders.
VI. SOCIAL WORKERS		
Social Worker (Associate's and Baccalaureate)[ll]		
Typical and atypical emotional growth and development; the impact of physical, mental, and cognitive impairment on human development; the interplay of biological, psychological, social, and spiritual factors; assessing types of information available from psychological and psychiatric educational records; process of referring the client for additional evaluations (e.g., psychological); The dynamics and effects of life stage and lifecycle crises; the impact of physical and mental illness on crises; dynamics and effects of trauma; dynamics and effects of loss, separation, and grief; indicators of and response to client danger to self and others; stages of crises; processes and techniques for cognitive and/or behavioral interventions.	Differentiating the use of, abuse of, and dependency on substances; the effects of addiction on the client; the effects of addiction on the family system and other relationships; eliciting sensitive information (e.g., substance abuse).	The co-occurrence of addiction and other disorders.
Social Worker (Master's)[mm]		
Behavioral, cognitive, and learning theories; impact of physical, mental, and cognitive disabilities on human development; interplay of biological, psychological, and social factors; dynamics of grief and loss; indicators and dynamics of abuse; psychopharmacology; components of a biopsychosocial history; symptoms of mental and emotional illness; indicators of psychosocial stress; indicators of traumatic stress and violence; current *Diagnostic and Statistical Manual* diagnostic framework and criteria; components and function of the mental status examination; indicators of client danger to self and others; use of cognitive behavioral techniques.	Addiction theories and concepts; indicators of substance abuse and other addictions.	None
Clinical Social Work[nn]		
Primary specialty.	Substance abuse and/or dependence; the effects of substance abuse and/or dependence on relationships; the effects of substance abuse and/or dependence; addiction theories;	Assessment and diagnosis of co-occurring disorders and conditions.

GERIATRIC POPULATION			
General Care	Mental Health (MH)	Substance Use (SU)	Co-occurring MH and SU
Older adult behavior and development; the interaction of age and/or disability with behaviors, attitudes, and identity.	The symptoms of mental and emotional illness across the life span; the indicators, dynamics, and impact of sexual abuse, emotional abuse, neglect, physical abuse, intimate partner violence, and other forms of exploitation across the life span; the dynamics and effects of life stage and lifecycle crises; the effect of the client system's life stage on the selection of an intervention.	None	None
Aging processes; influence of age on behaviors and attitudes.	None	None	None
N/A	Gerontology; differences in age and/or disability factors and characteristics; the influences of age and/or disability; the impact of age and/or disability on self-image; the effects of discrimination based on age and/or disability;	None	None

GENERAL POPULATION		
Mental Health (MH)	Substance Use (SU)	Co-occurring MH and SU
	the effects of drugs and alcohol on behavior; other addictions; the effects of other addictions on behavior and relationships.	
VII. PHARMACISTS[oo]		
None	Science foundation should include acute and chronic toxic effect of xenobiotics on the body, including drug or chemical overdose and toxic signs of drugs of abuse.	None
Psychiatric Pharmacy[pp]		
Primary specialty.	Substance-related disorders included in definition of psychiatric disorders; evaluate psychiatric services for compliance with standards established by national accrediting and regulatory agencies as related to practice in health care settings (e.g., mental health, substance abuse).	Knowledge of pharmacologic treatment of psychiatric and neurologic disorders in special populations (e.g., comorbidity).
VIII. OCCUPATIONAL THERAPISTS		
Occupational Therapy Assistant[qq]		
Curriculum must prepare students to work with a variety of populations including, but not limited to, children, adolescents, adults, and elderly persons in areas	None	None

GERIATRIC POPULATION			
General Care	Mental Health (MH)	Substance Use (SU)	Co-occurring MH and SU
	the methods used to assess needed level of care (e.g., geriatrics); the impact of aging parents on adult children.		
Science foundation should include principles of end-of-life care; pathophysiologic and pharmacotherapy alterations, dosage calculation, and adjustments, and drug monitoring for positive/negative outcomes specific for special population patients (e.g., geriatric) for prescription and nonprescription medications; advanced pharmacy practice experiences must include primary, acute, chronic, and preventive care among patients of all ages; in general, each site used for required pharmacy practice experiences should have a patient population that exhibits diversity in age.	None	None	None
N/A	Knowledge of pharmacologic treatment of psychiatric and neurologic disorders in special populations (e.g., age); disorders in the elderly (including medication use and other psychiatric disorders not included in general list of psychiatric disorders).	Substance-related disorders included in definition of psychiatric disorders.	Knowledge of pharmacologic treatment of psychiatric and neurologic disorders in special populations (e.g., comorbidity, age).
Demonstrate knowledge and understanding of human development throughout the life span	Curriculum must prepare students to work with a variety of populations, including	None	None

GENERAL POPULATION		
Mental Health (MH)	Substance Use (SU)	Co-occurring MH and SU
of physical and mental health; course content must include, but is not limited to, developmental psychology; demonstrate knowledge and understanding of the concepts of human behavior to include the behavioral and social sciences (e.g., principles of psychology, sociology, abnormal psychology); demonstrate knowledge and appreciation of the role of sociocultural, socioeconomic, and diversity factors and lifestyle choices in contemporary society (e.g., principles of psychology, sociology, and abnormal psychology); understand the effects of physical and mental health, heritable diseases and predisposing genetic conditions, disability, disease processes, and traumatic injury to the individual within the cultural context of family and society on occupational performance; express support for the quality of life, well-being, and occupation of the individual, group, or population to promote physical and mental health; consider client factors, including body functions (e.g., cognitive, mental) and body structures in occupational performance evaluation; interventions must address client factors, including body functions (e.g., cognitive, mental).		
Occupational Therapist (Master's[rr] and Doctoral[ss])		
The curriculum must prepare students to work with a variety of populations, including, but not limited to, children, adolescents, adults, and elderly persons in areas of physical and mental health; course content must include, but is not limited to, developmental psychology; demonstrate knowledge and understanding of the concepts of human behavior to include the behavioral and social sciences. Course content must include, but is not limited to, introductory psychology, abnormal psychology, and introductory sociology or introductory anthropology; analyze the effects of physical and mental health, heritable diseases, and predisposing genetic conditions, disability, disease processes, and traumatic injury to the individual within the cultural context of family and society on occupational performance; express support for the quality of life, well-being, and occupation of the individual, group, or population to promote physical and mental health; consider client factors, including body functions (e.g., cognitive, mental) and body structures in occupational performance evaluation; interventions must address client factors, including body functions (e.g., cognitive, mental).	None	None

GERIATRIC POPULATION			
General Care	Mental Health (MH)	Substance Use (SU)	Co-occurring MH and SU
(including elderly persons); recommended that the student be exposed to a variety of clients across the life span and to a variety of settings in Level II fieldwork.	elderly persons, in areas of physical and mental health.		
Demonstrate knowledge and understanding of human development throughout the life span (including elderly persons); select appropriate assessment tools based on client needs, contextual factors, and psychometric properties of tests. These must be relevant to a variety of populations across the life span, culturally relevant, based on available evidence, and incorporate use of occupation in the assessment process; recommended that the student be exposed to a variety of clients across the life span and to a variety of settings in Level II fieldwork.	The curriculum must prepare students to work with a variety of populations, including elderly persons, in areas of physical and mental health.	None	None

GENERAL POPULATION		
Mental Health (MH)	Substance Use (SU)	Co-occurring MH and SU
Gerontology[tt]		
N/A	N/A	N/A
Mental Health[uu]		
Primary specialty.	None	None
IX. DIRECT CARE WORKERS		
Certified Nursing Assistant[vv]		
Mental health and social service needs, including modifying aide's behavior in response to residents' behavior, awareness of developmental tasks associated with the aging process, how to respond to resident behavior, allowing the resident to make personal choices, providing and reinforcing other behavior consistent with the resident's dignity, and using the resident's family as a source of emotional support.	None	None
Home Health Aide[ww]		
None	None	None

[a] Step 2 Clinical Knowledge (CK) Content Description and General Information, USMLE 2011.
[b] Program Requirements for Graduate Medical Education in Family Medicine, ACGME 2007.
[c] Program Requirements for Graduate Medical Education in Geriatric Medicine, ACGME 2006.
[d] Program Requirements for Graduate Medical Education in Internal Medicine, ACGME 2009.
[e] Program Requirements for Graduate Medical Education in Geriatric Medicine, ACGME 2007.

GERIATRIC POPULATION			
General Care	Mental Health (MH)	Substance Use (SU)	Co-occurring MH and SU
Primary specialty.	Knowledge of relevant evidence, including theories regarding age-related changes or pathology that affect cognitive and psychological function.	None	None
N/A	Synthesizes knowledge of how occupational performance and context influence life satisfaction, quality of life, and mental health across the life span in the design and delivery of services.	None	None
	Mental health and social service needs, including awareness of developmental tasks associated with the aging process; care of cognitively impaired residents, including techniques for addressing the unique needs and behaviors of individuals with dementia (Alzheimer's and others), communicating with cognitively impaired residents, understanding the behavior of cognitively impaired residents, appropriate responses to the behavior of cognitively impaired residents; and methods of reducing the effects of cognitive impairments.	None	None
None	None	None	None

[f] Program Requirements for Graduate Medical Education in Psychiatry, ACGME 2007.
[g] Program Requirements for Graduate Medical Education in Geriatric Psychiatry, ACGME 2003.
[h] Program Requirements for Graduate Medical Education in Addiction Psychiatry, ACMGE 2003.

[i]American Osteopathic Association. 2011. Basic standards for fellowship training in geriatrics in osteopathic family medicine and manipulative treatment. http://www.osteopathic.org/inside-aoa/accreditation/postdoctoral-training-approval/postdoctoral-training-standards/Documents/basic-standards-for-fellowship-training-in-geriatrics-osteopathic-family-practice.pdf.

[j]NBOME 2009. Fundamental Osteopathic Medical Competencies: Guidelines for Osteopathic Medical Licensure and the Practice of Osteopathic Medicine. AOA. 2011. Specific Basic Standards for Osteopathic Fellowship Training in Internal Medicine Geriatrics. http://www.osteopathic.org/inside-aoa/accreditation/postdoctoral-training-approval/postdoctoral-training-standards/Documents/specific-requirements-for-fellowship-training-in-geriatric-medicine.pdf.

[k]NBOME 2011, Computer-Based COMLEX Content Outline, http://www.nbome.org/intro/m_outline.html.

[l]Basic Standards for Residency Training in Family Practice and Manipulative Treatment, AOA and ACOFP 2011.

[m]Basic Standards for Fellowship Training in Geriatrics in Family Practice and Manipulative Treatment, AOA and ACOFP 2011.

[n]Basic Standards for Fellowship Training in Addiction Medicine in Family Practice and Manipulative Treatment, AOA and ACOFP 2008.

[o]Basic Standards for Residency Training in Internal Medicine, AOA and ACOI 2011.

[p]Specific Basic Standards for Osteopathic Fellowship Training in Internal Medicine Geriatrics, AOA and ACOI 2011.

[q]Basic Standards for Residency Training in General Psychiatry, AOA and ACONP 2009.

[r]Basic Standards for Residency Training in Geriatric Psychiatry, AOA and ACONP 2008.

[s]Basic Standards for Addiction Psychiatry, AOA and ACONP 2007.

[t]Accreditation Standards for Physician Assistant Education, Fourth Edition, ARCEPA March 2010.

[u]2011 NCLEX-PN® Detailed Test Plan: Item Writer/Item Reviewer/Nurse Educator Version, NCSBN April 2011.

[v]2010 NCLEX-RN® Detailed Test Plan: Item Writer/Item Reviewer/Nurse Educator Version, NCSBN April 2010.

[w]Gerontological Nursing Board Certification Test Content Outline, ANCC 2010.

[x]Psychiatric and Mental Health Nursing Board Certification Test Content Outline, ANCC 2010.

[y]The Essentials of Master's Education for Advanced Practice Nursing, AACN 1996.

[z]The Essentials of Doctoral Education for Advanced Nursing Practice, AACN October 2006 (standards do not differ between Master's and Doctoral levels in these areas).

[aa]Acute Care Nurse Practitioner Competencies, National Panel for Acute Care Nurse Practitioner Competencies 2004.

[bb]National Panel for Psychiatric-Mental Health NP Competencies, September 2003, http://www.aacn.nche.edu/leading-initiatives/education-resources/PMHNP.pdf.

[cc]Adult-Gerontology Primary Care Nurse Practitioner Competencies, AACN 2010.

[dd]Adult-Gerontology Clinical Nurse Specialist Competencies, AACN March 2010.

[ee]ASPPB Information for EPPP Candidates: Examination for Professional Practice in Psychology (EPPP), ASPPB 2011.

[ff]Examination Manual for Board Certification in Clinical Psychology for the American Board Of Professional Psychology, ABPP 2011.

[gg]Examination Manual for Board Certification in Counseling Psychology for the American Board of Professional Psychology, ABPP 2010.

[hh]Manual for Obtaining Board Certification, American Board of Couple and Family Psychology 2011.

[ii]Certification Guidelines and Procedures Candidate's Manual, American Board of Rehabilitation Psychology 2011.

[jj]Accreditation Manual for Master's Level Rehabilitation Counselor Education Programs, CORE 2011.

[kk]Council for Accreditation of Counseling and Related Educational Programs 2009 Standards, CACREP 2009.
[ll]ASWB Examination program Knowledge, Skills and Abilities: Bachelor's Examination, ASWB 2011. (Note: Associate candidates also take Bachelor's Examination.)
[mm]Examination program Knowledge, Skills and Abilities: Masters Examination, ASWB 2011.
[nn]ASWB Examination program Knowledge, Skills and Abilities: Clinical Examination, ASWB 2011.
[oo]Accreditation Standards and Guidelines for the Professional Program in Pharmacy Leading to the Doctor of Pharmacy Degree, ACPE 2011.
[pp]Content Outline for the Psychiatric Pharmacy Specialty Certification Examination, Board of Pharmacy Specialties, May 2005.
[qq]Accreditation Standards for an Educational Program for the Occupational Therapy Assistant, ACOTE 2006.
[rr]Accreditation Standards for a Master's Degree-Level Educational Program for the Occupational Therapist, ACOTE 2006.
[ss]Accreditation Standards for a Doctoral Degree-Level Educational Program for the Occupational Therapist, ACOTE 2006 (standards do not differ between master's and doctoral levels in these areas).
[tt]Competencies, Criteria, and Client Outcomes: Gerontology Board Certification, AOTA 2009.
[uu]Competencies, Criteria, and Client Outcomes: Mental Health Board Certification, AOTA 2009.
[vv]C.F.R. Part 483 (Requirements for States and Long-Term Care Facilities), October 1, 2001.
[ww]C.F.R. Part 484 (Conditions of Participation: Home Health Agencies), October 1, 2001.

Appendix D

IOM Recommendations from *Retooling for an Aging America: Building the Health Care Workforce* (2008)

Recommendation 1-1: Congress should require an annual report from the Bureau of Health Professions to monitor the progress made in addressing the crisis in supply of the health care workforce for older adults.

Enhancing Geriatric Competence

Recommendation 4-1: Hospitals should encourage the training of residents in all settings where older adults receive care, including nursing homes, assisted-living facilities, and patients' homes.

Recommendation 4-2: All licensure, certification, and maintenance of certification for health care professionals should include demonstration of competence in the care of older adults as a criterion.

Recommendation 5-1: States and the federal government should increase minimum training standards for all direct-care workers. Federal requirements for the minimum training of certified nursing assistants (CNAs) and home health aides should be raised to at least 120 hours and should include demonstration of competence in the care of older adults as a criterion for certification. States should also establish minimum training requirements for personal-care aides.

Recommendation 6-2: Public, private, and community organizations should provide funding and ensure that adequate training opportunities are available in the community for informal caregivers.

Increasing Recruitment and Retention

Recommendation 4-3: Public and private payers should provide financial incentives to increase the number of geriatric specialists in all health professions.

Recommendation 4-3a: All payers should include a specific enhancement of reimbursement for clinical services delivered to older adults by practitioners with a certification of special expertise in geriatrics.

Recommendation 4-3b: Congress should authorize and fund an enhancement of the Geriatric Academic Career Award (GACA) program to support junior geriatrics faculty in other health professions in addition to allopathic and osteopathic medicine.

Recommendation 4-3c: States and the federal government should institute programs for loan forgiveness, scholarships, and direct financial incentives for professionals who become geriatric specialists. One such mechanism should include the development of a National Geriatric Service Corps, modeled after the National Health Service Corps.

Recommendation 5-2: State Medicaid programs should increase pay and fringe benefits for direct-care workers through such measures as wage pass-throughs, setting wage floors, establishing minimum percentages of service rates directed to direct-care labor costs, and other means.

Redesigning Models of Care

Recommendation 3-1: Payers should promote and reward the dissemination of those models of care for older adults that have been shown to be effective and efficient.

Recommendation 3-2: Congress and foundations should significantly increase support for research and demonstration programs that
- promote the development of new models of care for older adults in areas where few models are currently being tested, such as prevention, long-term care, and palliative care; and
- promote the effective use of the workforce to care for older adults.

Recommendation 3-3: Health care disciplines, state regulators, and employers should look to expand the roles of individuals who care for older adults with complex clinical needs at different levels of the health care system beyond the traditional scope of practice. Critical elements of this include

- development of an evidence base that informs the establishment of new provider designations reflecting rising levels of responsibility and improved efficiency;
- measurement of additional competence to attain these designations; and
- greater professional recognition and salary commensurate with these responsibilities.

Recommendation 6-1: Federal agencies (including the Department of Labor and the Department of Health and Human Services) should provide support for the development and promulgation of technological advancements that could enhance an individual's capacity to provide care for older adults. This includes the use of activity-of-daily-living (ADL) technologies and health information technologies, including remote technologies, that increase the efficiency and safety of care and caregiving.

Appendix E

Committee Biographies

DAN G. BLAZER, M.D., M.P.H., Ph.D. (*Chair*), is the J.P. Gibbons Professor of Psychiatry and Behavioral Sciences and vice chair for Education and Academic Affairs at Duke University Medical Center. Following 9 years in academic administration as chair of the Department of Psychiatry and Dean of Medical Education at Duke University School of Medicine, Dr. Blazer returned to teaching, research, and practice in 1999. In 2002-2003 he was a Fellow at the Center for Advanced Studies of the Behavioral Sciences at Stanford University. He is the author or editor of 34 books, and author or coauthor of more than 190 published abstracts and over 400 peer-reviewed articles. He is also the author or coauthor of over 180 book chapters. Many of the book chapters and scientific articles are on the topics of depression, epidemiology, and consultation liaison psychiatry, especially with the elderly. Dr. Blazer's research has focused on the prevalence of physical and mental illness in the elderly. Honors received by Dr. Blazer include a Research Career Development Award from the National Institute of Mental Health (NIMH); listing in *Who's Who in America, Who's Who in American Men and Women of Science*, and *The Best Doctors in America*; Fellowship in the American College of Psychiatry and Gerontological Society of America (GSA); Distinguished Life Fellowship in the American Psychiatric Association; Distinguished Faculty Member of Duke University School of Medicine; Jack Weinberg Award for research in geriatric psychiatry; Oscar Pfister Award for the integration of religion and psychiatry from the American Psychiatric Association; and the Pioneers in Geriatric Psychiatry Award from the American Association of

Geriatric Psychiatry. Dr. Blazer is past president of the American Association of Geriatric Psychiatry and the American Geriatric Society, and past chair of the membership committee of the Institute of Medicine (IOM). He is currently the editor of *Duke Medicine HealthNews* and a member of the editorial board of the *Archives of General Psychiatry*. Dr. Blazer was elected to the Institute of Medicine in 1995.

MARGARITA ALEGRÍA, Ph.D., is director of the Center for Multicultural Mental Health Research and a professor of psychology in the Department of Psychiatry at Harvard Medical School. Dr. Alegría researches mental health services for Latinos and other ethnic populations. She is currently the principal investigator of the Advanced Center for Mental Health Disparities, and the Latino arm of the National Latino and Asian American Study, as well as the co–principal investigator of the CHA-UPR Excellence in Partnerships for Community Outreach, Research on Health Disparities and Training (EXPORT) Center. Her published works focus on mental health services research, conceptual and methodological issues with minority populations, risk behaviors, and disparities in service delivery. Dr. Alegría received her Ph.D. from Temple University and was elected to the IOM in 2011.

MARÍA P. ARANDA, Ph.D., L.C.S.W., is an associate professor at the University of Southern California (USC) School of Social Work. She joined the faculty in 1995 and holds a joint appointment with the USC Leonard Davis School of Gerontology. She chairs the Scientific Governing Board of the Edward J. Roybal Institute on Aging and the Older Adult Subconcentration, both at USC. Dr. Aranda's research and teaching interests address the interplays among chronic medical conditions, psychiatric disorders, and sociocultural diversity among people from low-income, minority populations. Dr. Aranda has served as principal investigator or co-investigator on several key studies funded by and/or in collaboration with the National Institute of Mental Health, National Cancer Institute, the John A. Hartford Foundation/Gerontological Society of America, National Institute of Rehabilitation and Research, Los Angeles Basin Clinical and Translational Science Institute, Alzheimer's Association/Health Resources and Services Administration, Los Angeles County Department of Mental Health, Larson Endowment for Innovative Research and Teaching, and AltaMed Health Services Corp. She has experience in the ethnographic study of adherence factors in clinical trials as well as clinical and epidemiological research examining the relationships among health, stress, psychosocial resources, and mental health and service use outcomes. Dr. Aranda has worked specifically on problem-solving therapy with elderly and middle-aged minorities and its efficacy as treatment for depression in community-based settings. Overall, Dr. Aranda's interests address mental health intervention and services research for underrepresented populations, psychosocial care of late-life psychiatric disorders, sociocultural adaptations to evidence-based mental health care, and training of interventionists in evidence-based practice.

STEPHEN BARTELS, M.D., M.S., is the Herman O. West Professor of Geriatrics and Professor of Psychiatry, professor of Community & Family Medicine at Dartmouth Medical School, and professor of Health Policy at the Dartmouth Institute for Health Policy and Clinical Practice. He is director of the Dartmouth Centers for Health and Aging, where he oversees the Dartmouth Center for Aging Research, the Northern New England Geriatric Education Center, and the Dartmouth-Hitchcock Aging Resource Center. His research interests include health care management and rehabilitation for older persons with serious mental disorders, health promotion, integration of mental health and primary care, self-management, applied use of health management technology, Medicaid and Medicare costs of medical and mental disorders in older adults, shared decision making, community-based implementation research, and evidence-based geriatric psychiatry. He has published more than 130 peer-reviewed articles and book chapters and has served in national leadership roles in the field of geriatrics. He is a past president of the American Association for Geriatric Psychiatry and founding chair of the Geriatric Mental Health Foundation. Dr. Bartels served as the expert consultant and author for the Older Adult Subcommittee Report for the President's New Freedom Commission on Mental Health. He has also testified before Congress and has participated in congressional briefings on aging and health policy and on funding for research on mental disorders in older persons. Dr. Bartels is the recipient of a 5-year research mentoring award from the National Institutes of Health and is the principal investigator for a multisite, postdoctoral training program in geriatric mental health services research. He also serves on the Executive Committee and faculty for the NIMH-sponsored Summer Research Institute and Advanced Research Institute in Geriatric Psychiatry. He has numerous research and training grants, including funding from NIMH, the Centers for Disease Control and Prevention (CDC), Health Resources and Services Administration, Substance Abuse and Mental Health Services Administration (SAMHSA), and foundation support, and served on the NIMH Interventions Review Committee from 2003 to 2009. He was the lead expert and author for the SAMHSA Action Plan for Behavioral Health Workforce Development for Older Adult Mental Health Services. He also served as the scientific co-director for SAMHSA's Older Americans Substance Abuse and Mental Health Technical Assistance Center and is currently the scientific lead for SAMHSA's National Technical Assistance Center for the Older Adult Targeted Capacity Grant Program for Evidence-Based Practice Implementation. He was selected for the Health Services Research Senior Career Award by the American Psychiatric Association in 2003, the Mental Health and Aging Award by the American Society on Aging in 2005, and the Riverbend Rainbow Award and the Outstanding Psychiatrist Award from the National Alliance for the Mentally Ill of New Hampshire in 2010.

CHRISTINE E. BISHOP, Ph.D., is the Atran Professor of Labor Economics at the Heller School of Social Policy and Management at Brandeis University. She is a health economist who applies microeconomics to policy-related problems in health services supply, demand, and financing. Her studies in long-term services and supports (LTSS) have addressed provider and recipient behavior, considering costs, production efficiency, payment, financing, and use of nursing homes and home health services. Her current research on the LTSS workforce builds on her training as a labor economist and previous research on nursing labor markets. Because population health and disability are at the root of demand for LTSS, and because preventive interventions may save future health and LTSS costs, Dr. Bishop has undertaken investigations of the role of access to prescription drugs in affecting need for health services and thus trends in disability in the elderly. She received her Ph.D. from Harvard University.

FREDERIC C. BLOW, Ph.D., is professor and director of the Mental Health Services Outcomes and Translation Section in the Department of Psychiatry at the University of Michigan Medical School, and director of the National Serious Mental Illness Treatment Resource and Evaluation Center for the Department of Veterans Affairs, Ann Arbor, Michigan. His areas of research expertise include alcohol screening and diagnosis for older adults, serious mental illness and concurrent substance abuse, alcohol brief interventions in health care settings, and geriatric mental health services research. He is a national expert in mental health and substance abuse services research and policy, with a focus on evidence-based practices. Dr. Blow has been the principal investigator on numerous federal, state, and foundation grants, and has published extensively in the areas of substance abuse and alcoholism among the elderly, substance abuse screening/treatment, and mental health. From 1996 to 1998, Dr. Blow was panel chair for the Center for Substance Abuse Treatment's Treatment Improvement Protocol on Substance Abuse Among Older Adults. Additionally, he is the first Huss/Hazelden Research Chair for the Butler Center for Research at the Hazelden Center in Center City, Minnesota. Dr. Blow maintains an active role in both graduate and undergraduate teaching and the mentoring of pre- and postdoctoral students and junior faculty.

KATHLEEN C. BUCKWALTER, Ph.D., RN, FAAN, is codirector of the National Health Law and Policy Resource Center, University of Iowa College of Law and formerly Sally Mathis Hartwig Professor of Gerontological Nursing Research. She served as associate provost for Health Sciences at the University of Iowa from 1997 to 2004; and director of the John A. Hartford Center for Geriatric Nursing Excellence from 2005 to 2011; and deputy director of the University's Center on Aging. She held secondary appointments in the College of Medicine Departments of Psychiatry and Internal Medicine, College of Public Health, and College of Law at the University of Iowa. Dr. Buckwalter is recognized for her research in psychiatric nursing, aging, and long-term care, and has a sustained record of private and federal support related to the evaluation of clinical nursing interventions for geropsychiatric populations. Her particular interest is in behavioral management strategies for rural caregivers of persons with dementia and the effectiveness of community programs to prevent, minimize, and treat psychiatric problems in the rural elderly. With support from the NIMH and Administration on Aging, Dr. Buckwalter headed the Mental Health of the Rural Elderly Outreach Project and served as principal investigator of the Progressively Lowered Stress Threshold (PLST) Model: Effectiveness for Rural Alzheimer's Disease and Related Disorders (ADRD) Caregivers funded by the National Institute of Nursing Research (NINR). She was the first recipient of the National Gerontological Nursing Association Board of Directors Award, and in 2007 she received New York University College of Nursing's Distinguished Scholar in Nursing Award. She was honored by the Iowa Association of Homes and Services for Aging Advocacy Award and the Gerontological Society of America Distinguished Mentorship in Gerontology Award. In 2010 she received the American Psychiatric Nurses Association Psychiatric Nurse of the Year award, the GSA Doris Schwartz Gerontological Nursing Research award, and the Iowa Department on Aging Lifetime Achievement award. Dr. Buckwalter serves on numerous review committees, editorial boards, and advisory groups. She has authored more than 250 articles, more than 85 book chapters, 8 health policy and commission papers, more than 50 monographs/videos/media, and more than 90 editorials/reviews/commentaries. In addition, she has edited eight books on topics such as geriatric mental health, memory, aging, and dementia.

CHRISTOPHER M. CALLAHAN, M.D., is the Indiana University Cornelius and Yvonne Pettinga Professor of Medicine. His research, education, and clinical interests are in primary care geriatrics. He is a research scientist in the Regenstrief Institute and the founding director of the Indiana University Center for Aging Research. In 1999-2000 he was a visiting scholar in the History and Psychopathology Research Program in the Department of Psychiatry at Cambridge University in the United Kingdom. Dr. Callahan has received a Paul B. Beeson Physician Faculty Scholar in Aging Award from the American Federation for Aging Research and a Midcareer Mentorship Award from the National Institute on Aging. He is the Principal Investigator of the Indiana University Roybal Center. His research has also been supported by the John A. Hartford Foundation and the Agency for Healthcare Research and Quality. He also received the Teaching Excellence Recognition Award at Indiana University and the Tony and Mary Hulman Health Achievement Award for Excellence in Health Sciences Research. Dr. Callahan's research focuses on strategies to improve the care of older adults in primary care. This research explores systems-level interventions to enable primary care physicians to deliver excellent care to older adults. His specific research interests include the recognition and treatment of late-life depression and the care of older adults with dementia. Dr. Callahan graduated from St. Louis University School of Medicine in 1985. He completed his internal medicine residency at Baylor College of Medicine in 1988 and completed a fellowship in health services research at Indiana University School of Medicine in 1991. He has a Certificate of Added Qualifications in Geriatric Medicine.

ANNI CHUNG, M.S.W., has been the president and CEO of Self-Help for the Elderly (SHE) since 1981. She completed the Leadership America Program in 2007. In 1997, she graduated from the Gallup Leadership Institute and was a National Fellow with the Asian Pacific American Women Leadership Institute. She oversees and manages a community-based organization that provides a comprehensive range of health, educational, social, and recreational services to more than 35,000 seniors a year. SHE employs over 500 staff with an annual budget of approximately $18 million, serving seniors in San Francisco, San Mateo, Santa Clara, and Alameda counties. Ms. Chung is currently on the Board of Directors of St. Mary's Medical Center and the No Health Without Mental Health Foundation. She was on the San Francisco Alzheimer's Task Force, a group charged by Mayor Newsom to develop a long-range plan for San Francisco's aging population. She is a member of the University of California Community Partnership Council and also serves on the American Diabetes Association's Asian and Pacific American Diabetes Action Council. Since 1998, she has been a member of AT&T's Community Partnership Agreement Committee and Verizon's Community Citizen's Collaborative, which make technology grants to community groups. She was chair of San Francisco's Digital Inclusion Task Force from 2006 to 2008. In addition to her community involvement, she is the producer and host of a weekly public affairs program called *Chinese Journal* for KTSF-TV 26. She graduated from the School of Social Work at San Francisco State University.

GARY L. GOTTLIEB, M.D., M.B.A., is the president and CEO of Partners HealthCare. He is a professor of psychiatry at Harvard Medical School and was appointed to the IOM in 2010. He has served as president of Brigham and Women's/Faulkner Hospitals; as president of North Shore Medical Center; and as chair of Partners Psychiatry. Before moving to Boston, he spent 15 years in Philadelphia. He arrived at the University of Pennsylvania as a Robert Wood Johnson Foundation Clinical Scholar. He later established Penn Medical Center's first program in geriatric psychiatry and he rose to become executive vice chair and interim chair of Penn's Department of Psychiatry and the Health System's associate dean for managed care. He went on to become director and CEO of Friends Hospital in Philadelphia. He has published in geriatric psychiatry and health care policy. He is a past president of the American Association of Geriatric Psychiatry. He received his B.S. cum laude from the Rensselaer Polytechnic Institute and his M.D. from the Albany Medical College of Union University in a 6-year accelerated biomedical program. He completed his internship and residency and served as chief resident at New York University/Bellevue Medical Center. Dr. Gottlieb currently serves as chair of the Private Industry Council, the city's workforce development board. He is also a member of the Boards of Directors of the Federal Reserve Bank of Boston and Partners in Health.

MICHAEL A. HOGE, Ph.D., is a professor and director of Clinical Training in Psychology within the Department of Psychiatry at the Yale University School of Medicine. He also serves as Director of Yale Behavioral Health, which provides a broad array of mental health and addiction services to adolescents and adults. He is a founding member of the Annapolis Coalition on the Behavioral Health Workforce, which initiated a national, interprofessional effort to improve the recruitment, retention, and training of individuals who provide prevention and treatment services for persons with mental illnesses and substance use disorders. Dr. Hoge serves as the senior science and policy advisor for the Coalition and was the senior editor of the national *Action Plan on Behavioral Health Workforce Development* which was commissioned by SAMHSA. He is also the senior editor of the *Alaskan Core Competencies for Direct Care Workers in Health and Human Services*, which details essential cross-sector skills for frontline staff. He has consulted on behavioral health workforce issues to the President's New Freedom Commission on Mental Health, the IOM, and many states and organizations. He now directs the Yale Group on

Workforce Development and the Yale Program on Supervision, and is chair of the Connecticut Workforce Collaborative on Behavioral Health. Dr. Hoge is the past chair of the Behavioral Health Professional and Technical Advisory Committee of the Joint Commission on Accreditation of Healthcare Organizations (JCAHO) and a recipient of the Moffic Award for Ethical Practice in Public Sector Managed Behavioral Healthcare. He received his doctorate from Kent State University.

OCTAVIO N. MARTINEZ, M.D., M.P.H., M.B.A., is the fifth executive director and the first Hispanic to lead the Hogg Foundation for Mental Health since it was created in 1940. The foundation's grants and programs support mental health services, research, policy analysis, and public education projects in Texas. As CEO, he oversees the vision, mission, goals, strategic planning, and day-to-day operations of the Foundation. He is a clinical professor with an appointment at the University of Texas at Austin in the School of Social Work. His academic interests include minority health, health disparities, and workforce issues. Prior to joining the Foundation, Dr. Martinez was a clinical psychiatrist at the Albemarle Mental Health Center and an affiliate associate professor at the Brody School of Medicine in North Carolina. He was part of a team that created a 23-Hour Crisis Unit at Albemarle Hospital in Elizabeth City, North Carolina, to serve a 10-county catchment area. Before that he was an assistant professor and psychiatrist at the University of Texas Health Science Center at San Antonio (UTHSCSA) and a faculty associate with the Center for Medical Humanities and Ethics. In San Antonio he served as director of Psychiatric Consultation/Liaison Services for two major teaching hospitals and codirector of behavioral sciences for the UTHSCSA medical school. He developed two community psychiatric clinics for underserved areas of San Antonio. He is a Fellow of the American Psychiatric Association and a member of the Texas Society for Psychiatric Physicians, American College of Mental Health Administration, National Hispanic Medical Association, and Harvard Faculty Club. From 2002 to 2006, he served as a Special Emphasis Panel Member for the National Institutes of Health, National Center on Minority Health and Health Disparities. He is also a recipient of the Adolph Meyer, M.D., Research Award in recognition of contributions in minority health and efforts to improve the mental health of all citizens regardless of socioeconomic status. Dr. Martinez is licensed to practice medicine in Texas and North Carolina and is a diplomate of the American Board of Psychiatry and Neurology. He has bachelor's and master's degrees in business administration with a concentration in finance from the University of Texas at Austin, an M.P.H. from the Harvard School of Public Health, and an M.D. from Baylor College of Medicine. He also completed The Commonwealth Fund/Harvard University Fellowship in Minority Health Policy at Harvard Medical School.

WILLARD MAYS, M.A., has extensive experience at the state (Indiana) and national levels in aging, health, mental health, and substance use with a specialty in older adult public policy. He is past chair of the National Coalition on Mental Health and Aging, which includes more than 80 federal agencies, national organizations, and state and local mental health and aging coalitions. He currently chairs the Indiana Mental Health and Aging Coalition. He is past chair of the Older Persons Division of the National Association of State Mental Health Program Directors, and was founding president of the National Association of PASRR Professionals. He is chair of the Mental Health and Aging Network of the American Society on Aging (ASA) and was recipient of the 2005 ASA Mental Health and Aging Award. He gave invited testimony to the President's New Freedom Commission on Mental Health and was a congressionally appointed Delegate to the 2005 White House Conference on Aging. He was coeditor and coauthor of the SAMHSA publication "Community Integration for Older Adults with Mental Illnesses: Overcoming Barriers and Seizing Opportunities." He is a consultant for the Centers for Medicare & Medicaid PASRR Technical Assistance Center and the SAMHSA Older Adult Mental Health Targeted Capacity Expansion Grant Technical Assistance Center. In 2012 he played a lead role in forming the Aging and Mental Health Advocacy Network to coordinate advocacy efforts for older adult mental health and addiction.

PETER V. RABINS, M.D., M.P.H., is a professor and the Richman Family Professor for Alzheimer's and Related Disease in the Department of Psychiatry and Behavioral Sciences at the Johns Hopkins University School of Medicine. He is also the director, Division of Geriatric Psychiatry and Neuropsychiatry. Dr. Rabins has joint appointments in the Department of Medicine and the departments of health policy & management and mental health at the Johns Hopkins Bloomberg School of Public Health. Dr. Rabins has focused his career on the study of psychiatric disorders in the elderly. His current research focuses on the measurement of quality of life in persons with Alzheimer's disease, the care of patients with late-stage dementia, autism in the elderly, and phenotypic variation in frontotemporal dementia. Because diseases and disabilities that are prevalent in the elderly commonly cross traditional disciplinary and training boundaries, Dr. Rabins has championed the use of care providers with differing training backgrounds as a necessary component of care for the elderly.

MARK SNOWDEN, M.D., M.P.H., is an associate professor in the University of Washington School of Medicine, Department of Psychiatry and Behavioral Sciences. He is medical director for geriatric psychiatry services at Harborview Medical Center in Seattle. In this capacity he provides and supervises geriatric psychiatry services to several community-based nursing homes and clinics, as well as inpatient treatment and consultations at Harborview Medical Center. He supervises clinical training for geriatric psychiatry fellows and general psychiatry residents who work with him in his clinic service in the nursing home and geriatric medicine primary care clinics. His research focuses on delivery of evidence-based mental health services to community-dwelling older adults and nursing home residents. He has led several expert panels in the review of the literature and in formulating recommendations for the dissemination of evidence-based practices for depression and other mental health conditions. He has received funding from the Robert Wood Johnson Foundation, NIMH, and CDC. He received his M.D. from the University of Washington, where he also completed psychiatric residency training and the geriatric psychiatry fellowship. He worked as a Robert Wood Johnson Clinical Scholar from 1994 to 1996. During that time he received an M.P.H. from the University of Washington School of Public Health.

ROBYN STONE, Dr.PH., is executive director of the LeadingAge Center for Applied Research (formerly the Institute for the Future of Aging Services) and senior vice president for research at LeadingAge (formerly the American Association of Homes and Services for the Aging). The center is an applied research organization dedicated to bridging the worlds of policy, practice, and research to advance the development and diffusion of high-quality aging and long-term care services and supports. Prior to joining LeadingAge, Dr. Stone was executive director and chief operating officer of the International Longevity Center–USA in New York City. She has also worked for the Agency for Healthcare Research and Policy and served the White House as Deputy Assistant Secretary for Disability, Aging, and Long-Term Care Policy and as Assistant Secretary for Aging in the U.S. Department of Health and Human Services in the Clinton Administration. She is an internationally recognized expert in long-term care and aging services policy and has published extensively in the areas of quality, workforce development, financing, and organization of long-term care and senior housing with services. Dr. Stone holds a doctorate in public health from the University of California, Berkeley.